CONTEMPORARY CARDIOLOGY

CHRISTOPHER P. CANNON, MD
SERIES EDITOR

For further volumes:
http://www.springer.com/series/7677

W. Frank Peacock

Editor

Short Stay Management of Acute Heart Failure

Second Edition

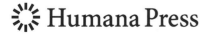 Humana Press

Editor
W. Frank Peacock
Department of Emergency Medicine
Cleveland Clinic Foundation
Cleveland, OH, USA

ISBN 978-1-61779-626-5   e-ISBN 978-1-61779-627-2
DOI 10.1007/978-1-61779-627-2
Springer New York Heidelberg Dordrecht London

Library of Congress Control Number: 2011946226

Humana Press is part of Springer Science+Business Media (www.springer.com)

Preface

My grandfather was a country doc, back in the first part of the twentieth century, in a small Florida town of a few hundred people. This was a time and place without electricity, cars, internet, or cell phones. And when I was a kid, he would tell me stories of how he walked or rode a horse for hours to get to a patient who had shortness of breath. Once there, crowded into a room surrounded by worried family, examinations were done under kerosene lantern and limited to touch, feel, and the stethoscope. With only history and physical exam, diagnosis was by the terms of Sir William Osler. No X-rays, no ECGs, no fancy echocardiograms, and no BNP levels.

In these years, because pneumonia was a death sentence, my grandfather would pray for signs of heart failure. For if the diagnosis was pneumonia, the only thing to do was to talk to the terrified spouse and tell them that it did not look good and that their loved one would probably be dead in 3 days. And while my grandfather would promise to do everything possible, the odds were long at best. Antibiotics did not exist. Pneumonia was a common final pathway. So this was the mantra of the country doctor. If the patient survived, the doctor was very good, but if not, it was simply fate. Other than providing comfort in their last days, there was little that could change fate.

In this bygone era, the physician could only hope their findings added up to a diagnosis of dropsy. With dropsy, the edematous condition known in today's vernacular as congestive heart failure, there was actually a treatment. This was because in 1785, the English physician William Withering described the use of foxglove for its treatment. As if a miracle, there was actually something that could be done. And thus, it says in my grandfather's textbook, handwritten at Rush Medical College, in his own careful script:

> For the treatment of edema with dyspnea due to dropsy, go to the place where foxglove plant grows and select several of the upper leaves. Roll them into a ball and place them into the pill compressor (it looks like a pair of pliers). Squeeze the handles with sufficient force so the result takes on the shape of a pill made from the leaves. Administer one pill by mouth on a daily basis. But (and this is the important part), don't squeeze the pill too tightly, otherwise it will be too hard and pass through the patient unchanged.

We have certainly come a long way in the last 100 years. The changes have been nothing short of astounding, but with irony that is inescapable. Today, pneumonia is curable, and heart failure is the irrevocable death sentence. How is it that congestive heart failure is now the veritable death sentence that slowly drowns its victims in their own secretions, filling the lungs with edema until the patient suffocates and slips into unconsciousness? This is the reality of the twenty-first century. With all our fancy medicines and technology, we can stall for time, but we still cannot change fate.

Congestive heart failure does not discriminate; it takes all with no regard to class, wealth, or age. And it continues to exact its toll on the human race, even though our species has been to the moon and back. From Dame Elizabeth Taylor to the guy who lives under a bridge in a cardboard box, for the last 20 years, the death rate from congestive heart failure has been historically consistent. Except for the lucky few who receive a heart transplant, like pneumonia at the turn of the century, today's diagnosis of heart failure is a death sentence. And while we have made great progress since the description of foxglove, we are only marginally closer to a cure than we were in my grandfather's era.

Heart failure is a diagnosis of deterioration, hospitalization, and discharge, repeating until death. And since a cure does not appear in the offing, what can we do? We can follow the mantra of the twentieth-century physician when faced with pneumonia. Provide comfort and maximize the quality of the patient's remaining days. That is the point of this book. This book outlines the opportunities to maximize the HF patient's quality of life. With rare exception, most people firmly state that days out of the hospital are better than days within. Returning for cyclic revisits to the emergency department and the hospital is a terrible stressor and robs the patient of any quality of life. So it is reasonable that a strategy whose goal is to improve a patient's few remaining days would focus on avoiding hospitalization, lengthening the time between rehospitalizations, and if hospitalization is absolutely necessary, shortening the time spent in the hospital.

This text presents strategies aimed at decreasing the length of time a patient spends engaged in the medical system, whether that be spending the night in the hospital, sitting in the emergency department undergoing evaluation and treatment, or calling an ambulance for a return visit. The goal is to make the patient feel better today while maximizing their quality time and independence outside of the hospital. Hopefully, we have served this mission.

Cleveland, OH, USA   W. Frank Peacock

Contents

Contributors

William Abraham, MD The Ohio State University, Columbus, OH, USA

Richard V. Aghababian, MD University of Massachusetts Medical School, Worcester, MA, USA

Nancy M. Albert, PhD, CCNS, CHFN, CCRN, FAHA Kaufman Center for Heart Failure, Cleveland Clinic, Cleveland, OH, USA

Ezra A. Amsterdam, MD Division of Cardiovascular Medicine, Department of Internal Medicine, Davis Medical Center, University of California, Sacramento, CA, USA

Khadijah Breathett, MD Department of Cardiology, The Ohio State University Medical Center, Columbus, OH, USA

Anna Marie Chang, MD Emergency Cardiac Care Fellow, Department of Emergency Medicine, University of Pennsylvania, Philadelphia, PA, USA

Michael Clarke, MD Department of Emergency Medicine, University of California, Davis Medical Center, Sacramento, CA, USA

Sean P. Collins, MSc, MD Department of Emergency Medicine, University of Cincinnati, Cincinnati, OH, USA

Ginger Conway, MSN, RN, CNP Division of Cardiovascular Disease, University of Cincinnati, Cincinnati, OH, USA

Shahriar Dadkhah, MD Swedish Covenant Hospital, Chicago, IL, USA

Chad E. Darling, MD Department of Emergency Medicine, University of Massachusetts Medical School, Worcester, MA, USA

Deborah B. Diercks, MD, MSc, FACEP Department of Emergency Medicine, University of California, Davis Medical Center, Sacramento, CA, USA

Arrash Fard, MD VA San Diego Healthcare System, San Diego, CA, USA

Gregory J. Fermann, MD Department of Emergency Medicine,
University of Cincinnati, Cincinnati, OH, USA

Patricia Fick, MD Department of Emergency Medicine, Vanderbilt University
Medical Center, Nashville, TN, USA

Brian Hiestand, MD, MPH, FACEP Department of Emergency Medicine,
Wake Forest University Health Sciences, Winston Salem, NC, USA

Judd E. Hollander, MD Department of Emergency Medicine,
University of Pennsylvania, Philadelphia, PA, USA

Kay Styer Holmes, RN, BSA, MSA Society of Chest Pain Centers,
Dublin, OH, USA

Navaid Iqbal, MD VA San Diego Healthcare System, San Diego, CA, USA

J. Douglas Kirk, MD, FACEP Department of Emergency Medicine, University
of California, Davis Medical Center, Sacramento, CA, USA

Karen Krechmery, RN, MSN Emory University Hospital Midtown,
Atlanta, GA, USA

Phillip D. Levy, MD, MPH Department of Emergency Medicine,
Wayne State University School of Medicine, Detroit, MI, USA

Alan Maisel, MD VA San Diego Healthcare System, San Diego, CA, USA

Arlene Mavko, BS, MA Society of Chest Pain Centers, Dublin, OH, USA

James McCord, MD Henry Ford Hospital, Detroit, MI, USA

Candace McNaughton, MD Department of Emergency Medicine,
Vanderbilt University Medical Center, Nashville, TN, USA

Vincent N. Mosesso Jr., MD Emergency Medicine, University of Pittsburgh
School of Medicine, Pittsburgh, PA, USA

Prehospital Care, University of Pittsburgh Medical Center,
Pittsburgh, PA, USA

L. Kristin Newby, MD, MHS Department of Medicine, Division
of Cardiovascular Medicine, Duke Clinical Research Institute,
Duke University Medical Center, Durham, NC, USA

Peter S. Pang, MD Department of Emergency Medicine, Center for
Cardiovascular Innovation - Department of Medicine, Northwestern University
Feinberg School of Medicine, Chicago, IL, USA

Rachel Rockford, MD Department of Emergency Medicine, University of
California, Davis Medical Center, Sacramento, CA, USA

Korosh Sharain, MA Stritch School of Medicine, Loyola University Chicago,
Chicago, IL, USA

Sandra Sieck, RN, MBA Sieck Healthcare Consulting, Mobile, AL, USA

Karina M. Soto-Ruiz, MD Baylor College of Medicine, Houston, TX, USA

Alan Storrow, MD Department of Emergency Medicine, Vanderbilt University Medical Center, Nashville, TN, USA

Richard Summers, MD Division of Cardiovascular Medicine, Department of Internal Medicine, University of Mississippi Medical Center, Jackson, Mississippi

Valorie Sweigart, RN, DNP Emory University Hospital Midtown, Atlanta, GA, USA

Kathleen L. Tong, MD Division of Cardiovascular Medicine, Department of Internal Medicine, Davis Medical Center, University of California, Sacramento, CA, USA

Robin J. Trupp, PhD, ACNP-BC, CHFN Society of Chest Pain Center, Columbus, OH, USA

Marvin A. Wayne, MD University of Washington, Seattle, WA, USA

EMS Medical Program Director, Whatcom County, WA, USA

Emergency Department, Peacehealth St. Joseph Medical Center, Bellingham, WA, USA

A. Keith Wesley, MD Medical Director, HealthEast Medical Transportation, St. Paul, MN, USA

Matthew A. Wheatley, MD Department of Emergency Medicine, Emory University School of Medicine, Atlanta, GA, USA

Yang Xue, MD VA San Diego Healthcare System, San Diego, CA, USA

Masood Zaman, MD Department of Emergency Medicine, Center for Cardiovascular Innovation - Department of Medicine, Northwestern University Feinberg School of Medicine, Chicago, IL, USA

Part I
Administrative and Regulatory Issues

Chapter 1
Society of Chest Pain Centers' Heart Failure Accreditation

Kay Styer Holmes and Arlene Mavko

Introduction

The Society of Chest Pain Centers (SCPC) is an international nonprofit organization dedicated to assisting healthcare facilities improve the care of their cardiac patients. It was established in 1998 by a group of cardiologists and emergency medicine physicians whose goals were to breakdown the silos in the care of the acute coronary syndrome (ACS) patient and to reduce cardiovascular mortality. SCPC has two primary strategies to accomplish these goals—education and accreditation.

SCPC introduced chest pain accreditation in 2003 as a vehicle to provide facilities with a road map to improve their processes and decrease variances in the care of the cardiac patient. The entire accreditation process is designed and built upon the principles of improvement science. It is important to approach the work of accreditation as a process improvement initiative. If approached in this manner, facilities will gain insight into the beginning of the process (gap analysis) and the direction they need to take (plan/charter) to improve their processes of care for cardiac patients.

SCPC recognized that heart failure is a leading cause of morbidity and mortality in the USA and is a growing burden for healthcare facilities and emergency departments. Thus, SCPC first offered Heart Failure Accreditation in 2009 as a natural transition from Chest Pain Accreditation, and because many of the underlying strategies and structure of accreditation work to improve the care of the heart failure patient. According to studies by [1] and [2], accredited chest pain centers performed significantly better on both their chest pain and heart failure CMS core measures, respectively. This suggested that Heart Failure Accreditation would have the same quality improvement outcomes as that established by accreditation of chest pain centers, in respect to patients presenting with suspected acute coronary syndromes.

K.S. Holmes, RN, BSA, MSA (✉) • A. Mavko, BS, MA
Society of Chest Pain Centers, Dublin, OH, USA
e-mail: kholmes@scpcp.org

W. Frank Peacock (ed.), *Short Stay Management of Acute Heart Failure*,
Contemporary Cardiology, DOI 10.1007/978-1-61779-627-2_1,
© Springer Science+Business Media, LLC 2012

Heart Failure Accreditation

Patients with a diagnosis of heart failure represent 20% of all hospital readmissions within 30 days of previous discharge [3]. This patient population is difficult to manage due to their chronic state and taxes our healthcare resources. Healthcare facilities could benefit from a standardized approach for this patient population to ensure appropriate patient placement and follow-up care, decreased hospital readmissions, and improved quality of life. In the latter part of 2007, SCPC brought together a team of nationally recognized healthcare professionals to write recommendations for the short stay management and evaluation of the heart failure patient. Collectively, these clinicians pooled their expertise and available research to provide the first written document describing the treatment of this patient population in an observation environment.

Heart Failure Accreditation encompasses the entire facility and is not a specification/inspection compliance–driven approach but rather an effort to engage facilities in an improvement process. The quality of care for the heart failure patient should be measured in some manner to demonstrate improvement. To the degree possible, the entire accreditation process is designed to be collegial and collaborative. The philosophy at SCPC is one of respect and realization of the uniqueness of facilities and the populations they serve.

The Process

The accreditation tool is laid out in tiers. A tier is a set of items arranged in rows. Items are specific features related to Heart Failure Accreditation. They are designed to be binary—that is, they are either present or absent. Items are categorized into four different tiers, each with a specific designation and color-coded as follows:

Tier I	Blue	Key elements	Main categories
Tier II	Yellow	Essential items	Detailed practices or processes related to the successful operation at the facility
Tier III	Green	Best practice items	Items based on research, guidelines, and current standards of care
Tier IV	Pink	Innovative items	Practices (ways of caring for patients and the organizational support for the care process) that are groundbreaking or pioneering

In order to achieve accreditation, when evaluated, facilities must receive a "Yes" for all tier I and tier II items and for some tier III items. Furthermore, facilities must provide documentation to support their achievement of the tier items marked "Yes." In addition to the documentation review, the accreditation review specialist will complete an onsite visit to validate the facility's documentation and processes. The accreditation review specialist also will submit a final report to an oversight committee (the Accreditation Review Committee), which makes the final determination to grant accreditation. Accreditation is for a 3-year period from the date that the Accreditation Review Committee makes its determination.

Key Elements

Key elements, all written on blue background, are items that represent the most general categories for Heart Failure Accreditation as follows:

Key Element 1: Emergency Department Integration with the Emergency Medical Services

- This key element encourages a formal relationship with the local emergency medical services to develop prehospital medication and airway protocols that will result in more timely and better outcomes for the patient.

Key Element 2: Emergency Assessment of Patients with Symptoms of AHF— Diagnosis

- This key element evaluates the facility's clinical processes as they relate to the initial presentation of the patient in the emergency department to facilitate rapid diagnosis and appropriate treatment.

Key Element 3: Risk Stratification of the Heart Failure Patient

- The intent of this key element is to provide guidance to assure that patients are placed in the most cost-effective environment within the hospital setting for their severity of illness or in an observation status.

Key Element 4: Treatment for Patients Presenting to the Emergency Department in Heart Failure

- The facility should have a streamlined standardized approach for patients presenting to the ED in acute decompensated heart failure. Treatment algorithms can be used as a tool to guide treatment modalities.

Key Element 5: Heart Failure Discharge Criteria from the Emergency Department and/or Observation Stay

- The decision to discharge the patient is made upon demonstrable clinical improvements as well as his/her ability to be managed as an outpatient.

Key Element 6: Heart Failure Patient Education in the Emergency Department and Observation Unit

- Over 70% of hospitalizations for heart failure in the USA have been linked to the patient's failure to follow medication regimens, dietary restrictions, and failure to seek care for worsening symptoms. The intent of Key Element 6 is to ensure that facilities educate patients thoroughly and consistently in all facets of self-care.

Key Element 7: Personnel, Competencies, and Training

- This key element is intended to ensure that there is a standard of care at facilities regarding physicians, nurses, technicians, and other healthcare providers who care for the heart failure patient. Physicians, nurses, techs, and other hospital personnel in contact with heart failure patients need ongoing education and training to keep current with standards of care, best practices, technology, and research literature.

Key Element 8: Process Improvement

- This key element helps facilities identify gaps in their processes and demonstrate improvements in both the processes of care and the outcomes for the heart failure patient. Their plan should integrate continuous improvement of all aspects of care, including quality monitoring and evaluation of processes for the care of the heart failure patient.

Key Element 9: Organizational Structure and Commitment

- Heart Failure Accreditation encompasses the entire facility. It is an operational model to improve processes of care for the heart failure patient. It is important for the entire facility that there is participation by administration and a commitment to work as a team and allocate resources to ensure the success of accreditation and demonstrate improvement in patient care.

Key Element 10: Community Outreach

- The intent of this key element is to ensure that all facilities with Heart Failure Accreditation are actively involved in educating the internal and external community on heart diseases, preventive measures, early heart attack care, risk factors for heart disease, signs and symptoms of heart failure, and self-care. It is SCPC's philosophy that facilities with Heart Failure Accreditation have an obligation and show a commitment to reducing heart-related deaths through public education.

Why Society of Chest Pain Centers and Providers Heart Failure Accreditation?

- Requires risk stratification protocols to ensure appropriate placement of patients based on their clinical presentation, comorbidities, and response to treatment
- Encourages facilities to identify gaps, revise processes of care, create standardization, and measure results
- Breaks down silos among departments to bring teams together to improve care
- Ensures that operational efficiencies gained meet clinical and financial goals, such as a decrease in 30-day readmissions and length of stay

- Engages emergency medical services in the process to include airway and medication protocol development as well as documentation to describe the patient's status prior to treatment that can support reimbursement
- Promotes the use of standardized order sets to improve patient safety, ensure appropriate documentation, and provide evidence-based care
- Avoids costly readmissions due to unclear medication discharge instructions, lack of posthospital follow-up care, and ineffective patient education
- Decreases exposure risk for audits from third-party providers and regulators through appropriate documentation and patient placement
- Decreases liability exposure when using protocol driven, evidence-based medicine
- Educates the community about recognizing symptoms of heart failure and provides a sense of partnership between patients, their families, and the healthcare team

Summary

SCPC has an international reputation as the leader in chest pain accreditation. Currently, there are over 650 accredited chest pain centers in the USA, which represents approximately 13% of all facilities available to become accredited. Once accredited, 93% of facilities choose to retain their accredited status, and the growth for accreditation continues at a rapid rate. Heart Failure Accreditation differs from Chest Pain Accreditation only because heart failure is more difficult to diagnosis and treat and the patient population tends to be more chronic than acute. SCPC has embraced this challenge to provide facilities with the means to improve both patient care and financial outcomes.

References

1. Ross MA, Amsterdam E, Peacock WF, Graff L, Fesmire F, Garvey JL, Kelly S, Holmes K, Karunaratne HB, Toth M, Dadkhah S, McCord J. Chest pain center accreditation is associated with better performance of center for medicare and medicaid services core measures for acute myocardial infarction. Am J Cardiol. 2008;102(2):120–4.
2. Peacock WF, Lesikar S, Ross MA, Diercks D, Graff L, Storrow A, McCord J, Ander D, Garvey JL. Chest pain center accreditation is associated with improved heart failure quality performance measures. Abstract presentation at the Society for Academic Emergency Medicine Annual Meeting, May 2008.
3. American Heart Association. Heart disease and stroke statistics 2010 update. Dallas, TX: American Heart Association; 2010.

Chapter 2
The Economics and Reimbursement of Congestive Heart Failure

Sandra Sieck

Introduction

Cardiovascular disease (CVD) remains entrenched as the leading cause of mortality in the USA [1]. Although the overall death rates due to CVD have been decreasing due to the increased incorporation of evidence-based therapies, the overall incidence of heart failure (HF) has remained relatively unchanged over the last two decades while the prevalence of HF has increased [2]. Innovative and exciting new treatment options offer the promise of improvement in activity-limiting symptoms, enhanced quality of life, and possibly, reduced mortality. Yet the economic burden of HF continues to impose a staggering challenge to all segments of the healthcare system. This challenge is particularly prominent for the acute care facility in the era of tightening budgets, diminishing reimbursements, quality of care mandates, government regulation, and an aging population.

While HF is indeed a chronic medical condition that physicians strive to optimally control, it is acute decompensated heart failure (ADHF) that most adversely affects the hospital's balance between providing effective acute care to patients and sustaining the economic viability of the institution. As hospitals are faced with the relentless shift toward caring for only the most acutely ill patients, they will be forced to develop more efficient, efficacious, cost-minimizing, and evidence-based treatment paths in order to remain viable and competitive in the rapidly changing healthcare market place.

S. Sieck, RN, MBA (✉)
Sieck Healthcare Consulting, Mobile, AL, USA
e-mail: ssieck@scpcp.org

W. Frank Peacock (ed.), *Short Stay Management of Acute Heart Failure*,
Contemporary Cardiology, DOI 10.1007/978-1-61779-627-2_2,
© Springer Science+Business Media, LLC 2012

Burden of Disease

Heart failure represents approximately 7% of the total burden of all cardiovascular diseases (CVD) [3]. The absolute incidence of HF is estimated at 670,000 new cases in a year and is age-related (Fig. 2.1) [4, 5]. Gains in survival with current therapies have resulted in an increase in the overall prevalence of HF [6]. In 2005, HF prevalence was 5.3 million [7]. By 2006, the prevalence of HF in the USA increased to 5.8 million or roughly 2.6% of the adult population [2] (Fig. 2.2). While the disease does occur in all ages, it is predominantly a disease of the elderly, with incidence and prevalence increasing with age. Among 40–59 year olds, 1–2% has HF. In the 60–79 age range, the prevalence increases to 4.8% for women and 9.3% for men [8]. With the aging US population, the number of people with HF is likely to continue to increase.

The increasing prevalence of HF also translates to substantial healthcare resource utilization. Almost 15 million office visits are attributable to HF [9]. HF is the most frequent Medicare diagnosis-related group (Medicare Severity or MS-DRG) payment system for hospital billing [10]. HF is responsible for more elderly hospitalizations than any other medical condition [11]. Hospital discharges for HF exceeded 1.1 million in 2006, up from nearly 1.08 million in 2005 and nearly one million in 2001 (Fig. 2.3). Total hospital days for HF are estimated at 6.5 million annually [9]. Although the average length of stay has decreased over the last decade to 6.3 days, the 30-day readmission rate has increased to 20% and is roughly 50% at 6 months [12].

HF represents a resource-intense and costly condition to treat. The total cost of care for HF continues to rise each year. HF is estimated to account for approximately $39.2 billion in total costs in 2010, up from $34.8 billion in 2008 [2]. Direct costs

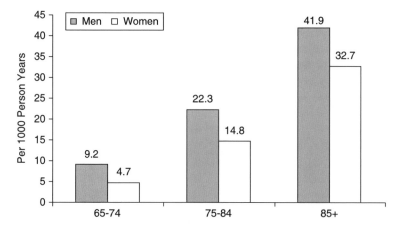

Fig. 2.1 The incidence of heart failure in the United States by age range and gender (From the American Heart Association Heart Disease and Stroke Statistics, Update 2010; Source: http://circ. ahajournals.org/cgi/reprint/CIRCULATIONAHA.109.192667)

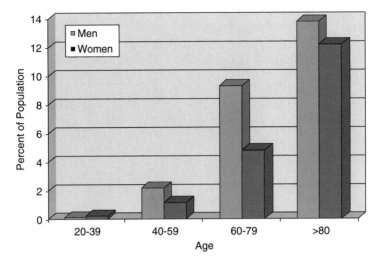

Fig. 2.2 Trends in the prevalence of heart failure in the United States by age range and gender (From the American Heart Association Heart Disease and Stroke Statistics, Update 2010; Adapted from http://circ.ahajournals.org/cgi/reprint/CIRCULATIONAHA.109.192667)

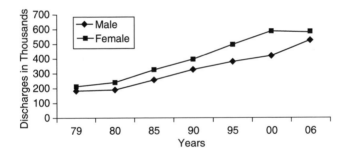

Fig. 2.3 Hospital discharges for heart failure in the USA (1979–2006). Trends in hospital discharges for heart failure in the United States (From the American Heart Association Heart Disease and Stroke Statistics, Update 2010; Source: http://circ.ahajournals.org/cgi/reprint/CIRCULATIONAHA.109.192667)

are estimated to be $33.7 billion and indirect costs $3.5 in 2009 [13] (Table 2.1). Heart failure costs represent 7–8% of the total care costs for all cardiovascular diseases. Of the subsets of healthcare costs, hospital charges account for 60% of the direct costs, with nursing home charges a distant second place at 13% (Fig. 2.4). These figures substantiate the importance of the hospital in the overall economic burden of HF. Hospitals bear both the brunt of the costs of care and the onus to provide more cost-efficient care to these patients.

Table 2.1 Cardiovascular disease costs in the United States: Breakdown of costs of cardiovascular care in the United States by disease type and category of care services (Adapted from American Heart Association Cardiovascular Diseases in the United States 2009)

	Heart diseases	Coronary heart disease	Stroke	Hypertensive disease	Heart failure	Total cardiovascular disease
Direct costs totals	$183.0	$92.8	$45.9	$54.2	$33.7	$313.8
Hospital	106.3	54.6	20.2	8.2	20.1	150.1
Nursing home	23.4	12.3	16.2	4.9	4.5	49.2
Physicians/other professionals	23.9	13.4	3.7	13.4	2.4	46.4
Drugs/other medical durables	22.1	10.3	1.4	25.4	3.3	52.3
Home health care	7.4	2.2	4.4	2.4	3.4	16.8
Indirect costs (totals)	$121.6	$72.6	$23.0	$192.2	$3.5	$161.5
Lost productivity/morbidity	24.0	10.6	7.0	8.4	–	30.1
Lost productivity/mortality	97.6	62.0	16.0	10.9	3.5	122.4
Grand totals	$304.6	$165.4	$68.9	$73.4	$37.2	$475.3

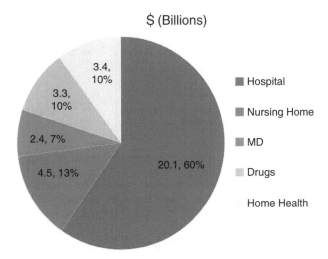

Fig. 2.4 Costs for heart failure in the United States (2009). Costs for heart failure in the United States by type of service (Data adapted from data in Table 1)

Hospital Care

Most ADHF patients are treated in the inpatient environment. The emergency department (ED) is the point of entry for three out of every four ADHF patients, and 75–90% of HF patients presenting to the ED are ultimately admitted to the hospital [14]. Since most HF patients are of Medicare age, facilities are reimbursed on a fixed inpatient payment under the current MS-DRG system effective since October 2008 and, therefore, must provide extremely efficient care in order to maintain financial viability. Today the average MS-DRG (291, 292, and 293) reimbursement is $5,759 for the acute care facility, which often does not receive sufficient reimbursement to cover the costs of care for the ADHF patient. Under the former DRG payment system for a typical hospital, the financial break-even point was roughly 5 days, but the average ADHF patient has a length of stay greater than 5 days, resulting in a fiscal loss for the hospital. A review of cost data in 2001 demonstrated an average loss of $2,104 per ADHF patient [15]. The new MS-DRG system was designed to more appropriately align financial compensation to severity and should offset some but not all of these losses.

In addition to the challenges of providing optimal efficiency in caring for the ADHF patient to avoid financial losses, CMS has placed further burdens on facilities by targeting inappropriate 1-day length of stay admissions and readmissions within 30 days. Review of such admissions could result in the hospital potentially losing reimbursement for such admissions, and thus further compounding an already fiscally austere situation. In light of the high readmission rates noted earlier, the hospital is vulnerable to even further losses as they could become fully financially responsible for the care of such patients. Facing such fiscal pressures in an already challenging overall economic environment, hospitals have been forced to reevaluate current practices and redesign care models for the ADHF patient.

The Observation Unit and Heart Failure

Over the last 10 years, emergency departments (ED) saw patient volume increasing substantially. In 2007, there were 117 million visits to the ED in the USA [16]. As the volume of ED visits continued to increase, admissions to acute care facilities increased, thus decreasing the access to inpatient beds. In an effort to improve access and reduce costs, hospitals have focused on efforts to further reduce length of stays and shift care from the inpatient to the outpatient arena.

In the 1990s, certain patients were often held in the ED for observation in an attempt to make a more clinically educated decision about the need for admission versus the safety of discharge after appropriate intensified treatment [17]. More formal chest pain centers (CPC) emerged and marked the initial attempts to evaluate low-risk chest pain patients for myocardial infarction in a short stay unit, often within the emergency department. This approach represented an operational mechanism to improve quality of care, enhance clinical outcomes, and reduce overall costs. The success of the CPC showed that quality of care was not compromised in this fiscally sound model. The CPC led the way for the development of a more formalized observation unit (OU) that could be expanded to treatment of other medical conditions, providing the same level of care in the outpatient setting as in the acute care setting.

As the OU evolved, the Centers for Medicare and Medicaid Services (CMS) initially targeted asthma, chest pain, and ADHF for efforts to reduce morbidity and mortality through use of efficient evaluation and intense treatment in nonacute care settings. CMS defines observation care as a "well defined set of specific, clinically appropriate services, which include ongoing short-term treatment, assessment, and reassessment before a decision can be made regarding whether a patient will require further treatment as hospital inpatients or if they are able to be discharged from the hospital" [18]. OU services are less than 48 h and often less than 24 h. Under unusual circumstances, it may exceed 48 h.

In the typical ED evaluation of the ADHF patients, over 75% of patients ended up being admitted to the acute hospital setting [19]. With intense and focused treatment, the OU affords the opportunity to reduce inpatient admissions. In a study of a hospitalist-run short stay unit, a heart failure diagnosis predicted stays longer than 72 h [20]. In this study, need for consultations and the lack of accessibility to diagnostic tests resulted in longer stays. OUs can accelerate accessibility to these services. Studies show that institution of evidence-based aggressive treatments in the OU, 75% of HF patients can be discharged home from the OU. Benefit also exists for those who require inpatient admission after OU treatment, as their overall hospital length of stay is shorter than for those admitted directly to the inpatient setting [21] (Fig. 2.5).

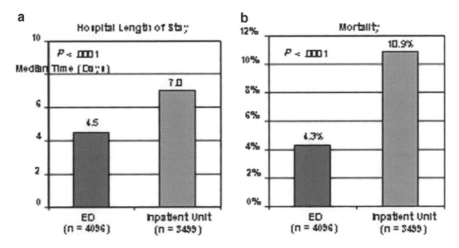

Fig. 2.5 Effect of site initiation of therapy on length of stay and mortality. ED, emergency department (From Emerman CL. Treatment of the acute decompensation of heart failure: efficacy and pharmacoeconomics of early initiation of therapy in the emergency department. *Rev Cardiovasc Med* 2003;3 (Suppl 7):S13–S20)

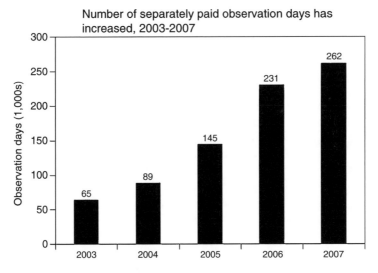

Fig. 2.6 Number of separately paid observation days has increased

Use of OU days has increased substantially over the decade (Fig. 2.6). Between 2003 and 2007, there was a 403% increase in OU separately payable observation days. The number of OU days increased from 65,000 in 2003 to over 262,000 in 2007 [22]. In 2007, 2.1% of the 111 million ED visits were admitted to the OU [23]. Use of the OU is likely to continue to increase in the current healthcare environment.

The high cost for patients with heart failure is attributed to high rates of hospital admissions and long lengths of stay for acute decompensation of this condition. The OU emerged as a viable strategy for putting into play efficient and aggressive diagnostic and therapeutic urgent services in an intensely monitored situation [24]. Addition of case management, disease management, and discharge planning activities has been shown to avoid subsequent hospitalizations.

Disease Management in Heart Failure

Disease management (DM) programs have targeted heart failure from their inception. Early DM programs focused on high-risk patients, predominantly those recently discharged from the hospital following decompensation in CHF. Programs subsequently expanded to those HF patients who were at high risk but who had not yet been hospitalized. The processes and interventions were similar for both target groups.

Patients in the acute care facility, whether as inpatients or in the OU, attentive and thorough discharge planning is a critical piece of the successful DM program [25].

From the societal point of view, DM programs in heart failure benefit the patient with respect to clinical outcomes and quality of life and perhaps in individual costs of care. Early studies on HF DM programs showed mixed clinical outcome results. Some DM programs have shown reductions in hospitalization and mortality in short-term efforts in high-risk patients [26, 27]. Most recent studies have suggested cost-effectiveness may be demonstrated over the long-term and in a broader risk patient [28, 29]. Overall program costs are often higher in the DM group, but the QALY (quality-adjusted life year) gained is beneficial. The cost savings in reduced hospitalizations are often offset or exceeded by the costs of the intervention [30]. Insurers benefit from lowered costs of readmission. Hospitals experience less revenue from readmissions, but they benefit on national quality measures by showing reduced readmissions. Those stakeholders responsible for the payment of the costs of the programs may or may not financially benefit; only if they too are financially responsible for future hospitalizations are they likely to benefit.

DM provides focused and evidence-based treatment approaches to patients with HF. Medically, it is the most appropriate comprehensive management approach for this group, and it shows improved outcomes. The healthcare system will have to evolve in its methods for paying for such program to put the burden for intervention costs on the stakeholders most likely to benefit from the outcomes.

Clinical Outcomes

The importance of the OU to the healthcare system is in the benefit on clinical and financial outcomes. The use of nationally recognized clinical guidelines and pathways for the treatment of ADHF is the first step toward optimizing HF care.

The Joint Commission on Accreditation of Healthcare Organizations (JCAHO) has created a set of quality performance indicators for HF. These indicators include objective measurement of ejection fraction, angiotensin-converting enzyme (ACE) inhibitor treatment if tolerated, provision of complete discharge instructions, and smoking cessation counseling.

Despite treatment advances in HF that include medications and device-based therapies, many HF patients do not receive treatment according to these guidelines [31]. The lack of adherence to guidelines may be related in part to a lack of knowledge, but more likely is the result of operational inefficiencies. Intense DM efforts to incorporate evidence-based treatments that focus on the accepted quality indicators can impact the ADHF patient. A study from the Veterans Affairs San Diego Healthcare System demonstrated significant improvement in nationally established performance measures for HF using a multidisciplinary, computerized care pathway [32]. The well-designed OU can provide the operational efficiencies necessary to put treatment guidelines into effect and thereby achieve optimal clinical outcomes.

Although OU management has been demonstrated to reduce morbidity and a trend toward reduced mortality, further studies are needed to assess the full impact of focused OU care—diagnosis, treatment, intensity of service, and staffing—on quality measures.

Cost-Effectiveness of the Observation Unit

The OU provides a location for the provision of intense medical therapy and services under close observation and frequent monitoring of response to such treatment. In the ADHERE data registry (a multicenter, observational database of patients discharged from the hospital with a DRG diagnosis for HF), the time to initiation of administration of certain intravenous medicines specifically directed at acute HF was 1.1 h if the patient's treatment was initiated in the ED compared with 22 h if therapy was begun in an inpatient unit [33]. The OU protocols for both treatment and timely adjustments in treatment plans lead to more intense and timely initiation of therapy, which can have remarkable differences in clinical outcomes, as well as a dramatic impact on financial implications.

Treatment of ADHF in an OU has resulted in reduced 30-day readmissions and hospitalizations and decreased LOS if a subsequent hospitalization is required [34]. The Cleveland Clinic experience with OU as a venue for treatment of the ADHF patient also reported positive 90-day outcomes [35].

- Revisits were reduced by 44%.
- ED observation discharges were increased by 9%.
- HF rehospitalizations were reduced by 36%.
- Observation rehospitalizations were reduced by 39%.

Limited studies on the direct cost-effectiveness of OU in ADHF treatment exist. In a study of cost-effectiveness of OU admission, a subset of low-risk ADHF patients admitted to OU demonstrated an acceptable societal marginal ratio when compared to discharge from the ED [36]. This benefit was related to the somewhat higher risk of readmission and early-after-discharge rate of death associated with ED discharge. Future cost-effectiveness studies are required to further delineate how cost-effective the OU is for ADHF.

Observation Services Reimbursement

In 2002, CMS developed a new coding and reimbursement rate specifically to cover OU services for chest pain, asthma, and heart failure. Ambulatory Patient Classification Code (APC) 0339 was designed to compensate for treating patients with these subsets of conditions aggressively on the front end versus admitting them to the acute care setting. In addition to the APC, hospitals could also bill for most diagnostic tests that were performed during the OU stay, if medically necessary. This marked a new direction in reimbursement.

In 2008, the rules on observation status changed as reported in the Federal Register CMS-1392-FC pages 66,905–66,907. In this, CMS deleted APC 0339 and created two composite APC codes for extended assessment and management, of which observation care is a component. CMS views this as "totality" of care provided for an outpatient encounter.

The new APC codes are:

Outpatient		Inpatient
APC 8002 FY 2011	APC 8003 FY 2011	MS-DRG FY 2011
OBS direct referrals	OBS with ED levels 4–5	291, 292, and/or 293
Any condition that meets medical necessity		ICD-9-CM specific
$394	$714	$7923 MCC[a], $5450 CC[a], $3903 no MCC or CC
8–24 (48) h	8–24 (48) h	5–7 days

[a] See Appendix

- *APC 8002 Level I* (HCPCS code G0378; see Appendix): Extended Assessment and Management Composite APC (observation following a *direct referral* or clinic visit). This APC requires a level 99205 or 99215 clinic visit on the day of or the day before observation or a direct referral to observation [37]. The payment for the OU with the clinic visit is $394.22. There is no longer a separate billing for each of these services.
- *APC 8003 Level II*: (HCPCS code G0384) Extended Assessment and Management Composite APC (observation following an *emergency level 4 or 5 visit*). This code includes both ED visit and observation visit. This APC requires a 99284 or 99285 ED visit or a 99291 critical care level visit on the day of or day before observation. The payment for the OU with the ED visit is $714.33.

Table 2.2 The new APC codes

Outpatient		Inpatient
APC 8002 FY 2011	APC 8003 FY 2011	MS-DRG FY 2011
OBS direct referrals	OBS with ED levels 4–5	291, 292, and/or 293
Any condition that meets medical necessity		ICD-9-CM specific
$394	$714	$7923 MCC[a], $5450 CC[a], $3903 no MCC or CC
8–24 (48) h	8–24 (48) h	5–7 days

[a] See Appendix

These new APC codes can be used for any condition requiring observation and noninvasive testing and lasting from 8 to 48 h. The APC coding can be financially beneficial to the hospital compared to the inpatient stay with MS-DRG payment (see Appendix). Most diagnostic tests that are performed during the OU stay are billable and reimbursable separately from the OU stay if deemed medically necessary. Another benefit of the APC coding for the hospital is that revisits occurring within 30 days or admissions to the hospital after an OU visit are all reimbursable. There is no restriction to the number of claims that can be submitted for a patient if billed under the APC outpatient system. Also, if a patient is admitted to an OU and then requires an inpatient hospital admission at that same point of contact, there is no "penalty." The hospital does not get the APC outpatient reimbursement, but instead receives the full MS-DRG inpatient reimbursement (Table 2.2).

While the new APC coding can be fiscally favorable to the hospital, there are more strict rules attendant to reimbursement. The updated Medicare Claims Processing Manual (Chap. 4, Sect. 290) and the Medicare Benefit Policy Manual (Chap. 6, Sect. 20.6) clarify key requirements for appropriate OU billing as follows:

- Observation care is an outpatient status that must be ordered as such by a physician and reported with a HCPCS code (see Appendix).
- The medical record must clearly verify that the physician has risk stratified the patient to determine the patient would be likely to benefit from OU care.
- A hospital begins billing for observation services, reported with HCPCS code G0378, at the clock time documented in the patient's medical record, which coincides with the time that observation services are initiated in accordance with a physician's order for observation services.
- The physician must clearly document in the progress notes the care plan for each hour of the stay.
- Reimbursements are only made for medically necessary hours, not just hours that a patient occupies a bed. OU is billed hourly to the payers and *reported as units of service*. Each hour must be deemed medically necessary with active and appropriate physician involvement for each billable hour. Observation time must be documented in the medical record.
- A beneficiary's time in observation (and hospital billing) ends when all clinical or medical interventions have been completed, including follow-up care furnished

by hospital staff and physicians that may take place after a physician has ordered the patient to be released or admitted as an inpatient.

- The number of units reported with HCPCS code G0378 [packaged under one of the two composite APCs (8002–8003)] must equal or exceed 8 h.
- Hospitals may bill for patients who are "direct referrals" to observation. A "direct referral" occurs when a physician in the community refers a patient to the hospital for observation, bypassing the clinic or emergency department (ED).
- Separate reimbursement may be made for all services with an S indicator and X ancillary services (see Appendix).
- The facility can bill for studies performed, but the patient is "clocked out" of the OU for the time spent having the study.

These are the current rules for Medicare patients. If a patient is not Medicare eligible, the rules for observation payment can differ for each payer, and the hospital must be aware of the contractual or standard payment processes for such care.

In order to optimize efficiency and revenues from an OU, the hospital must design its OU to operationally maximize its daily use. While the OU can be in any specific physical location within a facility, estimates of the potential volume of OU cases must be made in advance of planning the unit. There are several key operational variables that deserve consideration [38]. The three key operational variables are occupancy rate, duration of observation, and discharge home rate. Occupancy rate will never be 100% since there is significant variability in a patient's time of arrival and bed turnaround time. A realistic target in an efficient OU probably approaches 90%. The duration of observation must be a minimum of 8 h to attain reimbursement under the composite APC's 8002 or 8003. The probable duration is likely to be between 8 and 24 h. And finally, the current experience and literature suggest that a discharge home rate of 80% probably represents a maximum outcome. These three variables are linked as each one affects the others. Additionally, in order to maintain the OU in an optimal operational state requires critical patient selection with well-defined inclusion and exclusion criteria and identification of those patient characteristics that are ideal for the OU treatment venue.

Physician supervision rules for CY 2011 also impact OU services and reimbursements.

CMS has identified supervision requirements for the provision of both therapeutic and diagnostic services furnished to hospital outpatients. Medicare requires hospitals to provide direct supervision for the delivery of all outpatient therapeutic services.

- Therapeutic services and supplies which hospitals provide on an outpatient basis are those services and supplies (including the use of hospital facilities) which are "incident to" the services of physicians and practitioners in the treatment of patients. *All hospital outpatient services that are not diagnostic are services that aid the physician or practitioner in the treatment of the patient. Such therapeutic services include clinic services, emergency room services, and observation services.*
- Direct supervision means that the physician or nonphysician practitioner is immediately available to furnish assistance and direction throughout the performance of the procedure, but it does not mean that the supervising individual

needs to be present in the room when the procedure is performed. CMS defined a *set of 16 services* requiring direct supervision by a physician or nonphysician practitioner to begin the service (referred to as "initiation"), followed by "general" supervision for the remainder of the service. The services include *observation*, intravenous infusion, and therapeutic, prophylactic, or diagnostic injection.

- General supervision means that the procedure is furnished under the physician's overall direction and control, but the physician's presence is not required during the performance of the procedure.
- Personal supervision means a physician must be in attendance in the same room during the performance of the procedure.

Although the reimbursement levels for APC codes are smaller compared to the MS-DRG reimbursement for a hospitalization, the operational expense for an OU stay is also smaller. Overhead costs are generally less in the ED or outpatient units when compared to inpatient treatments because of the productivity and turnover rate of the beds. Thus, intense therapy for ADHF that results in a short stay in an OU can actually result in a profit for the hospital facility. But the ability to show a profit in the ADHF patient still requires a redesign of the current system and attention to an early risk-stratified, protocol-driven process in order to be successful.

Consolidated Versus Virtual Design

Reimbursement is likely to continue to change over time, and the design of the OU with respect to number of beds and physical layout will be impacted by these changes. The CMS are now targeting all diagnosis that meets medical necessity for observation services in an effort to increase quality, reduce cost, and reduce the number of inappropriate admissions. Consolidated units by design are concentrated resources in a common area designed to meet these strategic objectives. Virtual units are house wide lacking concentric resources proving difficult to follow the stringent policies and procedures released in the latest Federal Registry for observation services. However, the core of design of the OU must be optimal clinical management and provision of the "right care at the right time."

Emerging Trends

Despite the focus of health care reform efforts, costs of health care continue to increase at rates above the consumer price index (CPI) [39]. The most formidable factor in today's healthcare arena involves pushback from payers that are demanding cost-efficient quality care. Payers will no longer be willing to simply reimburse for absolute units of care, even if such care is deemed medically necessary. Payers are expecting value for their expenditures. Charges for care must be accompanied by measured demonstration of quality.

Centers for Medicare and Medicaid Studies, Moving to Value-based Purchasing System

Transforming Medicare from a passive payer to an active purchaser of higher quality, more efficient health care system

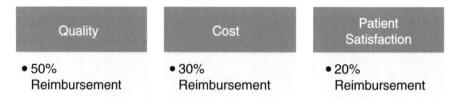

Quality	Cost	Patient Satisfaction
• 50% Reimbursement	• 30% Reimbursement	• 20% Reimbursement

Tools and Incentive for promoting better quality, while avoiding unnecessary costs
* Tools = Measurement and Public Reporting
* Incentives = Pay for Reporting and Pay for Performance

Fig. 2.7 CMS—moving to value-based purchasing system (Source: http://www.cms.gov/AcuteInpatientPPS/downloads/hospital_VBP_plan_issues_paper.pdf issued Jan. 17, 2007)

CMS has been moving forward in this regard on several fronts and is currently leading the way in value-based reimbursement. Historically, Medicare reimbursement has rewarded the quantity of healthcare services provided. Recognizing that this perverse system indirectly rewards potential overutilization and unnecessary services, a redirection toward value-based purchasing (VBP) emerged to transform the current system into one that will reward providers for delivering high quality and efficient care in an integrated delivery system (Fig. 2.7). CMS believes this program will represent a critical piece in its evolution from a passive payer to an active purchaser of quality care.

CMS has actively piloted quality-based programs in different treatment venue settings. Although subsequent alteration of the hospital VBP details are anticipated as results emerge after implementation, the final rule for the Medicare Hospital Inpatient VBP Program became effective on July 1, 2011.[1] This program will begin in fiscal year (FY) 2013 and will be applied to discharges occurring on or after October 1, 2012.

Hospitals will continue to receive payments for care provided to Medicare patients based on the Medicare Inpatient Prospective Payment System. However, hospitals will see overall payment reductions from 2013 through 2017. These payment reductions (across the board cuts of 1 percent to start) will provide funding for

[1] Department of Health and Human Services, Centers for Medicare and Medicaid Services, 42 CFR Parts 422 and 480, Medicare Program: Hospital Inpatient Value-Based Purchasing Program. Federal Register/Vol.76, No. 88/Friday, May 6, 2001/Rules and Regulations.

the VBP program. In FY 2013, this amount is estimated to be $850 million, which will then be used for the new incentive payments. The reduction in payment increases by 0.25%/yr to FY 2017 and maxes out at 2%.

Facilities will be able to 'earn back' these funds through the VBP performance measures. CMS has selected 13 measures which will be the foundation of the initial hospital VBP program in 2013 (Table 2.3). This first set includes primarily process of care measures and a patient experience of care measure. This set is comprised of currently used measures that are considered standard evidence-based reflections of quality care and measures that haven't yet 'topped out.' FY 2014 measures will include mortality measures, AHRQ patient safety indicators and hospital acquired condition measures (Table 2.4).

Benchmarks have been developed for these indicators and a scoring methodology was created that assigns an achievement and improvement score to each hospital for each of the measures. Thus, either attainment of target goal or improvement in a score compared to the baseline period will result in higher reimbursement levels. While the ability of the hospital VBP method to alter the way healthcare is provided, result in improved outcomes, and reduce overall costs is unknown, its introduction clearly represents an important shift in future provider reimbursements.

Another emerging payment model focuses on a shift in responsibility away from physician and hospital to a shared responsibility between the physician and the hospital. The new healthcare reform act unveiled the concept of the accountable healthcare

Table 2.3 Final Measure Set for Fiscal Year 2013 Hospital Value Based Purchasing Program

Measure	Measure Description
	Clinical Processes of Care Measures
	Acute Myocardial Infarction
AMI-7a	Fibrinolytic therapy received within 90 minutes of hospital arrival
AMI-8a	Primary PCI received within 90 minutes of hospital arrival
	Heart Failure
HF-1	Discharge instructions
	Pneumonia
PN-3b	Blood cultures performed in the ER prior to antibiotic received in the hospital
PN-6	Initial antibiotic selection for CAP in immunocompromised patients
	Healthcare-Associated Infections
SCIP-Inf-1	Prophylactic antibiotic received within one hour prior to surgical incision
SCIP-Inf-2	Prophylactic antibiotic selection for surgical patients
SCIP-Inf-3	Prophylactic antibiotics discontinued within 24 hours after surgery end time
SCIP-Inf-4	Cardiac surgery patients with controlled 6AM postoperative serum glucose
	Surgeries
SCIP-Card-2	Surgery patients on a beta-blocker prior to arrival that received a beta blocker during the perioperative period
SCIP-VTE-1	Surgery patients with recommended venous thromboembolism prophylaxis ordered
SCIP-VTE-2	Surgery patients who received appropriate venous thromboembolism prophylaxis within 24 hours prior to surgery to 24 hours after surgery
	Patient Experience of Care Measures
HCAHPS	Hospital Consumer Assessment of Healthcare Providers and Systems Survey

PCI percutaneous coronary intervention, *ER* emergency room, *CAP* community acquired pneumonia

Table 2.4 FY 2014 Outcome Measures for VBP Program

Category	Measures
Mortality Measures	Acute Myocardial Infarction 30 day mortality
	Heart Failure 30 day mortality
	Pneumonia 30 day mortality
AHRQ Patient Safety Indicators	Complication/patient safety for selected indicators
	Mortality for selected medical conditions
Hospital Acquired Condition Measures	Foreign object retained after surgery
	Air embolism
	Blood incompatibility
	Pressure ulcers Stages III-IV
	Falls and trauma
	Vascular catheter-associated infections
	Catheter-associated urinary tract infection
	Manifestations of poor glycemic control

organization to prompt collaboration between groups of doctors and hospitals to provide more integrated and coordinated care. While some managed care organizations already practice this model, it will involve some creativity in nonmanaged areas of the country to come to full fruition

Health plans have introduced pay-for-performance programs that reward providers and facilities for providing higher quality care. While quality appears to be the focus of such efforts, there is an underlying belief that such care will also reduce overall costs. Thus, marrying cost and quality is becoming an entrenched theme in today's healthcare environment.

CMS is also focusing efforts on reducing fraud and abuse in the healthcare system. According to CMS officials, new rules would give federal health officials more power to identify fraud early and help them reduce an estimated $55 billion in improper payments made annually through Medicare and Medicaid [40]. It is estimated that over $60 billion is lost annually by Medicare from fraud. The Federal Bureau of Investigation estimates that 3–10% of the public and private healthcare dollar is lost to fraud, amounting to $75–250 billion annually [41]. Some estimates go as high as $100 billion.

The hospital setting is in the midst of more intense scrutiny. In 2009, the federal RAC program (Recovery Audit Contractors) was created to recover monies related to inappropriate admissions. The third-party contractors review 1-day hospitalizations that are deemed unnecessary as services could have safely been provided in the outpatient setting [42]. Unfavorable reviews can result in significant loss of monies for hospitals. Observation services targets 24 h length of stay (LOS). One-day stay = 24 h. What is the difference? The main difference is the ability to provide safe, cost-effective care in the most resource appropriate setting. With the LOS remaining constant in this equation, medical necessity is the deciding factor. If a patient truly meets inpatient criteria, then the inpatient setting is the appropriate environment for care. Any issues with this decision can be alleviated through proper documentation. One-day stays are not the only objective of the RAC program. Excessive readmission and several MS-DRGs known to have historical high error rates are also targets. This is best demonstrated in the Program for Evaluating Payment Patterns Electronic Report (PEPPER) developed by the Texas Medical Foundation which provides hospital-specific Medicare data statistics for discharges vulnerable to improper payments.

These reimbursement initiatives make it critical for acute care facilities to enhance data-capturing capabilities, improve coding accuracy, apply risk stratification to care pathways, and focus on clinical outcomes in order to remain financially sound.

The acute care facility can survive in this ever-changing environment, but only if particular attentions to efficient processes and sound fiscal operation are maintained. For OU success in ADHF, this means creating and adhering to evidence-based guidelines, prompt and diligent physician oversight of care on an hourly basis, pristine medical record documentation, and redesign of the acute care model.

The Y-Model

In reviewing CMS' plan for value-based purchasing, hospitals must merge quality, finance, and patient satisfaction to create a viable plan of operation. While this is a common concept in the business world, it has not yet been fully incorporated throughout the healthcare arena. The Y-model is an innovative approach that allows facilities to closely examine different aspects of operations within their systems [43]. It encompasses the concept of healthcare delivery along a continuum from the point of entry into the "system" through to discharge. This Y-model can be applied to the overall operations of these systems or to one specific disease such as HF. By applying variations of the Y-model which all focus on three end points, quality, cost, and patient satisfaction facilities, can recognize ways to turn HF from a negative contribution margin to one that breaks even or contributes favorably.

Using the Y-model in the healthcare setting can be compared to an industrial setting. Industrial facilities can detail the exact route from raw material to finished product with detailed accuracy. The end product is priced to the market based on the operating costs within the process. If the manufacturing process varies greatly over time, costs of production rise and are passed on in a higher market price. In order to keep prices down, actions must be taken to get the variances under control. If not, the contribution margin is eroded and eventually could become negative. The objective is to keep the contribution margin at its maximum without compromising quality.

This model can be similarly applied to an ADHF patient routing through the healthcare delivery setting. Patients receive services within different "care units" within the acute hospital setting. These care units are analogous to the industrial setting's business units. By understanding how each care unit's operational strategies affect each subsequent care unit from point of entry to discharge, a seamless transfer of patient care in both outpatient and inpatient settings can optimize quality improvement and positive economic value. Without each care unit providing vital information to others in this holistic approach, moving patients efficiently through the system is challenged.

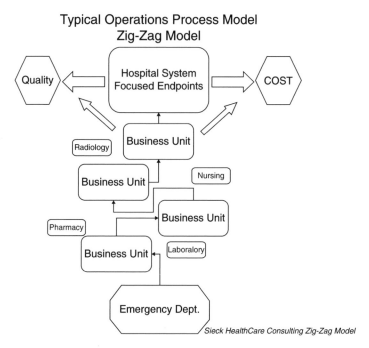

Fig. 2.8 Zigzag model of care (2008 Update: Sieck S. Cost effectiveness of chest pain units. Cardiol Clin 2005; 23(4):598)

The current processes in the healthcare delivery to the ADHF patient are more characteristic of a "zigzag model" (Fig. 2.8). An ADHF patient enters through the ED and receives treatments and evaluations through multiple disconnected service sectors or "care units" (known as business units in the commercial sector). These care units are represented by nursing, radiology, pharmacy, laboratory, etc. Each of the care units is viewed and acts as a single independent business unit from the standpoint of the hospital. The outputs of these care units' activities are collated by the provider, usually once the patient has been admitted to the acute hospital bed. It is then—at the "back end" of the process that care treatment plans are decided upon. The zigzag model is a disconnected and fragmented model.

The Y-model represents a different approach and provides a template to facilities on optimizing covering costs of care by placing the proper resources at the "front end" of the point of care entry. This concept begins at the point of entry and ends at discharge and marries a clinical and financial strategy that meets quality indicators while producing desirable profit margins. Beginning in the ED, this concept emphasizes an efficient, rapid assessment and action centered on a seamless integration of ancillary services such as the laboratory, diagnostic imaging, and skilled nursing while understanding the economic impacts on decisions made as the patient is directed through the system.

Using this template can impact quality, costs, efficiency, and clinical outcomes. This model provides drill down on the exact volume by ICD-9 codes instead of the inpatient MS-DRG to give a more accurate picture of the number of patients that are

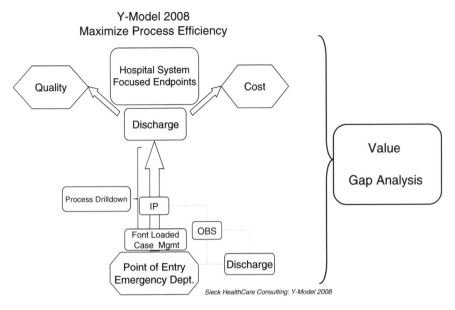

Fig. 2.9 Y-model using risk stratification and ABC approach

passing through the hospital door within a system. With this, granular level analysis and the proper guidance facilities can target this and other diseases more effectively. Patients who require an inpatient admission are properly admitted, and those who could be effectively treated in the outpatient setting (OU) are treated and properly released. The placement of more critical patients in the inpatient acute care setting impacts the case mix index positively because the patients are simply sicker and require more resources.

Creating a new care delivery system for the ADHF patient that is based on the Y-model can positively impact the contribution margins when ADHF patients are carefully identified, risk stratified, and given appropriate early treatment during the interaction. This model emphasizes a multidisciplinary accountability model to align the "care units" that affect an ADHF patient's progress through the current system. The emphasis is on front-end compliance that sets up the pathway the patient will follow. A patient is not "arbitrarily" admitted to an inpatient bed, treated, and then discharged. A decision is made up front on the most ideal care venue for the risk-stratified patient to be admitted to and undergo tailored treatment. It also initiates the financial pathway with identified markers throughout the patient inter-action that allow facilities to know the ramifications of making random decisions versus following a protocol designed to emphasize quality while optimizing eco-nomic results. The Y-model places an emphasis on process improvement while tar-geting the end points of quality and contribution margin (Fig. 2.9).

This variation of the model was recently used successfully at an 850+-bed medi-cal center in Florida for an initiative on ADHF. Prior to the initiative, the hospital had a "zigzag" model of care. Patients entered through the ED, were admitted to the acute care bed, and labs completed and treatment initiated several hours into the process. With initiation of the Y-model, a general consensus of appropriate clinical and cost-efficient processes began at the point of entry and continued through discharge. The new design resulted in improvements in turnaround time for therapy, reduced LOS, enhanced patient placement in the most appropriate bed venue (e.g., CCU, telemetry, or Clinical Decision Unit), and improved patient satisfaction.

Improvements demonstrated in the redesign can be translated to multiple high-risk diagnoses. Similar to the ACS patient, not every ADHF absolutely requires a CCU or OU bed, and similarly, not all ADHF patients are candidates for the OU. Point-of-entry triaging to the most appropriate care unit where an individualized treatment plan is rendered allows a facility to better merge quality care with positive financial outcomes.

Conclusion

The US healthcare system is in the midst of seismic shifts. Continuing pressures to increase access to care, increase coverage to a greater number of patients, enhance quality, and reduce costs will result in a healthcare delivery model that is vastly more efficient than the model seen at the end of the last century. ADHF is a disease state that accounts for a significant portion of the total costs for treatment of cardio-vascular diseases. As such, changes in the delivery model surrounding HF are likely to evolve more rapidly over the next decade. Payers will increasingly shift to value-based reimbursement, further impacting an already challenged hospital delivery system. The hospital's survival will be dependent upon how well it addresses these financial and logistical forces. Although financial aspects of care play a vital role in the new model of care, economics cannot be considered a higher priority than clinical outcomes. These two parameters are equally important to the successful implementation of a redesigned care process for the ADHF patient population.

Appendix

What Is MS-DRG? Medicare Severity Diagnosis-Related Group

Under the inpatient prospective payment system, each case is categorized into a diagnosis-related group depending on the patient's diagnosis, the procedures performed, complicating conditions, age, and discharge status. Each DRG has a payment weight assigned to it based on the average resources used to treat Medicare patients in that DRG compared to the cost of cases in other DRGs. The weights are calibrated annually.

On October 1, 2008, CMS replaced its 538 DRGs with 745 new, severity-adjusted DRGs. The new DRG system requires a greater level of documentation and related coding specificity (identification of complications and comorbidities) in order for hospitals to be reimbursed properly for critically ill patients.

What Are MCC and CC Specific?

In the FY 2008 hospital inpatient prospective payment system final rule, CMS revised the existing complication/comorbidity (CC) listing and established three different levels of severity into which diagnosis codes would be divided. The three levels are *MCC (major CC), CC,* and non-CCs. while non-CCs reflect the lowest. It was noticed that non-CC diagnosis codes do not significantly affect severity of illness or resource use.

Per the hospital IPPS final rule, the overall statistics by CC group are as follows:

MCC: 22.2% of patients
CC: 36.6% of patients
Non-CC: 41.1% of patients

A complication is defined as a condition that arises during the hospital stay, and a comorbid condition is a preexisting condition. Both of these conditions have been identified as potentially extending the length of hospital stay by at least 1 day in 75% of the cases.

MCC: Major Complication or Comorbidity

- MCCs reflect the highest level of severity

CC: Complication or Comorbidity and CMI

- *Complication (medicine)* is an infrequent and unfavorable evolution of a disease, a health condition, or a medical treatment.
- *Comorbidity* is either the presence of one or more disorders (or diseases) in addition to a primary disease or disorder or the effect of such additional disorders or diseases.
- *Case mix index* (CMI) is the average diagnosis-related group weight for all of a hospital's Medicare volume. A mix of cases in a hospital reflects the diversity, clinical complexity, and the needs for resources in the population of patients in a hospital.

What Is HCPCS?

- HCPCS stands for Healthcare Common Procedure Coding System. *(est. 1978; Centers for Medicare and Medicaid Services).*
- For Medicare and other health insurance programs to ensure healthcare claims are processed in an orderly and consistent manner, standardized coding systems

are essential. The HCPCS level II code set is one of the standard code sets used by medical coders and billers for this purpose.

Separate Reimbursement May Be Made for All Services with an S Indicator and X Ancillary Services

What is an S indicator, and what are X ancillary services?

X: ancillary services		
X	Ancillary services	Paid under OPPS; separate APC payment
S: significant procedure, multiple not discounted		
S	Significant procedure, not discounted when multiple	Paid under OPPS; separate APC payment

References

1. Lloyd-Jones D, Adams RJ, Brown TM, et al. Heart disease and stroke statistics 2009 update. A report from the American Heart Association Statistics Committee and Stroke Statistics Committee. Circulation 2010;121(7):e46–215.
2. Lloyd-Jones D, Adams RJ, Brown TM, et al. Heart disease and stroke statistics. 2010 Update-at-a-Glance. 2010. http://www.americanheart.org/downloadable/heart/1265665152970DS-32 41%20HeartStrokeUpdate_2010.pdf. Accessed 29 Aug 2010.
3. American Heart Association. Cardiovascular disease statistics. Dallas: AHA; 2010. http://www.americanheart.org/presenter.jhtml?identifier=4478. Accessed 1 Dec 2010.
4. Horwich TB, Fonarow GC. Glucose, obesity, metabolic syndrome, and diabetes relevance to incidence of heart failure. J Am Coll Cardiol. 2010;55:283–93.
5. Fonarow GC, Horwich TB. Glucose, obesity, metabolic syndrome, and diabetes. Relevance to incidence of heart failure. J Am Coll Cardiol. 2010;55:283–93.
6. Curtis LH, Whellan DJ, et al. Incidence and prevalence of heart failure in elderly persons, 1994–2003. Arch Intern Med. 2008;168:418–24.
7. Rosamund W, Flegal K, Furie K, et al. Heart disease and stroke statistics. 2008 Update-at-a-Glance. http://www.americanheart.org/downloadable/heart/1200082005246HS_Stats%202008.final.pdf Accessed 30 Aug 2010.
8. NHANES:2005–2005. Source: NCHS and NHLBI. Heart disease and stroke statistics. 2010 Update-at-a-Glance. http://www.americanheart.org/downloadable/heart/1265665152970DS-3241%20HeartStrokeUpdate_2010.pdf. Accessed 29 Aug 2010.
9. O'Connell JB, Bristow MR. Economic impact of heart failure in the United States: time for a different approach. J Heart Lung Transplant. 1994;13:S107–12.
10. Massie BM, Shah NB. Evolving trends in the epidemiologic factors of heart failure: rationale for preventive strategies and comprehensive disease management. Am Heart J. 1997;133:703–12.
11. Peacock WF, Albert NM. Observation unit management of heart failure. Emerg Med Clin North Am. 2001;19:209–32.
12. Bueno H, Ross JS, et al. Trends in length of stay and short-term outcomes among medicare patients hospitalized for heart failure, 1993–2006. JAMA. 2010;303(21):2141–7.

13. Cardiovascular Disease Costs in the United States. 2009 American Heart Association. http://www.americanheart.org/downloadable/heart/1238516653013CVD_Stats_09_final%20single%20pages%20(2).pdf. Accessed 30 Aug 2010.
14. ADHERE Registry data on file January 2004.
15. American Hospital Directory. Statistics for the Top 20 Base MS-DRGs: an online source for cost report data. http://www.ahd.com.
16. Niska R, Bhulya F, et al. National hospital ambulatory medical care survey: 2007 emergency department summary. National Health Statistics Report, Number 26, August 6, 2010.
17. Graff LG. Observation medicine. The healthcare system's tincture of time. Irving, TX: ACEP; 2010. p. 134.
18. Medicare benefit policy manual, Chapter 6. Hospital services covered under part B. https://www.cms.gov/manuals/Downloads/bp102c06.pdf. Accessed 12 Jan 2010.
19. Peacock WF, Emerman CL. Emergency department management of patients with acute decompensated heart failure. Heart Failure Rev. 2004;9(3):187–93.
20. Lucas BP, Kumapley R, et al. A hospitalist-run short stay unit: features that predict length-of-stay and eventual admission to traditional inpatient services. J Hosp Med. 2009;4(5):276–84.
21. Emerman CL. Treatment of the acute decompensation of heart failure: efficacy and pharmacoeconomics of early initiation of therapy in the emergency department. Rev Cardiovasc Med. 2003;3 Suppl 7:S13–20.
22. MedPAC analysis our outpatient prospective payment system claims that CMS uses to set payment rates, 2003–2007: A data book: healthcare spending and the Medicare program, June 2009.
23. National Health Statistics Report. National Hospital Ambulatory Medical Care Survey:2007 Emergency Department Summary. Number 26. August 6, 2010 US Department of Health and Human Services.
24. Peacock WF, Collins YJ, et al. Heart failure observation units: optimizing care. Ann Emerg Med. 2006;47(1):22–33.
25. Phillips CO, Wright SM, et al. Comprehensive discharge planning with postdischarge support for older patients with congestive heart failure: a meta-analysis. JAMA. 2004;29(11):1358–67.
26. Gonseth J, Guallar-Castillon P, et al. The effectiveness of disease management programmes in reducing hospital re-admission in older patients with heart failure: a systematic review and meta-analysis of published reports. Eur Heart J. 2004;25(18):1570–95.
27. Roccaforte R, Demers C, et al. Effectiveness of comprehensive disease management programmes in improving clinical outcomes in heart failure patients. A meta-analysis. Eur Heart J. 2005;7(7):1133–44.
28. Chan DC, Heidenreich PA, et al. Heart failure disease management programs: a cost-effectiveness analysis. Am Heart J. 2008;155:332–8.
29. Miller G, Randolph S, et al. Long-term cost-effectiveness of disease management in systolic heart failure. Med Decis Making. 2009;29:325–33.
30. Gregory D, Kimmelsteil C, et al. Hospital cost effect of a heart failure disease management program: the specialized primary and networked care in heart failure (SPAN-CHF) trial. Am Heart J. 2006;15(5):1013–8.
31. Fonarow GC. How well are chronic heart failure patients being managed? Rev Cardiovasc Med. 2006;7 Suppl 1:S3–11.
32. Gardetto NJ, Greaney K, et al. Critical pathway for the management of acute heart failure at the Veterans Affairs San Diego Healthcare System: transforming performance measures into cardiac care. Crit Pathw Cardiol. 2008;7(3):153–72.
33. Fonarow GC, for the ADHERE Scientific Advisory Committee. The Acute Decompensated Heart Failure Registry (ADHERE): opportunities to improve care of patients hospitalized with acute decompensated heart failure. Rev Cardiovasc Med. 2003;4:S21–30.
34. Peacock WF, Remer EE, Aponte J, et al. Effective observation unit treatment of decompensated heart failure. Congest Heart Fail. 2002;8:68–73.
35. Peacock F. Management of acute decompensated heart failure in the emergency department. J Am Coll Cardiol. 2003;4:336A.

36. Collin SP, Schauer DP, et al. Cost-effectiveness analysis of ED decision-making in patients with non-high-risk heart failure. Am J Emerg Med. 2009;30:293–302.
37. Observation Care Payments to Hospitals FAQ. http://www.acep.org/practres.aspx?id=30486. Accessed 12 Sept 2010
38. Observation Medicine Section Newsletter. American College of Emergency Physicians. 2008 June; 18(1).
39. Kaiser Family Foundation. http://facts.kff.org/chart.aspx?ch=212. Accessed 4 Dec 2010.
40. CMS to Unveil Proposed Regulations to Combat Health Program Fraud. California HealthCare Foundation. http://www.californiahealthline.org/articles/2010/9/20/cms-to-unveil-proposed-regulations-to-combat-health-program-fraud.aspx#ixzz1067vyvsj. Accessed 12 Jan 2010.
41. Morris L. Combating fraud in health care: an essential component of any cost containment strategy. Health Affairs. 2009;28(5):1351–6.
42. Graff LG. Observation medicine. The healthcare system's tincture of time. Irving, TX: ACEP; 2010. p. 9.
43. Sieck Healthcare Consulting. http://www.sieckhealthcare.com. Accessed 12 Jan 2010.

Chapter 3
Regulatory Requirements in Acute Heart Failure

Nancy M. Albert

Regulatory requirements of acute heart failure services affect two areas supporting care delivery: coverage determination and performance management, both of which could affect accreditation of physicians, health-care organizations, and healthcare plans. While the former affects reimbursement of the costs of care by the third-party payor, the latter represents clinical care quality and healthcare provider conformity to national guideline-recommended acute heart failure care assessment and management services. For both coverage determination and performance management regulations and indicators, some are globally applied across the environment of care settings (emergency care, short stay care, hospital care, or ambulatory care), and others are directed toward specific healthcare providers and/or care settings. The purpose of this chapter is to describe regulatory requirements for acute heart failure, many of which were designed to promote optimal use of and minimize gaps in evidence-based heart failure care and regulate cost of care.

Acute heart failure care regulatory requirements have developed over time for two primary reasons. First, after hospitalization for acute heart failure, patients remain at high risk for morbidity and mortality. When all-cause 30-day risk-standardized rehospitalization rates were assessed in patients discharged with decompensated heart failure, the trend from mid-2006 through mid-2009 was unchanged, at a median of 24.5% [1]. In a study of patients using Medicare fee-for-service benefits that were hospitalized for decompensated heart failure, while mortality was on the decline over a 4- and 13-year period respectively, 30-day rehospitalization rose over time, even after adjustments were made for confounding factors [2, 3]. Even with the decline in the death rate from cardiovascular diseases in recent years, one in 8.6 deaths mentioned heart failure, and for patients who survive the acute decompensated event, 54% of men and 40% of women will die within 5 years [4]. Second, despite compelling clinical trial

N.M. Albert, PhD, CCNS, CHFN, CCRN, FAHA (✉)
Kaufman Center for Heart Failure, Cleveland Clinic,
9500 Euclid Avenue, J3-4, Cleveland, OH 44195, USA
e-mail: albertn@ccf.org

W. Frank Peacock (ed.), *Short Stay Management of Acute Heart Failure*,
Contemporary Cardiology, DOI 10.1007/978-1-61779-627-2_3,
© Springer Science+Business Media, LLC 2012

evidence and evidence-based guideline-recommended care documents available to healthcare providers, underutilization of evidence-based care is routinely reported for drug therapy prescriptions [5–7], cardiac device utilization, [8] and patient education [9], in both hospital [10, 11] and cardiology practice [12] settings. Further, this lack of uniformity in heart failure care was found based on hospital size, hospital setting, patient characteristics (including age, ethnicity, gender, and depression history) and day of hospital admission [13–17]. Attention to systems, structure and process components of healthcare delivery and documentation during the acute hospital episode may overcome current barriers to delivery of evidence-based, individualized heart failure care. In addition, early collaborative care that involves cardiologist and primary care [18] or multidisciplinary care services that include ongoing education [19] after discharge from an emergency department or hospital may help facilitate evidence-based guideline-recommended care and reduce rehospitalization and mortality.

Coverage Determination Regulations in Acute Heart Failure

Coverage regulations for acute heart failure encompass medication, cardiac devices, testing modalities, and therapies aimed at improving outcomes. In September 2010, Medicare published revised national coverage determinations, and in December 2010, some new programs and program revisions became effective (Table 3.1) [20, 21]. Summarizing these new determinations is as follows: reimbursement for nesiritide used for acute decompensated heart failure is unchanged, as is reimbursement for implantable cardioverter-defibrillator implantation, cardiac output monitoring by electrical impedance, cardiac rehabilitation, and external counterpulsation. Intensive cardiac rehabilitation programs have been added, and while they require the same cardiac diagnoses as II or III (outpatient) services that do not include a diagnosis of heart failure, one-half of patients hospitalized for heart failure have a diagnosed etiology of coronary artery disease [22] and may meet cardiac rehabilitation qualifications. Since cardiac rehabilitation programs provide medical evaluation, prescribed exercise, cardiac risk factor modification, diet education, and counseling in psychosocial, lipid, and stress management to restore active and productive lives, every patient who meets medical history qualifications should have postdischarge orders and be strongly encouraged to attend. In a Cochrane review of exercise program uptake and patient adherence, three programs developed to increase uptake of cardiac rehabilitation were effective, and two of seven programs to increase patient adherence to cardiac rehabilitation were effective [23]. In patients with heart failure who participated in a randomized controlled trial of a 12-week cardiac rehabilitation program, intervention group patients had reduced all-cause and major acute coronary event rehospitalizations, improved 12-month survival, improved 3-month quality of life, and performed better on 6-minute walk tests compared to control group patients [24]. Moreover, in a Cochrane review and meta-analysis of 19 randomized controlled trials of 3647 primarily male patients with

Table 3.1 Centers for Medicare and Medicaid national coverage determinations

Category	Factor	Details of coverage	Implementation date/reference
Drug therapies			
	Nesiritide	• Must be inpatient and have a claim for acutely decompensated HF, not chronic HF and another cause of hospitalization	05/22/2006
		• Short-term intravenous treatment in patients with dyspnea at rest	
Cardiac rehabilitation programs			
	Physician-supervised	• Phase II (outpatient immediate posthospitalization recuperation phase)	Revised: 12/01/2010
	(1) Intensive cardiac rehabilitation services	• 72 1-h sessions, up to 6 sessions per day, over a period of up to 18 weeks that includes physician-prescribed exercise, cardiac risk factor modification, psychosocial assessment, and outcomes assessment	
	(2) Pritikin Programs for Diet and Exercise	• Demonstrate through peer-reviewed, published research that it has accomplished one or more of the following for its patients: (a) positively affected the progression of coronary heart disease; (b) reduced the need for CAB surgery; and (c) reduced the need for PCI	New: 10/25/2010
	(3) Ornish Program for Reversing Heart Disease		New: 10/25/2010
		• Demonstrate through peer-reviewed, published research that it accomplished a statistically significant reduction in 5 or more of the following measures for patients from their levels before cardiac rehabilitation services to after cardiac rehabilitation services: (a) low-density lipoprotein; (b) triglycerides; (c) body mass index; (d) systolic blood pressure; (e) diastolic blood pressure; and (f) need for cholesterol, blood pressure, and diabetes medications	
		• Patient populations: (a) within 12 months after MI; (b) post-CAB surgery; (c) heart valve repair or replacement; (d) stable angina with exercise stress test positive for exercise-induced ischemia within 6 months of starting program; and (e) post-heart or heart/lung transplant	
	Physician-supervised cardiac rehabilitation	• Individualized treatment plan: a written plan tailored to an individual patient that includes (a) description of the diagnosis; (b) type, amount, frequency, and duration of the items and services furnished; and (c) goals set for the individual patient	Revised: 12/01/2010
		• Patient populations: see last bullet above	

(continued)

Table 3.1 (continued)

Category	Factor	Details of coverage	Implementation date/reference
Cardiac devices			
	Implantable cardioverter-defibrillator placement	• Patient populations: (a) documented episode of cardiac arrest due to VF, not due to a transient or reversible cause; (b) documented sustained VT, either spontaneous or induced by an EP study, not associated with an acute MI and not due to a transient or reversible cause; (c) documented familial/inherited conditions with a high risk of life-threatening VT, such as hypertrophic cardiomyopathy; (d) prior MI with left ventricular ejection fraction ≤35% and inducible, sustained VT or VF at EP study within 40 days of MI and did not have NYHA FC IV HF, cardiogenic shock, or symptomatic hypotension while in a stable rhythm; had CAB surgery or PCI within past 3 months; had an enzyme positive MI within the past 40 days; had clinical symptoms or findings that would prompt candidacy for coronary revascularization; or any noncardiac disease associated with <1 year survival; (e) ischemic dilated cardiomyopathy and documented prior MI, NYHA FC II and III HF, and LVEF ≤35%; (f) Nonischemic dilated cardiomyopathy >9 months, NYHA FC II and III HF and LVEF ≤35%; (g) meet coverage requirements for CRT device and have NYHA FC IV HF • Be enrolled in either a Food and Drug Administration approved Category B investigational device exemption clinical trial, a trial under the CMS Clinical Trial Policy or a qualifying data collection system including approved clinical trials and registries	Version 3: 01/27/2005
	Implantable cardioverter-defibrillator interrogation (in-person and remote)	• Electronic analysis (interrogation, evaluation of pulse generator status, evaluation of programmable parameters at rest/during activity, interpretation of ECG recordings at rest/exercise, and derived data elements, analysis of event markers, and device response) • Reprogramming • Monitoring period: in-person, 30 days; remote, 90 days • Professional and technical component codes	
	Wearable cardioverter-defibrillator interrogation	• Electronic analysis (interrogation, evaluation of pulse generator status, evaluation of programmable parameters at rest and during activity, interpretation of ECG recordings, analysis of event markers and device response) • Same as above with reprogramming • Monitoring period: in-person, 30 days or 90 days • Professional and technical component codes	

Cardiac output monitoring by electrical impedance	• Patient populations: (a) differentiation of cardiogenic from pulmonary causes of acute dyspnea when medical history, physical examination, and standard assessment tools provide insufficient information, and the treating physician has determined that TEB hemodynamic data are necessary for appropriate management of the patient; (b) optimization of atrioventricular (A/V) interval for patients with A/V sequential cardiac pacemakers when medical history, physical examination, and standard assessment tools provide insufficient information; (c) monitoring of continuous inotropic therapy for patients with terminal congestive HF at home or for patients waiting at home for a heart transplant; (d) evaluation for acute or chronic cardiac rejection post–heart transplant as an alternative to myocardial biopsy; and (e) optimization of fluid management in patients with congestive HF when medical history, physical examination, and standard assessment tools provide insufficient information, and the treating physician has determined that TEB hemodynamic data are necessary for appropriate management • Frequency: daily	Version 3: 01/06/2007
Implantable cardiovascular monitor – in-person or remote interrogation	• Interrogation device evaluation for analysis of one or more recorder physiologic cardiovascular data element from external and internal sensors • Monitoring period: 30 days • Professional and technical component codes	
Transtelephonic ECG transmission	• Indications: (a) detect, characterize, and document symptomatic transient dysrhythmias; (b) initiate, revise, or discontinue dysrhythmic drug therapy; or (c) early (24-h coverage must be provided) monitoring of patients discharged after MI • Requirements: (a) capable of transmitting EKG Leads I, II, or III; and (b) tracing must be sufficiently comparable to a conventional ECG	03/01/1980
External counterpulsation	• Not covered for AHF or postdischarge after AHF episode; only disabling angina	Version 2: 04/03/2006

AHF acute heart failure, *CAB* coronary artery bypass, *CMS* Centers for Medicare and Medicaid Services, *CRT* cardiac resynchronization therapy, *ECG* electrocardiographic, *EP* electrophysiology, *MI* myocardial infarction, *NYHA FC* New York Heart Association functional class, *PCI* percutaneous coronary interventions, *TEB* thoracic electrical bioimpedance, *VF* ventricular fibrillation, *VT* ventricular tachyarrhythmia

systolic heart failure and New York Heart Association class II–III status, all-cause short- and long-term survival and rehospitalization were similar between groups at follow-up; however, heart failure-related hospitalizations were lower, and health-related quality of life improved with exercise therapy [25]. Thus, while cardiac rehabilitation is not a component of acute heart failure care during emergency or hospital admission, postdischarge, it may improve efficacy of exercise programs that have been associated with decreases the subsequent cost of care and disease morbidity.

Observation Unit Regulations in Acute Heart Failure

Observation care includes ongoing short-term assessment, treatment, and reassessment in order to make a decision about whether a patient will require a hospital admission or if discharge and outpatient care are feasible [26]. Observation services are common for patients with acute heart failure who present for emergency care and who then require a significant period of monitoring or treatment before a decision concerning admission or resolution of dyspnea and other acute symptoms that may allow for discharge can be made. Generally, observation services should not exceed 48 h, and the majority of patients should have a decision as to whether hospital admission is needed in less than 24 h, based on the clock time documented in the medical record that coincides with the time the physician creates a written order for observation services. To receive reimbursement for observation services by Medicare, a minimum of 8 h of service is required, and if over 24 h are used, Medicare will not pay separately for the excess hours used; with all costs included in a composite payment as discussed below.

Regulations specific to observation services of patients with acute heart failure include physician billing and hospital billing. Physician billing is linked to service type for initial services rendered when placing a patient in observation status and observation care following initiation of observation services. Medicare has specific documentation requirements for billing observation care services and admission to hospital service (inpatient status) following observation care. Table 3.2 provides the CPT codes used specifically for physician payment of observation services [26], based on the January 2010, Centers for Medicare and Medicaid Services revised consultation services payment policy for observation care and documentation requirements [26].

Observation services coding also involves criteria hospitals must meet to receive Medicare payment, separate from physician payment. Coding for observation services encompasses an ambulatory payment classification (APC) code, which is the coding used by Medicare to bill for hospital outpatient services. An APC includes Current Procedural Technology (CPT) codes developed by Medicare, and Healthcare Common Procedure Coding System (HCPCS) level II codes developed by the American Medical Association. An HCPCS number is assigned to every task and service a healthcare provider may use to deliver services to a Medicare patient including medical, surgical, and diagnostic services. Uniformity in coding ensures

Table 3.2 Medicare national coverage for medical management of heart failure in observation status

Time period	Rules	CPT codes

Initial observation period	• Contractors pay for initial observation care billed by a physician who ordered hospital outpatient observation services:
	  – Contractor is responsible during the observation period
	  – May be a physician with or without admitting privileges
	  – Physician must be authorized to furnish outpatient services
		99221
		99222
		99223

Following initiation of observation services	• Physician coding reflects the amount of time the patient receives observation care on the same calendar day as the initial observation care: – If <8 h, a discharge service CPT code is not reported	99218 99219 99220
	• When a patient is discharged on a different calendar day, the codes above are used to designate care received, and the discharge code is also used to designate discharge	Discharge CPT code: 99217
	• When a patient receives ≥8 h of care and <24 h and is discharged on the same calendar day, codes used include admission and discharge services	99234 99235 99236

Admission to inpatient status *following* observation care	• If the same physician who ordered observation services also admits the patient for inpatient status before the end of the same calendar day observation status began, only the initial hospital visit for evaluation and management services provided on that date can be billed
	• If the patient is admitted for inpatient status subsequent to the date of initiation of observation services, the physician must bill an initial hospital visit for the services provided on that date:
	  – The physician may not bill hospital observation discharge management code
	  – The physician may not bill an outpatient/office visit for care provided while the patient received hospital outpatient observation services on the date of admission to inpatient status
		NA

Documentation require-ments *including* admission and discharge services	• History, examination, and medical decision-making in the medical record, including:
	  – Stating the stay for observation care involves 8 h, but <24 h
	  – Identification that the billing physician was present and personally performed services
	  – Identification that an order for observation services, progress notes, and discharge notes were written by the billing physician
		NA

CPT Current Procedural Terminology, *NA* not applicable, *HCPCS* Healthcare Common Procedure Coding System

consistency in billing and payment for specific services. Thus, if no payable HCPCS code is assigned to a claim, no payment will be received.

There are two composite APC codes used by Medicare to pay hospitals for observation care: (1) APC 8002 – level 1 "extended assessment and management composite" requires a clinic visit prior to observation services, at least 8 h of observation care, and no procedure with a status indicator of T (reflecting a significant procedure subject to multiple procedure discounting); (2) APC 8003 – level II "extended assessment and management composite" requires an emergency care visit or critical care services, at least 8 h of observation care, and no procedure with a status indicator of T. When composite codes are used, reimbursement reflects a single payment that includes the combination of the emergency/critical care service or the clinic service plus observation care. The claim for observation services that includes an emergency department visit, a clinic visit, or critical care service must occur on the same day or the day before the date reported for observation.

Alternately, the patient can be directly referred for observation care on the same date of service as the date reported for observation services. A direct referral for observation services is defined as a referral by a community physician to the hospital for observation without receiving hospital clinic, emergency room, or critical care services on the day observation care began. In order for a hospital to receive separate payment for a direct referral for observation care, the claim must show HCPCS numbers for hourly observation (HCPCS code GO378 that reflects a minimum of 8 h of observation care) and direct admit to observation with the same date of service (APC 0604), and that no services with status indicators for clinic or emergency department visit or critical care were provided on the same day of service. A direct referral to observation services does not qualify for separate payment under APC.

Unlike in the past, specific diagnosis codes, such as heart failure, chest pain, or asthma, are no longer needed for observation care reimbursement. Likewise, criteria for specific diagnostic services that were previously needed to receive facility payment are no longer required. In addition to physician and hospital payments, hospital facilities may report intravenous infusions or injections separate from observation service codes to payers, including Medicare. Finally, non-Medicare payers may have different payment policies that may require different coding.

Quality Regulations in Acute Heart Failure Linked to Medicare Payment

The Joint Commission on Accreditation of Healthcare Organizations (JCAHO), a private nonprofit organization, sets standards for health-care delivery programs and facilities requirements. The Center for Medicare Services (CMS) has legal oversight over the JCAHO's Medicare criteria since the CMS agreed to accept certification by the JCAHO as proof of compliance. All acute care hospitals must be Medicare compliant to receive reimbursement from the CMS for services in patients 65 years or older, and compliance with Medicare requirements is an expectation of JCAHO

Table 3.3 Hospital quality measures with reports linked to Medicare payment

Area	Measure	Year[a]	Data source
Heart failure	Evaluation of left ventricular systolic function[b]	2005	Chart abstraction
	Angiotensin-converting enzyme inhibitor or angiotensin receptor blocker for left ventricular dysfunction[b]	2005	Chart abstraction
	Discharge instructions[b]	2007	Chart abstraction
	Adult smoking cessation advice or counseling	2007	Chart abstraction
	Risk-standardized HF 30-day mortality rate[b]	2008	Medicare claims
	Risk-standardized 30-day all-cause readmission rate following HF hospitalization[b]	2010	Medicare claims
Patient experience	Hospital Consumer Assessment of Healthcare Providers and Systems (HCAHPS) survey	2008	Patient survey
Outcomes and complications	Complication/patient safety for selected indicators (composite)	2010	Medical claims
(AHRQ Quality Measures)	Mortality for selected medical conditions (composite)	2010	Medical claims

[a]Year linked to Medicare payment
[b]Endorsed by National Quality Forum
AHRQ Agency for Healthcare Research and Quality, *HF* Heart failure

accreditation. The JCAHO collects data from hospitals in ten areas of quality measurement and reports the findings to CMS. Of the ten, all involve inpatients except one area, outpatient measures, and none of the specific 11 outpatient measures involve medical heart failure care. Of the nine inpatient areas, one is specific to heart failure and has six measures (Table 3.3) [27] and another, patient experience, has 1 measure, the Hospital Consumer Assessment of Healthcare Providers and Systems (HCAHPS) survey. The HCAHPS survey solicits patients' views, comments, and ratings on their hospital experiences in 18 areas and includes the themes of medical care quality, customer service, clinician-patient interaction, cleanliness and quietness of the hospital environment, pain management, communication about medicines, and discharge information [28]. The final area that involves patients with acute heart failure is a newly developed area linked to Medicare payment in 2010. Called outcomes and complications, it reflects the Agency for Healthcare Research and Quality (known as AHRQ, of the Department of Health and Human Services) quality measures that involve complications (Table 3.3). Most measures are graded based on performance, but in a few, the focus is that centers should lack problems that signify egregious errors or compromised patient care.

Of the hospital quality measures linked to Medicare payment, five heart failure-specific cardiovascular measures are endorsed by the National Quality Forum (Table 3.3), for public reporting and quality improvement. These five heart failure measures were endorsed in May 2008 and have undergone the public comment phase of review (through December 14, 2010) for continued endorsement [29]. The National Quality Forum was created in 1999 by a coalition of public- and private-sector leaders in response to a recommendation that an organization was needed to promote and ensure patient protections and healthcare quality through measurement and public reporting. The Department of Health and Human Services contracted the National Quality Forum in 2009 to develop a portfolio of quality and efficiency measures that will allow the federal government to determine if healthcare spending on quality initiatives achieves the best results for patients and taxpayers [29].

In general, performance measures for acute heart failure have undergone rigorous review by volunteer experts of many national organizations before endorsement and use in national reporting. As the focus on quality of care, in terms of adherence to nationally recognized treatment guidelines, continues to grow in importance, quality-reporting expectations will also continue to expand. Hopefully, more reports will be forthcoming that provide a positive link between reaching or exceeding benchmark goals for specific performance measures and important clinical patient- and hospital-centered outcomes.

In conclusion, regulatory requirements for acute heart failure services include those that influence coverage (and ultimately payment) and quality of care. Payment of acute heart failure care services involving diagnosis-related group payment to hospitals for inpatient care was not described; however, regulations for services provided as outpatient observational care regarding hospital and physician reimbursement, based on packaging of related services, were discussed. As newer drug, device, and monitoring therapies become available for acute heart failure management, regulations for coverage and performance monitoring will be updated, requiring healthcare provider and administrator vigilance.

References

1. Bernheim SM, Grady JN, Lin Z, et al. National patterns of risk-standardized mortality and readmission for acute myocardial infarction and heart failure. Update on publicly reported outcomes measures based on the 2010 release. Circ Cardiovasc Qual Outcomes. 2010;3: 459–67.
2. Heidenreich PA, Sahay A, Kapoor JR, Pham MX, Massie B. Divergent trends in survival and readmission following a hospitalization for heart failure in the Veterans Affairs health care system 2002 to 2006. J Am Coll Cardiol. 2010;56:362–8.
3. Bueno H, Ross JS, Wang Y, et al. Trends in length of stay and short-term outcomes among Medicare patients hospitalized for heart failure, 1993–2006. JAMA. 2010;303:2141–7.
4. Lloyd-Jones D, Adams RJ, Brown TM, et al. Heart disease and stroke statistics 2010 update: a report from the American Heart Association. Circulation. 2010;121:e45–e215.
5. Fonarow GC, Abraham WT, Albert NM, et al. Dosing of beta-blocker therapy before, during, and after hospitalization for heart failure (from Organized Program to Initiate Lifesaving Treatment in Hospitalized Patients with Heart Failure). Am J Cardiol. 2008;102(11):1524–9.
6. Fonarow GC, Abraham WT, Albert NM, OPTIMIZE-HF Investigators and Coordinators, et al. Influence of beta-blocker continuation or withdrawal on outcomes in patients hospitalized with heart failure: findings from the OPTIMIZE-HF program. J Am Coll Cardiol. 2008;52(3):190–9.
7. Albert NM, Yancy CW, Liang L, et al. Use of aldosterone antagonists in heart failure. JAMA. 2009;302(15):1658–65.
8. Shah B, Hernandez AF, Liang L, Get With The Guidelines Steering Committee, et al. Hospital variation and characteristics of implantable cardioverter-defibrillator use in patients with heart failure: data from the GWTG-HF (Get With The Guidelines-Heart Failure) registry. J Am Coll Cardiol. 2009;53(5):416–22.

9. Albert NM, Fonarow GC, Abraham WT, et al. Predictors of delivery of hospital-based heart failure patient education: a report from OPTIMIZE-HF. J Card Fail. 2007;13(3):189–98.
10. Fonarow GC, Abraham WT, Albert NM, OPTIMIZE-HF Investigators and Hospitals, et al. Association between performance measures and clinical outcomes for patients hospitalized with heart failure. JAMA. 2007;297(1):61–70.
11. O'Connor CM, Stough WG, Gallup DS, Hasselblad V, Gheorghiade M. Demographics, clinical characteristics, and outcomes of patients hospitalized for decompensated heart failure: observations from the IMPACT-HF registry. J Card Fail. 2005;11(3):200–5.
12. Fonarow GC, Albert NM, Curtis AB, et al. Improving evidence-based care for heart failure in outpatient cardiology practices: primary results of the registry to improve the use of evidence-based heart failure therapies in the outpatient setting (IMPROVE HF). Circulation. 2010; 122(6):585–96.
13. Walsh MN, Yancy CW, Albert NM, et al. Equitable improvement for women and men in the use of guideline-recommended therapies for heart failure: findings from IMPROVE HF. J Cardiac Fail. 2010;16:940–9.
14. Yancy CW, Fonarow GC, Albert NM, et al. Influence of patient age and sex on delivery of guideline-recommended heart failure care in the outpatient cardiology practice setting: findings from IMPROVE HF. Am Heart J. 2009;157:754–762.e2.
15. Hernandez AF, Fonarow GC, Liang L, et al. Sex and racial differences in the use of implantable cardioverter-defibrillators among patients hospitalized with heart failure. JAMA. 2007; 298(13):1525–32.
16. Horwich TB, Hernandez AF, Liang L, Get With Guidelines Steering Committee and Hospitals, et al. Weekend hospital admission and discharge for heart failure: association with quality of care and clinical outcomes. Am Heart J. 2009;158(3):451–8.
17. Albert NM, Fonarow GC, Abraham WT, et al. Depression and clinical outcomes in heart failure: an OPTIMIZE-HF analysis. Am J Med. 2009;122(4):366–73.
18. Lee DS, Stukel TA, Austin PC, et al. Improved outcomes with early collaborative care of ambulatory heart failure patients discharged from the emergency department. Circulation. 2010;122(18):1806–14.
19. Ferrante D, Varini S, Macchia A, GESICA Investigators, et al. Long-term results after a telephone intervention in chronic heart failure: DIAL (Randomized Trial of Phone Intervention in Chronic Heart Failure) follow-up. J Am Coll Cardiol. 2010;56(5):372–8.
20. Medicare National Coverage Determinations Manual. https://www.cms.gov/manuals/downloads/ncd103c1_Part1.pdf. Accessed 8 Oct 2010.
21. Centers for Medicare and Medicaid Services. Medicare Approved Facilities/Trials/Registries. http://www.cms.gov/MedicareApprovedFacilitie/. Accessed 13 Dec 2010.
22. Rossi JS, Flaherty JD, Fonarow GC, et al. Influence of coronary artery disease and coronary revascularization status on outcomes in patients with acute heart failure syndromes: a report from OPTIMIZE-HF (Organized Program to Initiate Lifesaving Treatment in Hospitalized Patients with Heart Failure). Eur J Heart Fail. 2008;10:1215–23.
23. Davies P, Taylor F, Beswick A, et al. Promoting patient uptake and adherence in cardiac rehabilitation. Cochrane Database Syst Rev. 2010;7:CD007131.
24. Davidson PM, Cockburn J, Newton PJ, et al. Can a heart failure-specific cardiac rehabilitation program decrease hospitalizations and improve outcomes in high-risk patients? Eur J Cardiovasc Prev Rehabil. 2010;17:393–402.
25. Davies EJ, Moxham T, Rees K, et al. Exercise training for systolic heart failure: Cochrane systematic review and meta-analysis. Eur J Heart Fail. 2010;12:706–15.
26. Centers for Medicare and Medicaid services. Pub 100-04 Medicare Claims Processing. http://www.cms.gov/transmittals/downloads/R1875cp.pdf. Accessed 8 Oct 2010.
27. Centers for Medicare and Medicaid Services. http://www.cms.gov/hospitalqualityinits/01_overview.asp? Accessed 8 Oct 2010.
28. Hospital Consumer Assessment of Healthcare Providers and Systems Hospital Survey. http://www.hcahponline.org/home.aspx. Accessed 7 Dec 2010.
29. National Quality Forum. http://www.qualityforum.org/. Accessed 7 Dec 2010.

Chapter 4
Quality and Operational Metrics in Heart Failure

Phillip D. Levy and Matthew A. Wheatley

Quality and Its Measurement

Quality in health care is an idealized yet elusive goal. This can, in large part, be attributed to the inherent difficulty associated with establishing a precise definition of quality—a circumstance derived from the existence of multiple stakeholders (e.g., health-care providers, local administrators, patients, community, insurers, government) each with differing perspectives on what constitutes the deliverables of "good" health care. At its core, however, quality is generally regarded as an attribute of provider care, specifically technical performance (or lack thereof) as viewed through the lens of "best-practice" medicine [1]. The latter represents the summation of those actions (or inactions) that have either proven effective or are, by virtue of consensus expert opinion, considered de facto to contribute to better outcomes (e.g., smoking cessation).

Quality is thus a comparative construct which measures variance from a benchmark set by what is considered to be best care as identified by a consensus standard. But what exactly is being measured and how can one be sure that the metric is relevant at the individual patient level and attributable to the provider (or system) in question? Moreover, to what standard is the assessment held: maximal, which does not consider health benefits within the context of related cost or optimal, which places a cost-effective value on care? Understanding these issues in an era of performance measures [2] and increased accountability for health outcomes is critical.

More than two decades ago, Avedis Donabedian championed the notion that quality can and should be assessed as a function of the relationship between three essential elements termed "structure," "process," and "outcome" [1]. As shown in

P.D. Levy, MD, MPH (✉)
Department of Emergency Medicine, Wayne State University School of Medicine, Detroit, MI, USA
e-mail: plevy@med.wayne.edu

M.A. Wheatley, MD
Department of Emergency Medicine, Emory University School of Medicine, Atlanta, GA, USA

W. Frank Peacock (ed.), *Short Stay Management of Acute Heart Failure*,
Contemporary Cardiology, DOI 10.1007/978-1-61779-627-2_4,
© Springer Science+Business Media, LLC 2012

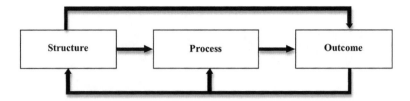

Fig. 4.1 Relationship between structure, process, and outcome in health care

Fig. 4.1, each can exist as both a precondition for (e.g., identification of a disparate outcome at an institution leading to a change in culture or practice) and a consequence of (e.g., inability to meet time-dependent goals for therapeutic intervention because of resource limitations) the others. These relationships, however, are far from linear and can be strongly influenced by confounding variables, especially case mix.

All of this has particular relevance to acute heart failure (HF), where, despite significant advances in medicine, postdischarge outcomes remain poor [3–5]. In the following pages, we discuss the specifics of quality as they relate to HF and highlight, using the Donabedian framework, those measures being used to differentiate performance.

Structure and Process: The Language of Operational Metrics

Structure

The definition for health-care structure is broad, including everything from geographic location and physical layout of health-care facilities, medical equipment and information technology systems, and personnel qualifications, certification, and training. This breadth leads to a lack of consensus and evidence as to what structural elements contribute to high-quality health-care process and thus high-quality outcomes. Based primarily on expert opinion, a former American College of Cardiology/ American Heart Association (ACC/AHA) Heart Failure Working Group [6] recommended four structural elements be considered as indicators of quality: clinical practice guidelines, monitoring of patient care and outcomes, disease management programs, and coordinated systems of care. Initially published in 2000, excellence in these areas, particularly the latter two, has come to define centers that consistently provide high-quality HF care.

Disease Management Programs

These are multidisciplinary, patient-focused programs that cover matters such as education about the disease and its treatment, dietary counseling, efforts to improve patients' compliance with medical regimens, and interventions to help patients achieve and maintain control of their volume status. These programs have been shown to reduce readmissions and improve functional status but not necessarily affect mortality rates [7, 8]. Further study is needed to define their overall cost-effectiveness and the optimal strategy [9, 10], as not all approaches (e.g., postdischarge telemonitoring in those recently hospitalized with acute HF) appear to provide clinical benefit [11].

Coordinated Systems of Care

As originally written by the ACC/AHA HF Working Group, this element involved the specific decision to refer medically refractory HF patients to specialty and transplant centers. It called for health-care facilities to establish a relationship with a specialty center and coordinate a plan for transfer that is predetermined and not in response to patient crisis. In such coordinated systems, patients would be referred based on their overall prognosis and response to medical care. Indeed, the literature has shown that patients with symptoms for >3 months and a more severe initial presentation are less likely to respond to therapy and may benefit from referral to specialty centers, including transplant centers [12]. Moreover, in medically refractory patients, referral to specialty centers has been reported to result in a 98% 1-year survival rate [13, 14] and reduce readmissions by 50%.

Though initially centered on referral, the concept of coordinated systems has morphed into one increasingly focused on greater linkage throughout the entire continuum of HF care. [15, 16] Such systems, termed accountable care organizations (ACOs), would provide continuity for patients across different institutional settings (including ambulatory and inpatient hospital visits) and, if possible, during episodes of acute decompensation. While prospective experience with structured, shared accountability, and related outcome data in HF are lacking, there is relatively strong evidence from the OPTIMIZE-HF (Organized Program to Initiate Lifesaving Treatment in Hospitalized Patients With Heart Failure) registry which suggests a relationship between readmission rate and early outpatient follow-up after an index HF hospitalization [17]. Among patients with acute HF who were discharged from the emergency department (ED) in the Canadian National Ambulatory Care Reporting System, an association between early collaborative HF care and increased use of drug therapies, cardiovascular diagnostic testing, and better outcomes has also been reported [18].

Process

Processes of care are the interventions made in the hospital or outpatient setting that will lead to a desired health-care outcome. They can be pharmacologic (e.g., the use of angiotensin-converting enzyme inhibitors [ACEI], beta-adrenergic blockers), diagnostic (the assessment of left ventricular dysfunction), or patient-focused (providing discharge instructions and encouraging daily weight measurement).

Ideal process measures have a well-defined outcome link, are broadly applicable to a defined group of patients, and are easily measured. Adherence to such interventions serves as a marker of quality of care and forms a foundation for quality improvement.

There are several challenges in defining ideal process of care measures for HF patients. First, HF is a clinical syndrome rather than a single disease entity. Patients' symptoms and left ventricular (LV) function can vary greatly, and with minimal apparent correlation. This makes it difficult to define process measures that are applicable to all HF patients. For instance, the majority of HF patients are known to have preserved systolic function; however, most diagnostic and therapeutic interventions have not been studied in this population [6]. In addition, patients at more advanced stages of disease are less likely to be receiving evidence-based therapy [19]. This is largely due to increased contraindications to therapy as mortality risk rises and decreased use of medication in eligible patients. More research is needed to define which therapies are beneficial to patients with early versus advanced stages of disease.

A second challenge is the lack of consensus as to what constitutes the ideal processes of care. A number of leading health-care organizations, including the AHA's Get With the Guidelines Heart Failure (GWTG-HF) program [20], have attempted to define processes (Table 4.1) which, based on the best available evidence or, in its absence, consensus opinion, should either be utilized in every patient (unless contraindicated) or at the least be tracked. While there is a considerable amount of overlap in the recommendations, there are also differences that make it difficult to set national or international goals and benchmarks for quality care. For instance, the Joint Commission on Accreditation of Healthcare Organizations (JCAHO), ACC/AHA, and AHA GWTG-HF each recommend ACEI or angiotensin receptor blocker (ARB) therapy for patients with LVEF <40%, evaluation of LV function, discharge instructions incorporating activity level, diet, discharge medications, follow-up appointments, weight monitoring, and what to do if symptoms worsen, and smoking cessation counseling. However, GWTG lists initiation of beta-blocker therapy for patients with LVEF <40% as an achievement measure, while the ACC/AHA recommends anticoagulation in patients with atrial fibrillation.

Furthermore, it is unknown which of the recommended processes are beneficial to HF patients presenting to the ED or the observation unit (OU). This is due, for the most part, to an absence of evidence regarding the causal relationship between ED or OU processes of care and specific outcomes. Previously proposed measures, such as door-to-treatment (i.e., diuretic) time, make empirical sense but have been insufficiently explored. The ideal processes of care, and thus the markers of quality, could be substantially different for patients with acute decompensation who are treated in a short-stay setting than for patients following a prolonged hospitalization, but at present, there is simply not enough data.

A final issue is ensuring that processes of care are carried out equally across socioeconomic, racial, ethnic, and gender groups. In OPTIMIZE-HF, it was found that African American patients admitted for HF were more likely to receive evidence-based medications while in hospital but less likely to receive discharge instructions or smoking cessation counseling [21].

Table 4.1 American Heart Association Get With The Guidelines Heart Failure process of care metrics [20]

Achievement (performance) measures—processes or aspects of care for which the evidence is so strong that failure to act on it reduces the likelihood of an optimal patient outcome (required for performance recognition by the GWTG program)

ACEI/ARBs at discharge for patients with LVEF <40%[a,b]

Beta-blocker at discharge for patients with LVEF <40%[a]

Discharge instructions addressing activity level, diet, discharge medications, follow-up appointment, weight monitoring, what to do if symptoms worsen[b]

Measurement of LV function prior to or during hospitalization or planned following discharge[b]

Smoking cessation counseling[b]

Quality measures—processes and aspects of care strongly supported by science but not universally indicated as achievement measures (not required for performance recognition)

Aldosterone antagonist at discharge for patients with LVEF <40%[a]

Anticoagulation for atrial fibrillation

Cardiac resynchronization therapy (CRT) employed or prescribed at discharge for patients with LVEF ≤35% and a QRS duration ≥120 ms

DVT prophylaxis by the end of hospital day 2

Evidence-based use of specific beta-blockers (bisoprolol, carvedilol, metoprolol)

Hydralazine/nitrate combination at discharge for African American patients with LVEF <40%[a]

Implantable cardioverter-defibrillator (ICD) placed or prescribed at discharge for patients with LVEF ≤35%

Pneumococcal vaccination prior to discharge

Influenza (during active season) vaccination prior to discharge

Reporting measures—additional processes or aspects of care that are reported as data elements and may be beneficial to subpopulations but are not generalizable (not required for performance recognition)

Blood pressure control at discharge (% with SBP <140 mmHg and DBP <90 mmHg)

Diabetes treatment[a]

Diabetes teaching

Follow-up visit within 7 days

Lipid-lowering medications at discharge for patients with CAD, CVA, or PVD[a]

Omega-3 fatty acid supplement use at discharge

Descriptive measures—other processes or aspects of care captured by reporting of descriptive data elements (not required for performance recognition)

Educational materials provided to patient or caretaker during hospitalization or at discharge addressing: activity level, diet, weight, follow-up, discharge medications, and what to do if symptoms worsen

---

[a]Metrics which, along with mortality and rehospitalization rates, are used by GWGT-HF to monitor performance at 30-days postdischarge

[b]Metrics which also serve the core performance measures for the Joint Commission on Accreditation of Healthcare Organizations (JCAHO) and the Center for Medicare and Medicaid Services (CMS)

Outcomes: Quality in Action

Good outcomes are the ultimate goal of any health-care system and the essence of quality. Ideal outcome measures should be measurable, sensitive to modifications in the structure and process of care, and practical to use and should take into account

Table 4.2 Outcomes of importance in heart failure [6]

Survival
Mortality rates
Quality-adjusted life years (QALYs)
Days out of the hospital and alive[a]
Resource utilization
Index visit
Admission rate
Admission location (floor, telemetry, ICU)
Length of stay
Postdischarge
Outpatient clinic visits
Emergency department visits
Hospital readmissions
Symptom resolution
Dyspnea scores
Health status and quality of life
Short form (SF) 8, 12, or 36
Minnesota living with heart failure
Kansas City cardiomyopathy
6-minute walk test
Patient knowledge and compliance
Perceived self-efficacy (diet, medications, lifestyle)
Illness-belief scales
Health literacy
Health numeracy

[a]May be considered a metric of both survival and resource utilization

patients' underlying risk for good or bad outcomes. The main challenge in using outcomes as a marker of quality is that they do not depend solely on the health care provided. Age, severity of cardiac dysfunction, presenting hemodynamic profile, degree of comorbidity, and socioeconomic status have all been shown to affect outcomes for acute HF patients [22].

An additional challenge specific to the ED setting is the relative absence of data linking ED or OU acute HF processes of care with postdischarge outcome. Consequently, it is unknown which of the commonly used outcome measures (Table 4.2) constitute a meaningful representation of what can reasonably be attributable to ED and OU management of HF patients. Thus, while a recent review of more than 50,000 acute HF patients in Ontario, Canada, found a slightly higher 90-day mortality rate (11.9% versus 9.5%; log-rank $P=0.016$) among those who were discharged from the ED versus admitted to the hospital, its interpretation within the context of health-care quality is difficult [23]. Moreover, while 90 days is a relatively short follow-up period, it is probably long enough to introduce substantial confounding. Shorter (i.e., 30-day) postdischarge event rates were favored in the AHA's recent Scientific Statement on Acute Heart Failure Syndromes in the emergency department [16] and are utilized by GWTG-HF [20] and may be more reflective of an ED, OU, or even inpatient treatment period. Perhaps of greater importance, 30-day mortality and readmission data for acute HF are publicly reported by the Centers for Medicare and Medicaid Services (CMS) as a measure of comparative hospital quality. Regardless of the sampling period, there may be added value through use of more time-sensitive metrics such as days out of hospital and alive [15], which provide a clearer signal of causality than measurement of dichotomous (and equally weighted) outcomes that occur at any point within a prespecified time frame.

Survival

Mortality rates are classically used for quality improvement within a health-care system. Though often considered the poorest of outcomes, it should be recognized that death is not always an unexpected event and, in some cases, particularly those with preterminal end-stage HF, may be an acceptable end point to the patient or their caregiver (ideally stipulated as such in advanced directives) [24–26]. This notwithstanding, mortality rate is a requisite indicator which, from a statistical perspective, should be measured from the patients' index hospitalization or at the point of initial diagnosis. Failure to do so may result in resampling of the same individual at multiple time points (i.e., episodes of recidivism) and create confounding due to competing risk for survival. Though difficult, differentiating death due to HF (i.e., sudden cardiac arrest or worsening ventricular function) from other causes is also important to provide the level of granularity needed to accurately estimate relationships within the Donabedian framework.

In terms of process to outcome link, it was found in OPTIMIZE-HF that none of the ACC/AHA performance measures resulted in reduced mortality risk and only ACEI/ARB prescription at discharge was shown to diminish the composite outcome of 60–90 days postdischarge death or rehospitalization [27]. Beta-blockade at the time of discharge on the other hand, a process not currently listed as an ACC/AHA performance measure but recommended by the GWTG-HF program, was strongly associated with a reduction in both mortality and the composite of death or rehospitalization. While the benefits of such therapy have not been specifically shown for acute HF patients treated in an ED or OU, broader utilization of ACEI/ARB and beta-blockers at discharge from either of these settings offers promise as an approach to improvement of postdischarge survival [28].

Resource Utilization

Health-care resource utilization is another important and often cited outcome measure. Because HF is a disease of recidivism with rehospitalization rates that approach 25–30% at 30 days [29], much of the focus on resource utilization remains appropriately fixed on postdischarge outcomes. The need to reduce postdischarge ED visits and the rate of readmission for those with acute HF is considered fundamental to both institutional quality improvement efforts and future research endeavors [6, 16].

Cost is also a primary driver of the interest in terms of resource utilization, and in addition to recidivism, there is growing interest in the disposition of patients with acute HF from the ED. At present, more than 80% of those with acute HF get admitted to the hospital in the USA, many of whom are directed to a monitored bed [16]. There is little data and no clinical policies or decision rules that dictate what type of patients may go home from the ED, which can be managed in an OU setting, and who should be admitted to an inpatient unit. Using decision-analytic model simulations, it has been shown that, in comparison to ED discharge among low-risk ED patients, the marginal cost-effectiveness ratio is reasonable for OU admission ($44, 249 per quality-adjusted life year) but unacceptably high for hospital admission ($684,101 per quality-adjusted life year). Sensitivity analyses demonstrated that as the risk of early (within 5 days) and late (within 30 days) readmission and mortality rose, OU admission became less costly and more effective than ED discharge, and with an increase in postdischarge event rates among those discharged from the OU, hospital admission was more cost-effective [30]. As evidenced, however, by the 15-year trend toward decreasing hospital length of stay, increasing use of skilled nursing facilities at discharge, and higher rates of readmission rate among Medicare beneficiaries with acute HF [31], point-in-time decisions do not exist in isolation and may have untoward downstream consequences.

A growing area of interest with respect to resource utilization (and the potential for reduction) is variation in practice at the regional, institutional, and individual practitioner levels. Such variation contributes to de facto differences in resource consumption and may be associated with divergent outcomes [32]. Presumably, this represents a combination of over-, under-, and misuse of clinical care, each of which offers the opportunity to improve upon practice patterns. Appropriate-use criteria have been developed to examine the rational use of radiographic testing in HF [33], and such scrutiny could be (but has not been) more broadly applied to identify ineffective or wasteful processes of care.

Patient-Centered

The final three outcome measures listed are patient-centered. They involve patient perceptions of symptom severity (predominantly dyspnea), overall health status, and illness beliefs/knowledge about compliance with diet and medication regimen.

During the acute phase of treatment, dyspnea resolution is paramount and may be the thing that matters most to patients. Though dyspnea is often not measured systematically, repeat assessment of severity using validated scales is possible, and identification of a differential response has emerged as an important end point for HF therapeutic trials [34–36]. However, what constitutes a meaningful change over time, and the lasting value of dyspnea as an outcome measure beyond response to ED or OU intervention, is not known.

Measures of health status and quality of life have become increasingly recognized as highly meaningful outcomes of cardiovascular care [37]. Those listed in Table 4.2 have been validated as tools for self-assessment of HF disease progression in chronic outpatient settings, but their direct applicability to patient care in the ED or OU is uncertain. Nonetheless, they can provide an important means to objectively compare postdischarge perceptions of wellness (or illness) which, in turn, may reflect the adequacy (or inadequacy) of seemingly sufficient treatment. Due to a lack of definitional standards for quality of life and variability in what may constitute a clinically significant improvement, comparative interpretation within and across scales is difficult.

Despite a rich history in the social science literature, metrics focused on disease-specific knowledge and understanding, as well as general health literacy and numeracy, have achieved incomplete uptake in the world of clinical medicine. An appraisal of such aspects, however, offers the unique opportunity to evaluate often overlooked potential contributors to poor disease self-management and assess (in a pre–post fashion) the relative effectiveness of educational interventions.

Toward Quality Improvement

Clinical Practice Guidelines

Removing variation in clinical care through adherence to established, evidence-based best practices forms the basis of the contemporary quality improvement initiative. To this end, HF specific clinical practice guidelines have been published by the ACC/AHA [13], the Heart Failure Society of America (HFSA) [38], the European Society of Cardiology (ESC) [39], and the Society of Chest Pain Centers (SCPC) [40]. Individually and collectively, these represent a combination of the best available evidence and consensus expert opinion as they pertain to various aspects of the overall process of care. Clinical practice guidelines have been shown to improve health-care processes and outcomes in general as well as specifically for HF. Institutional adoption of clinical practice guidelines has been promoted as a structural mechanism to improve the quality of care delivered to HF patients [6].

Unfortunately, many of the HF guideline-based recommendations put forth have been designed for longitudinal patient care in the clinical setting or following hospital admission. Less well-defined are the necessary process measures for patients with acute decompensated heart failure, particularly in the ED and OU setting. While the ACC/AHA has included some information on acute HF in the most recent-focused update of their 2005 Guidelines for the Diagnosis and Management of Heart Failure in Adults, and the Heart Failure Society of America (HFSA) has given recommendations for acute HF care in their 2010 Comprehensive Heart Failure Practice Guideline, only the SCPC has published clinical guidelines that are focused on the ED and OU phases of care [40]. Use of the SCPC guidelines to identify acute HF patients at low risk of adverse outcomes has recently been validated using the HEARD-IT (HEart failure and Audicor Technology for Rapid Diagnosis and Initial Treatment) database [41]. Whether the SCPC or any other guidelines can affect acute HF patient outcome, however, remains to be seen.

Performance Measures

Whereas clinical guidelines are meant to serve as an evidentiary review of the literature and provide the scientific background for specific patient care recommendations, performance measures function as tools of accountability [2]. They focus on discrete processes of care for which there is evidence of the highest quality (class I, level A) showing unequivocal benefit and consensus that a failure to provide the therapy would meaningfully reduce the likelihood of a positive outcome. As alluded to in a preceding section, specific performance measures (Table 4.1) for HF have been developed by organizations with a vested interest in health-care quality including the JCAHO, the ACC/AHA, CMS, and, most recently, GWTG-HF. To enhance awareness and increase recognition of those institutions which achieve a higher standard, the GWTG-HF program confers performance awards to hospitals when they reach certain milestones (bronze = 90 consecutive days of 85% adherence to performance measures, silver = 12 consecutive months of 85% adherence to performance measures, and gold = 24 or more consecutive months of 85% adherence to performance measures). The GWTG-HF program recently added a performance "plus" designation for those gold and silver award centers which achieve 75% compliance over 12 months in at least 4 out of 9 second-tier (i.e., "quality") measures.

While there is evidence supporting clinical benefit from adherence to the ACC/AHA performance measures for HF [42] and a modest mortality reduction for hospitals receiving performance awards from GWTG-HF [43], there is also concern about the ramifications associated with utilizing performance measures to standardize quality [44]. Hospital adherence to the CMS core measures is now publicly reported, and increasingly, these reports are being used to distinguish providers and systems that deliver high-quality care from those who are marginal or deficient. Additionally, reimbursement at all levels is now closely tied to related, performance-based initiatives [44]. Such use of payment thresholds to incentivize performance, however, is not without consequence and may serve to reward paper compliance rather than encourage practice which results in actual substantive improvements in patient care (e.g., simple documentation of smoking cessation counseling versus initiation of a quantifiable, behavioral encounter) [2]. Furthermore, pay-for-performance initiatives tend to be absolute without consideration of incremental cost-effectiveness (i.e., maximal rather than optimal perspective on health care) [2, 44] and, in some instances, may even create misalignment between financial incentives for the institution itself (i.e., by inducing performance measure achievement through relative increases in payment which are offset by declining reimbursement from reduced hospital admissions).

Table 4.3 Society of Chest Pain Centers' key elements for heart failure accreditation

1. Emergency department integration with the emergency medical services
2. Emergency assessment of patients with symptoms of acute decompensated heart failure—diagnosis
3. Risk stratification of the heart failure patient
4. Treatment of patients presenting to the emergency department in heart failure
5. Heart failure discharge criteria from the emergency department, observation stay or inpatient stay
6. Heart failure patient education in the emergency department, observation and inpatient unit
7. Personnel, competencies, and training
8. Process improvement
9. Organizational structure and commitment
10. Heart failure community outreach

To ensure that relevant information is accurate, proper documentation of performance and, perhaps more importantly, exceptions (i.e., medical, patient-level, or systematic reasons why the measure cannot or should not be performed) is needed. This may require prospective recording of additional data elements by providers during a clinical encounter or, absent this, reliance on often imperfect administrative data. Electronic medical records could facilitate data collection through exportation of quality metric information (though most systems would require extensive software upgrades to enable this) or use of provider-directed automated prompts (which may be problematic as clinicians tend to develop "alert fatigue") [2].

Accreditation

Meeting (or striving to meet) the various aspects of care stipulated by guidelines and performance measures can be a daunting task. However, cataloging, understanding, and quantifying baseline practice (and outcomes) are critical steps in this process and central tenets of quality improvement. The intensive data gathering required can be facilitated by seeking accreditation—an unbiased approach to assessment of institutional performance which serves to recognize those centers which conform to a predefined (higher) standard of care. Rooted in the principles of improvement science, accreditation involves a thorough review of site-specific quality elements. It is another way of replicating best practices which, at the same time, encourages institutional innovation and creativity to achieve optimal outcomes. The SCPC has been a driving force in the development of HF accreditation, creating an "accreditation tool" that includes ten "key elements" (Table 4.3), each of which is supported by lower tier item groupings (termed "essential," "best practice," and "innovation").

Purported benefits of accreditation include the introduction of critical process improvement tools, integration of care processes across departments, provision of a road map for strategic planning, enhancement of patient care, development of pathways to reduce medical errors, and streamlining of third-party analysis through use of uniform operational definitions and common language. Though experience with

HF accreditation is evolving, SCPC (Society of Chest Pain Center Accreditation) has been associated with increased ACC/AHA evidence-based guideline adherence in the first 24 h of care [45].

Conclusions

Using the best available evidence and expert opinion, measurable quality and operational metrics for HF have been defined by a number of prominent organizations. To be in better position to achieve these metrics, health-care systems will ideally be structured around patient-focused, multidisciplinary disease management programs that focus on coordination of care across providers and institutions. Adherence to specific performance measures has been associated with improvements in patient outcomes, including increased survival and decreased recidivism, and has profound implications for reimbursement. These metrics, however, were developed for admitted patients, and whether or not they can be extended to the ED or OU is still to be determined. Rather than an impediment, this gap in knowledge provides a unique opportunity to prospectively evaluate the validity of existing practice guidelines and performance measures under differing circumstances and improve upon them in a manner that enhances their applicability to ED and OU settings.

References

1. Donabedian A. The quality of care. How can it be assessed? JAMA. 1988;260(12):1743–8.
2. Spertus JA, Bonow RO, Chan P, et al. ACCF/AHA new insights into the methodology of performance measurement. J Am Coll Cardiol. 2010;56(21):1767–82.
3. Ko DT, Alter DA, Austin PC, et al. Life expectancy after an index hospitalization for patients with heart failure: a population-based study. Am Heart J. 2008;155(2):324–31.
4. Setoguchi S, Stevenson LW, Schneeweiss S. Repeated hospitalizations predict mortality in the community population with heart failure. Am Heart J. 2007;154(2):260–6.
5. Gheorghiade M, Pang PS. Acute heart failure syndromes. J Am Coll Cardiol. 2009;53(7): 557–73.
6. Krumholz HM, Baker DW, Ashton CM, et al. Evaluating quality of care for patients with heart failure. Circulation. 2000;101(12):E122–140.
7. Gwadry-Sridhar FH, Flintoft V, Lee DS, et al. A systematic review and meta-analysis of studies comparing readmission rates and mortality rates in patients with heart failure. Arch Intern Med. 2004;164(21):2315–20.
8. Levy P, Nocerini R, Grazier K. Paying for disease management. Dis Manag. 2007;10(4): 235–44.
9. Ashton CM. Care of patients with failing hearts: evidence for failures in clinical practice and health services research. J Gen Intern Med. 1999;14(2):138–40.
10. Philbin EF. Comprehensive multidisciplinary programs for the management of patients with congestive heart failure. J Gen Intern Med. 1999;14(2):130–5.
11. Chaudhry SI, Mattera JA, Curtis JP, et al. Telemonitoring in patients with heart failure. N Engl J Med. 2010;363(24):2301–9.

12. Steimle AE, Stevenson LW, Fonarow GC, et al. Prediction of improvement in recent onset cardiomyopathy after referral for heart transplantation. J Am Coll Cardiol. 1994;23(3): 553–9.
13. Hunt SA, Abraham WT, Chin MH, et al. 2009 Focused update incorporated into the ACC/AHA 2005 Guidelines for the Diagnosis and Management of Heart Failure in Adults A Report of the American College of Cardiology Foundation/American Heart Association Task Force on Practice Guidelines Developed in Collaboration With the International Society for Heart and Lung Transplantation. J Am Coll Cardiol. 2009;53(15):e1–e90.
14. Rickenbacher PR, Trindade PT, Haywood GA, et al. Transplant candidates with severe left ventricular dysfunction managed with medical treatment: characteristics and survival. J Am Coll Cardiol. 1996;27(5):1192–7.
15. Peacock WF, Braunwald E, Abraham W, et al. National Heart, Lung, and Blood Institute working group on emergency department management of acute heart failure: research challenges and opportunities. J Am Coll Cardiol. 2010;56(5):343–51.
16. Weintraub NL, Collins SP, Pang PS, et al. Acute heart failure syndromes: emergency department presentation, treatment, and disposition: current approaches and future aims: a scientific statement from the American heart association. Circulation. 2010;122(19):1975–96.
17. Hernandez AF, Greiner MA, Fonarow GC, et al. Relationship between early physician follow-up and 30-day readmission among Medicare beneficiaries hospitalized for heart failure. JAMA. 2010;303(17):1716–22.
18. Lee DS, Stukel TA, Austin PC, et al. Improved outcomes with early collaborative care of ambulatory heart failure patients discharged from the emergency department. Circulation. 2010;122(18):1806–14.
19. Peterson PN, Rumsfeld JS, Liang L, et al. Treatment and risk in heart failure: gaps in evidence or quality? Circ Cardiovasc Qual Outcomes. 2010;3(3):309–15.
20. American Heart Association (2010) Get with the guidelines—heart failure overview. http://www.heart.org/HEARTORG/HealthcareResearch/GetWithTheGuidelinesHFStroke/GetWithTheGuidelinesHeartFailureHomePage/Get-With-The-Guidelines-Heart-Failure-Overview_UCM_307806_Article.jsp. Accessed 20 Oct 2010.
21. Yancy CW, Abraham WT, Albert NM, et al. Quality of care of and outcomes for African Americans hospitalized with heart failure: findings from the OPTIMIZE-HF (Organized Program to Initiate Lifesaving Treatment in Hospitalized Patients With Heart Failure) registry. J Am Coll Cardiol. 2008;51(17):1675–84.
22. Collins SP, Storrow AB. Acute heart failure risk stratification: can we define low risk? Heart Fail Clin. 2009;5(1):75–83.
23. Lee DS, Schull MJ, Alter DA, et al. Early deaths in patients with heart failure discharged from the emergency department: a population-based analysis. Circ Heart Fail. 2010;3(2):228–35.
24. Formiga F, Chivite D, Ortega C, et al. End-of-life preferences in elderly patients admitted for heart failure. Q J Med. 2004;97(12):803–8.
25. Goodlin SJ, Hauptman PJ, Arnold R, et al. Consensus statement: palliative and supportive care in advanced heart failure. J Card Fail. 2004;10(3):200–9.
26. Krumholz HM, Phillips RS, Hamel MB, et al. Resuscitation preferences among patients with severe congestive heart failure: results from the SUPPORT project. Study to Understand Prognoses and Preferences for Outcomes and Risks of Treatments. Circulation. 1998;98(7):648–55.
27. Fonarow GC, Abraham WT, Albert NM, et al. Association between performance measures and clinical outcomes for patients hospitalized with heart failure. JAMA. 2007;297(1):61–70.
28. Fermann GJ, Collins SP. Observation units in the management of acute heart failure syndromes. Curr Heart Fail Rep. 2010;7(3):125–33.
29. Jencks SF, Williams MV, Coleman EA. Rehospitalizations among patients in the Medicare fee-for-service program. N Engl J Med. 2009;360(14):1418–28.
30. Collins SP, Schauer DP, Gupta A, et al. Cost-effectiveness analysis of ED decision making in patients with non-high-risk heart failure. Am J Emerg Med. 2009;27(3):293–302.

31. Bueno H, Ross JS, Wang Y, et al. Trends in length of stay and short-term outcomes among Medicare patients hospitalized for heart failure, 1993–2006. JAMA. 2010;303(21):2141–7.
32. Ong MK, Mangione CM, Romano PS, et al. Looking forward, looking back: assessing variations in hospital resource use and outcomes for elderly patients with heart failure. Circ Cardiovasc Qual Outcomes. 2009;2(6):548–57.
33. White CS, Davis SD, Aquino SL, et al. American College of Radiology Appropriateness Criteria® congestive heart failure. http://www.guideline.gov/content.aspx?id=9604. Accessed 27 Dec 2010.
34. Gheorghiade M, Follath F, Ponikowski P, et al. Assessing and grading congestion in acute heart failure: a scientific statement from the acute heart failure committee of the heart failure association of the European Society of Cardiology and endorsed by the European Society of Intensive Care Medicine. Eur J Heart Fail. 2010;12(5):423–33.
35. Hogg KJ, McMurray JJ. Evaluating dyspnoea in acute heart failure: progress at last! Eur Heart J. 2010;31(7):771–2.
36. Mebazaa A, Pang PS, Tavares M, et al. The impact of early standard therapy on dyspnoea in patients with acute heart failure: the URGENT-dyspnoea study. Eur Heart J. 2010;31(7): 832–41.
37. Spertus JA. Evolving applications for patient-centered health status measures. Circulation. 2008;118(20):2103–10.
38. Lindenfeld J, Albert NM, Boehmer JP, et al. HFSA 2010 comprehensive heart failure practice guideline. J Card Fail. 2010;16(6):e1–194.
39. Dickstein K, Cohen-Solal A, Filippatos G, et al. ESC Guidelines for the diagnosis and treatment of acute and chronic heart failure 2008: the Task Force for the Diagnosis and Treatment of Acute and Chronic Heart Failure 2008 of the European Society of Cardiology. Developed in collaboration with the Heart Failure Association of the ESC (HFA) and endorsed by the European Society of Intensive Care Medicine (ESICM). Eur Heart J. 2008;29(19):2388–442.
40. Peacock WF, Fonarow GC, Ander DS, et al. Society of Chest Pain Centers recommendations for the evaluation and management of the observation stay acute heart failure patient-parts 1–6. Acute Card Care. 2009;11(1):3–42.
41. Collins SP, Lindsell CJ, Naftilan AJ, et al. Low-risk acute heart failure patients: external validation of the Society of Chest Pain Center's recommendations. Crit Pathw Cardiol. 2009; 8(3):99–103.
42. Maeda JL. Evidence-based heart failure performance measures and clinical outcomes: a systematic review. J Card Fail. 2010;16(5):411–8.
43. Heidenreich PA, Lewis WR, LaBresh KA, et al. Hospital performance recognition with the Get With The Guidelines Program and mortality for acute myocardial infarction and heart failure. Am Heart J. 2009;158(4):546–53.
44. Ghali JK, Massie BM, Mann DL, et al. Heart failure guidelines, performance measures, and the practice of medicine mind the gap. J Am Coll Cardiol. 2010;56(25):2077–80.
45. Chandra A, Glickman SW, Ou FS, et al. An analysis of the Association of Society of Chest Pain Centers Accreditation to American College of Cardiology/American Heart Association non-ST-segment elevation myocardial infarction guideline adherence. Ann Emerg Med. 2009;54(1):17–25.

Chapter 5
Interaction of Performance Measurements, Staffing, and Facility Requirements for the Heart Failure Observation Unit

Valorie Sweigart and Karen Krechmery

Research into existing observation units can provide a valuable starting point for establishing a heart failure center. Site visits are one common method. Obtaining protocols that can be adapted and individualized for your facility is also common. Establishing a multidisciplinary team can assist in providing needed expertise. Decisions such as an open, closed, or mixed unit should be made before establishing heart failure guidelines.

Performance Measurements

Evidence-based clinical practice guidelines for the care of heart failure patients guide providers, individual units, and hospitals in developing their own best practice measures [1]. Identifying best practice measures can integrate both administrative practices such as staffing, with clinical outcomes such as patient length of stay. Benchmarking is a method used to compare your own practice with those of like hospitals. Establishing best practice levels of performance is the goal of benchmarking.

Well-known organizations that have established guidelines also known as core measures for best practice include The Joint Commission, The American College of Cardiology, and The American Heart Association [2–4]. These organizations provide published data that can be used as a benchmark for establishing individualized patient outcome goals. While some of these guidelines are intended for inpatient use,

V. Sweigart, RN, DNP (✉) • K. Krechmery, RN, MSN
Emory University Hospital Midtown, Atlanta, GA, USA
e-mail: valorie.sweigart@emoryhealthcare.org

W. Frank Peacock (ed.), *Short Stay Management of Acute Heart Failure*,
Contemporary Cardiology, DOI 10.1007/978-1-61779-627-2_5,
© Springer Science+Business Media, LLC 2012

they reflect evidence-based standards of care for heart failure patients. Ambulatory care guidelines can also contribute to the development of observation medicine management goals, which is considered outpatient care.

Performance improvement measures need to be established by each institution based on the overall mission of the observation unit. These measures are used by the unit to determine the effectiveness of the heart failure protocol. Length of stay and discharge rates are common indicators of success. If the standard for the observation unit is a length of stay of less than 24 h, then length of stays greater than 24 h would indicate inefficiency either with treatment protocols, patient selection, or patient response to treatment. Discharge rates assist in identifying appropriate patient selection. The patient may have comorbidities that would have precluded effective treatment in this time frame. Therefore, exclusion criteria can be established or modified based on this data. Other data that may assist in refining protocol and patient selection may be examining time of day of admission and length of stay. Considerations such as time of discharge for elderly patients may be a factor. Based on time of admission, you may not be able to achieve the desired outcome for discharge within a 24-h time frame.

All patients admitted for heart failure must have realistic goals defined at the time of admission. Patient selection is key to the process. Placing a patient in observation must have a high probability of success within the observation time frame. Patients with multiple goals and/or comorbidities most likely will not be ready for discharge in less than 24 h.

Valuable feedback of unit/staff performance can be obtained directly from patients. Patient telephone surveys by the unit staff have been shown to provide valuable information regarding the operations of the department. A simple standardized questionnaire can be developed by the staff and physicians related to key aspects of care. Telephone calls placed at a decided interval after discharge can obtain information that can guide the department in developing their own best practices based on their patients' perspectives. This information can also be incorporated into the unit's performance improvement plan.

Health-care organizations benchmark administrative measures in which common hospital characteristics are compared to like organizations. There are many organizations or consortiums that provide these services such as Press Ganey, well known for patient satisfaction measurements. According to Press Ganey, positive patient experiences have been linked with positive clinical and financial outcomes for the organization. Therefore, measurement of patient satisfaction done with standardized methodology can be used to reflect the hospital performance and areas that can be targeted for improving patient's perception of quality [5].

Another key measure to an institution's success is staff and physician satisfaction. The Gallup Company is an organization that has demonstrated through research that organizations with a high level of staff and physician engagement or commitment report higher levels of patient satisfaction [6]. Staff that is actively engaged in the care of the patient will go above and beyond the basic standards required to provide care to the patient. One such example would be a nurse that leaves discharge materials at the bedside related to patient education vs. a nurse that reviews the materials with the patient and then assesses the patient's understanding of the information provided. Having engaged staff ultimately leads to better patient satisfaction and optimum unit level operations.

Staffing

Observation unit staffing is composed of physicians, associate providers (AP) such as nurse practitioners or physician assistants, registered nurses, support staff such as nursing assistants and unit clerks, as well as social workers. Typical models utilize an AP that is responsible for directing the care during the patient visit 24 h per day 7 days per week. A physician is responsible for patient rounds. This ensures that all patients are examined by a physician prior to discharge and provides for collaboration with the AP. Registered nurses provide direct patient care and are present 24 h per day 7 days per week.

Nursing staffing models vary with the needs of each unit. All units must have a registered nurse responsible for the overall care of the patient. Typical nurse/patient ratios vary with each state/institution but generally are in the range of 4:1 or 6:1. This can be adjusted based on patient acuity or volume. The numbers of nurses required in an observation unit can be calculated using worked hours per unit of service (WHUOS). This is a common financial unit of measurement and can be benchmarked with like institutions. It is derived from the total number of hours worked by staff divided by the total number of units of service or visits. This number can then be used to more accurately predict the required budget by incorporating the number of days of the month and adjusting for seasonal or temporal fluctuating patient volumes. Many units also supplement nurses with nursing assistants. The number of nurses and support staff for each unit is dependent on the size of the unit and staffing decisions at that institution. Larger units may require clerical staff to answer phones, direct unit activities such as testing schedules, assist family members, etc. Nursing assistants may be required for phlebotomy, transport of patients to and from tests, and obtaining vital signs or ECGs. Finally, social services, discharge planning, nutritionists, and transplant coordinators may be on call for specialized patient needs.

As within all hospitals, basic life support (BLS) training is considered mandatory for all staff involved in patient care. Advanced life support (ALS) is also required for all registered nurses in the emergency department. Most heart failure patients go directly from the emergency department to the observation unit and will require ongoing cardiac monitoring, therefore necessitating that the RN staff in the unit to also be ACLS certified. Dysrhythmia training is also a basic competency that is a unit requirement, and other annual competencies may be needed depending on unit/hospital standards and the breadth of pathologies routinely managed in the specific OU.

Facility Requirements

Physical requirements for building a unit, or remodeling an existing area, can be found in the National Fire Protection Association 101: Life Safety Code 2009 which establishes a minimum threshold of safety for patients in new and existing structures. Guidelines for building codes are also available through the American Institute of Architects (AIA). Square footage requirements, utilities requirements, sinks, etc., for individual rooms are outlined as well as federal and state requirements for Medicare and/or Medicaid facilities.

The numbers of beds needed for an observation unit can be calculated based on the current number of emergency department beds. In a 2007 observational study by Ross et al., they were able to arrive at a common bed utilization characteristic based on emergency department observation unit (EDOU) beds per ED visit of 1 EDOU bed/7,461 ED visits or a daily number of EDOU patients per EDOU bed of 1.14 patients per bed per day [7].

Basic equipment for care of heart failure patients would include oxygen, air sources, and suction available in each room. Many of these patients receive ongoing oxygen as well as nebulizer treatments periodically. Cardiac monitoring is also required for heart failure patients. Decisions at each institution would need to include hardwire monitoring with bedside monitors or telemetry monitoring. The advantage to hardwire monitoring is having the ability to do a 12-lead ECG at the bedside at any time that a change in patient condition warrants one. ST segment monitoring capability is another advantage of bedside monitoring.

Heart failure patients should be weighed upon admission and prior to discharge. A patient scale, preferably portable, is needed for the unit. Although scales are available to weigh up to 1,000 lb, a 600-lb scale is adequate for an OU. It should have a wide base for standing and handrails to assist the patient to stand. Further, since diuresis is a common goal with heart failure patients, toilets in each room are desirable, otherwise bedside commodes or urinals can be utilized for these patients.

Emergency equipment should be readily available if needed. This should include a defibrillator/AED and airway management equipment. A crash cart with emergency drugs and suction equipment is also necessary to perform ACLS protocols in the event of a cardiac arrest. Again, ACLS certified staff is needed to implement emergency procedures.

In summary, because of the wide variety of and unknown severity of illness of many OU heart failure patients, the OU requires staffing and physical supply needs similar to that of the ED. Furthermore, the availability of on-site expertise in cardiac monitoring and airway management is necessary to prevent complications from unexpected events. Finally, because patients may spend considerably longer periods in the OU, the dietary and bathroom needs will exceed that of the ED. Thus, the OU ultimately represents a hybrid between the ED and the inpatient environment in terms of physical plant and staffing requirements.

References

1. Albert N. Evidence-based nursing care for patients with heart failure. AACN Adv Crit Care. 2006;17(2):170–83.
2. Specifications Manual for Joint Commission National Quality Core Measures Page. http://www.jointcommission.org/specifications_manual_for_joint_commission_national_quality_core_measures/. Updated October 20, 2010. Accessed 15 Dec 2010.
3. Practice Guidelines and Quality Standards Page. http://www.cardiosource.org/Science-And-Quality/Practice-Guidelines-and-Quality-Standards/2009/Heart-Failure-in-Adults-Guidelines-for-the-Diagnosis-and-Management-of.aspx. Updated 2009. Accessed 3 Dec 2010.
4. Heart Failure Statements and Guidelines Page. http://my.americanheart.org/professional/StatementsGuidelines/ByTopic/TopicsD-H/Heart-Failure_UCM_321545_Article.jsp. Accessed 18 Dec 2010.
5. Quality PerformerSM: Reporting and Analysis for Hospital Performance Improvement. http://www.pressganey.com/ourSolutions/hospitalSettings/clinicalSuite/qualityPerformer.aspx. Accessed 20 Dec 2010.
6. Employee Engagement: A Leading Indicator of Financial Performance Page. http://www.gallup.com/consulting/52/Employee-Engagement.aspx. Accessed 28 Dec 2010.
7. Ross MA, Wilson AG, McPherson M. The impact of an ED observation bed on inpatient bed availability. Acad Emerg Med. 2001;8:576.

Part II
Pathophysiology and Demographics

Chapter 6
Heart Failure: Epidemiology and Demographics

Karina M. Soto-Ruiz

Abbreviations

ABC	Aging and body composition
ACC	American College of Cardiology
ACEI	Angiotensin-converting enzyme inhibitors
AHA	American Heart Association
CHD	Coronary heart disease
EF	Ejection fraction
GFR	Glomerular filtration rate
HF	Heart failure
ICD	Implantable cardioverter defibrillator
JCAHO	Joint Commission on Accreditation of Healthcare Organization
LVH	Left ventricular hypertrophy
MDRD	Modification of diet in renal disease
SBP	Systolic blood pressure

Heart failure (HF) is defined by the American Heart Association/American College of Cardiology (AHA/ACC) as a "complex clinical syndrome that can result from any structural or functional cardiac disorder that impairs the ability of the ventricle to fill or eject blood," and it underscores that "it is a largely clinical diagnosis that is based on a careful history and physical examination" [1]. The burden of heart failure is its enormous cost, both in human and financial measures. Heart failure affects over five million people in the USA and accounts for nearly $39.2 billion annually in health-care expenditures [2]. It is the most frequent cause of hospitalizations in patients 65 years of age or older. Heart failure is a disease of the elderly. It has an annual incidence of 10 cases per 1,000 after age 65 (Fig. 6.1), which then doubles

K.M. Soto-Ruiz, MD (✉)
Baylor College of Medicine, Houston, TX, USA
email: sotoruiz@bcm.edu

W. Frank Peacock (ed.), *Short Stay Management of Acute Heart Failure*,
Contemporary Cardiology, DOI 10.1007/978-1-61779-627-2_6,
© Springer Science+Business Media, LLC 2012

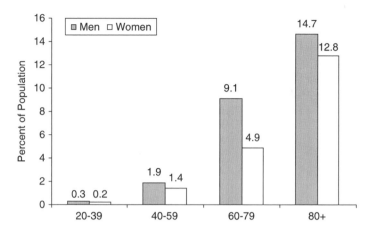

Fig. 6.1 Percentage of population with the diagnosis of heart failure according to age group (From the Heart Disease and Stroke Statistics—2010 Update)

every decade thereafter [3]. Subjects older than 65 years represent more than 75% of prevalent HF cases in the USA [4].

With the aging of 78 million baby boomers, 1 in 5 Americans is expected to be older than 65 years by 2050 and at risk for HF. This is projected to impact health care and health-care economics [5]. It is clear that the burden of heart failure is already increasing. In earlier studies from Framingham, the incidence of HF diagnosed with standardized criteria was between 1.4 and 2.3 per 1,000 patients annually, among people 29–79 years old [6]. Data from the Kaiser Permanente system comparing the incidence of HF from 1970 to 1974 and from 1990 to 1994 in persons 65 years old or older indicated that the age-adjusted incidence increased by 14% over this time and was greater for older persons and for men [7]. Conversely, reports from the Framingham Heart Study [8] and the Olmsted County Study [9], including outpatient heart failure data, indicate that over time, the incidence remained stable [9] or even declined in women [8]. Overall, the Framingham and Olmsted County studies have shown trends of increasing HF incidence among older persons; this pattern is important given the aging of the population.

Hospitalization

There are nearly 658,000 annual emergency department (ED) encounters primarily for acute HF in the USA; almost 20% of the total HF specific ambulatory care is delivered each year [10]. Ultimately, nearly 80% of patients treated in the ER are admitted to the hospital [11]. Heart failure is the single most frequent cause of hospitalization in persons 65 years of age or older, and hospital discharges for heart failure increased 175% between 1979 and 2004 [3]. The annual hospitalization rate for these patients now exceeds one million in the USA, 80% of whom are older than

65 years, and readmission rate as high as 50% within 6 months of discharge has been reported [12].

National Hospital Discharge Survey data from 1979 to 2004 showed the number of hospitalizations with any mention of heart failure tripled from 1,274,000 in 1979 to 3,860,000 in 2004 and that heart failure was the first-listed diagnosis for 30–35% of hospitalizations [13]. Unfortunately, incidence cannot be obtained from this data, as the statistics were event-based (allowing multiple hospitalizations for the same individual). However, despite the large impact of HF, its burden may be inadequately assessed. In a random sample of all incident HF in Olmsted County from 1987 to 2006, hospitalizations were common after HF diagnosis, with 83% of patients hospitalized at least once [14].

Hospitalizations for HF are likely to increase due to an aging population, improved survival after myocardial infarction, and more effective therapies to prevent sudden death, such as beta-blockers and implantable cardioverter defibrillators (ICD). Despite current management options, postdischarge mortality and rehospitalization at 60–90 days are as high as 15% and 30%, respectively [15]. This suggests that interventions to avoid readmissions are necessary. It has been shown that patients who have a 1-week follow-up after hospital discharge are less likely to be readmitted within 30 days than those that did not [16].

Mortality

Heart failure prognosis is poor, with a survival rate estimated at 50% and 10% over 5 and 10 years [17–19]. After age adjustment, 5-year mortality was 59% in men and 45% in women during 1990–1999 in the Framingham data [8] and 50% in men and 46% in women during 1996–2000 in Olmsted County [9]. Survival improvement in the elderly population was shown in data from the Kaiser Permanente system [7]; survival after diagnosis of HF improved by 33% in men and 24% in women and was primarily associated with beta-blocker therapy. Data suggests a relative improvement in survival after development of HF [8, 9], but others challenge this, especially in the elderly [20]. Overall, the absolute survival rate after a heart failure diagnosis remains low, and death has increased by 20.5% in the past decade. In patients older than 67 years old, median survival is less than 3 years after hospitalization for HF [21, 22].

Overall, improvement in survival of the hospitalized HF population is unclear but has been reported by some [17]. In one study, the median survival increase was associated with the effectiveness of angiotensin-converting enzyme inhibitors (ACEI) therapy, increasing from 1.2 to 1.6 years in a sample size of 66,547 patients. These results have been criticized because they were measured in hospitalized patients without validation; thus, improvement outcomes may be biased by coding trends. Administrative data from the Henry Ford Health System that included outpatient encounters reported a median survival of 4.2 years without discernible improvement over time [23]. Finally, the mortality rate after hospitalization for HF in the Health ABC (health, aging, and body composition study) was 18.0%, similar to other studies [5, 9, 22].

Diagnosis

Several diagnostic criteria exist, including the Framingham criteria [6] (Table 6.1), the Boston criteria [24] (Table 6.2), the Gothenburg criteria [25], and the European Society of Cardiology criteria [26]. When the Boston and Framingham criteria were

Table 6.1 Framingham criteria

Major criteria	Minor criteria
Paroxysmal nocturnal dyspnea	Bilateral ankle edema
Neck vein distention	Nocturnal cough
Rales	Dyspnea on ordinary exertion
Hepatojugular reflex	Hepatomegaly
Acute pulmonary edema	Pleural effusion
Third sound gallop	Tachycardia ($\geq$120 beats/min)
Increased central venous pressure (>16 cm water at the right atrium)	Decrease in vital capacity by 33% from maximal value recorded
Radiographic cardiomegaly (increasing heart size on chest X-ray film)	
Pulmonary edema, visceral congestion, or cardiomegaly at autopsy	
Weight loss $\geq$4.5 kg in 5 days in response to treatment of CHF	

The diagnosis of CHF required that two major or one major and two minor criteria be present concurrently. Minor criteria were acceptable only if they could not be attributed to another medical condition

Table 6.2 Boston criteria

History	
• Rest dyspnea	4
• Orthopnea	4
• Paroxysmal nocturnal dyspnea	3
• Dyspnea on walking on level	2
• Dyspnea on climbing	1
Physical examination	
• Heart rate (91–110 min, 1; >110/min, 2)	1/2
• Elevated jugular venous pressure	2/3
– (>6 cm H_2O 2; >6 cm H_2O, plus hepatomegaly or edema 3)	
• Rales (basilar 1; >basilar 2)	1/2
• Wheezing	3
• S_3 gallop	3
Chest X-ray	
• Alveolar pulmonary edema	4
• Interstitial pulmonary edema	3
• Bilateral pleural effusion	3
• Cardiothoracic ratio >0.5	3
• Upper-zone flow redistribution	2

No more than four points allowed from each of the three categories
No possible or definite heart failure if score equals 0–4, 5–7, 8–12 points respectively

compared blindly [27], their sensitivity was 100%; however, the specificity and positive predictive value of the Framingham criteria were lower than the Boston criteria for definite heart failure. Some authors recommend use of the Boston criteria in older adults as it has been shown to improve adverse outcome predictability [28]. The comparison of the Cardiovascular Health Study criteria and the Framingham criteria offered similar results [29]. The Framingham criteria offer good performance and are well suited for secular trends as the criteria are unaffected by time and usage of diagnostic test. In earlier Framingham and Olmstead County studies, no survival improvement was reported when heart failure was validated using the Framingham criteria [30].

Once the HF diagnosis is established, further classification is determined by the presence of preserved or reduced ejection fraction (EF). A cutoff of 50% is recommended by the AHA and ACC, and 55% is recommended by the American Society of Echocardiography guidelines [31]. Heart failure with an EF of 50% or greater in the absence of major valve disease is defined as heart failure with preserved systolic function [32]. With this threshold, ejection fraction is preserved in more than half of heart failure cases in the community [33, 34]. Assessment of diastolic function, done with Doppler echocardiography, is a class I indication in the heart failure guidelines [1]. Further, left ventricular function assessment is considered a performance measure for heart failure under the Joint Commission on Accreditation of Healthcare Organizations (JCAHO) [35] as left ventricular dysfunction is associated with an increase in risk of sudden death [36].

Recently, the ACC/AHA guidelines adopted the term "heart failure with preserved ejection fraction" rather than "diastolic heart failure" [1]. It was found that the prevalence of heart failure with preserved ejection fraction in patients discharged between 1987 and 2001 increased. Prevalence increased from 38% to 47% and then to 54% in three consecutive 5-year periods. This was more common in community patients versus referral patients (55% vs. 45%). Prevalence of preserved ejection fraction in patients with a discharge diagnosis of heart failure was 49% in patients 65 years or older and 40% among those under the age of 65 [37]. There raises concern regarding potential misdiagnosis of heart failure in patients with preserved ejection fraction and mild symptoms not requiring hospital admission [37].

Risk Factors

The risk factor profile for cardiovascular disease is changing with increasing prevalence of obesity, metabolic syndrome, and diabetes mellitus [38]. In the Health ABC Study (Table 6.3), nine variables were associated with heart failure and included (1) age, (2) left ventricular hypertrophy (LVH), (3) a history of smoking, (4) coronary heart disease (CHD), (5) systolic blood pressure (SBP), (6) heart rate, (7) serum glucose, (8) albumin, and (9) creatinine. SBP was dichotomized as controlled versus uncontrolled at 140 mmHg, fasting glucose level at 125 mg/dL, resting heart rate at 75 beats/min [39], and albumin level at 3.8 g/dL [40]. Creatinine levels were

Table 6.3 Health ABC Study risk factors

1. Age
Modifiable risk factors
2. CHD
3. LVH
4. Smoking
5. Glucose level (125 mg/dL)
6. SBP (140 mmHg)
Potentially modifiable risk factors
7. Heart rate (75 beats/min)
8. Albumin level (3.8 g/>dL)
9. Renal function (GFR 60 mL/min/1.73 m^2)

ABC aging and body composition, *CHD* coronary heart disease, *LVH* left ventricular hypertrophy, *SBP* systolic blood pressure, *GFR* glomerular filtration rate

converted to glomerular filtration rate (GFR) using MDRD (modification of diet in renal disease) formula [41], and cutoff at 60 mL/min/1.73 m^2 was used to define impaired GFR. Smoking and CHD status were collapsed into binary predictors. Independent risk factors were classified as modifiable (CHD, LVH, smoking, glucose level, and SBP) and potentially modifiable (heart rate, albumin level, and renal function). In this study, most modifiable risk factors were significantly more prevalent among Black participants (when compared with White participants). Blood pressure and coronary heart disease were the leading causes of HF. A substantial proportion is attributed to metabolic and cardiorenal factors, including glucose level, renal abnormalities [42], and low albumin levels. It remains unclear whether a low albumin level signifies cachexia, inflammation or comorbidity burden, or if hypoalbuminemia precipitates symptoms due to fluid extravasation [43]. Increased heart rate has been reported as a risk factor as it may represent a surrogate of vasovagal imbalance or a physiologic response to worsening cardiac function [44].

There seems to be a higher prevalence of LVH in Blacks, which is consistent with the high prevalence of uncontrolled blood pressure in this population. LVH was encountered in 8.6% of participants with systolic blood pressure of less than 140 mmHg. A higher incidence of heart failure among Black participants [5] has also been described. Patients with preserved EF were older, more likely to be female, had a higher BMI, and were more likely to be obese, and hemoglobin levels were lower than those with reduced EF [37]. Heart failure can be conceptualized as a chronic disease epidemic with an increase in prevalence related to the aging of the population and the improvement of survival with heart failure [23].

It is important to characterize recurrent outcomes, like hospitalizations, in chronic diseases; these have the potential of providing new insight on the outcome of heart failure by characterizing patterns of hospitalizations and identifying subjects at risk for recurrent hospitalizations that should be offered aggressive preventive strategies [35].

Conclusion

Heart failure is a public health problem with an ever increasing incidence and prevalence. The most affected population is older than 65 years of age and male. Heart failure is the most frequent cause of hospitalizations in this population, and mortality rate increases after hospitalizations due to heart failure. Risk factors that increase probability of developing heart failure have been identified, such as hypertension and coronary heart disease. Although scientific advances have been made in identifying laboratory parameters (glucose, albumin, and creatinine levels) that aid in the risk stratification of heart failure, validated diagnostic criteria/guidelines that utilize laboratory parameters to complement the clinical picture are needed. And while the economic burden of this disease is enormous, it will only increase as population ages, life expectancy increases, and new therapeutic measures emerge improving a somewhat grim prognosis for patients already with this disease.

References

1. Hunt SA. ACC/AHA 2005 guideline update for the diagnosis and management of chronic heart failure in the adult: a report of the American College of Cardiology/American Heart Association Task Force on Practice Guidelines (Writing Committee to Update the 2001 Guidelines for the Evaluation and Management of Heart Failure). J Am Coll Cardiol. 2005;46: e1–82.
2. Lloyd-Jones D, Adams RJ, Brown TM, et al. Heart disease and stroke statistics–2010 update: a report from the American Heart Association. Circulation. 2010;121:e46–215.
3. Rosamond W, Flegal K, Friday G, et al. Heart disease and stroke statistics–2007 update: a report from the American Heart Association Statistics Committee and Stroke Statistics Subcommittee. Circulation. 2007;115:e69–171.
4. Ammar KA, Jacobsen SJ, Mahoney DW, et al. Prevalence and prognostic significance of heart failure stages: application of the American College of Cardiology/American Heart Association heart failure staging criteria in the community. Circulation. 2007;115:1563–70.
5. Kalogeropoulos A, Georgiopoulou V, Kritchevsky SB, et al. Epidemiology of incident heart failure in a contemporary elderly cohort: the health, aging, and body composition study. Arch Intern Med. 2009;169:708–15.
6. McKee PA, Castelli WP, McNamara PM, et al. The natural history of congestive heart failure: the Framingham study. N Engl J Med. 1971;285:1441–6.
7. Barker WH, Mullooly JP, Getchell W. Changing incidence and survival for heart failure in a well-defined older population, 1970–1974 and 1990–1994. Circulation. 2006;113:799–805.
8. Levy D, Kenchaiah S, Larson MG, et al. Long-term trends in the incidence of and survival with heart failure. N Engl J Med. 2002;347:1397–402.
9. Roger VL, Weston SA, Redfield MM, et al. Trends in heart failure incidence and survival in a community-based population. JAMA. 2004;292:344–50.
10. Schappert SM, Rechtsteiner EA. Ambulatory medical care utilization estimates for 2006. Natl Health Stat Rep. 2006;2008:1–29.
11. Januzzi JL, van Kimmenade R, Lainchbury J, et al. NT-proBNP testing for diagnosis and short-term prognosis in acute destabilized heart failure: an international pooled analysis of 1256 patients: the International Collaborative of NT-proBNP Study. Eur Heart J. 2006;27: 330–7.

12. Haldeman GA, Croft JB, Giles WH, et al. Hospitalization of patients with heart failure: National Hospital Discharge Survey, 1985 to 1995. Am Heart J. 1999;137:352–60.
13. Fang J, Mensah GA, Croft JB, et al. Heart failure-related hospitalization in the U.S., 1979 to 2004. J Am Coll Cardiol. 2008;52:428–34.
14. Dunlay SM, Redfield MM, Weston SA, et al. Hospitalizations after heart failure diagnosis a community perspective. J Am Coll Cardiol. 2009;54:1695–702.
15. Gheorghiade M, Abraham WT, Albert NM, et al. Systolic blood pressure at admission, clinical characteristics, and outcomes in patients hospitalized with acute heart failure. JAMA. 2006;296:2217–26.
16. Hernandez AF, Greiner MA, Fonarow GC, et al. Relationship between early physician follow-up and 30-day readmission among Medicare beneficiaries hospitalized for heart failure. JAMA. 2010;303:1716–22.
17. MacIntyre K, Capewell S, Stewart S, et al. Evidence of improving prognosis in heart failure: trends in case fatality in 66 547 patients hospitalized between 1986 and 1995. Circulation. 2000;102:1126–31.
18. Mosterd A, Cost B, Hoes AW, et al. The prognosis of heart failure in the general population: the Rotterdam study. Eur Heart J. 2001;22:1318–27.
19. Cowie MR, Wood DA, Coats AJ, et al. Survival of patients with a new diagnosis of heart failure: a population based study. Heart. 2000;83:505–10.
20. Curtis LH, Whellan DJ, Hammill BG, et al. Incidence and prevalence of heart failure in elderly persons, 1994–2003. Arch Intern Med. 2008;168:418–24.
21. Croft JB, Giles WH, Pollard RA, et al. Heart failure survival among older adults in the United States: a poor prognosis for an emerging epidemic in the Medicare population. Arch Intern Med. 1999;159:505–10.
22. Kosiborod M, Lichtman JH, Heidenreich PA, et al. National trends in outcomes among elderly patients with heart failure. Am J Med. 2006;119:e611–617.
23. McCullough PA, Philbin EF, Spertus JA, et al. Confirmation of a heart failure epidemic: findings from the Resource Utilization Among Congestive Heart Failure (REACH) study. J Am Coll Cardiol. 2002;39:60–9.
24. Carlson KJ, Lee DC, Goroll AH, et al. An analysis of physicians' reasons for prescribing long-term digitalis therapy in outpatients. J Chronic Dis. 1985;38:733–9.
25. Eriksson H, Caidahl K, Larsson B, et al. Cardiac and pulmonary causes of dyspnoea–validation of a scoring test for clinical-epidemiological use: the Study of Men Born in 1913. Eur Heart J. 1987;8:1007–14.
26. Swedberg K, Cleland J, Dargie H, et al. Guidelines for the diagnosis and treatment of chronic heart failure: executive summary (update 2005): The Task Force for the Diagnosis and Treatment of Chronic Heart Failure of the European Society of Cardiology. Eur Heart J. 2005;26:1115–40.
27. Mosterd A, Deckers JW, Hoes AW, et al. Classification of heart failure in population based research: an assessment of six heart failure scores. Eur J Epidemiol. 1997;13:491–502.
28. Di Bari M, Pozzi C, Cavallini MC. The diagnosis of heart failure in the community. Comparative validation of four sets of criteria in unselected older adults: the ICARe Dicomano Study. J Am Coll Cardiol. 2004;44:1601–8.
29. Schellenbaum GD, Rea TD, Heckbert SR, et al. Survival associated with two sets of diagnostic criteria for congestive heart failure. Am J Epidemiol. 2004;160:628–35.
30. Senni M, Tribouilloy CM, Rodeheffer RJ, et al. Congestive heart failure in the community: trends in incidence and survival in a 10-year period. Arch Intern Med. 1999;159:29–34.
31. Lang RM, Bierig M, Devereux RB, et al. Recommendations for chamber quantification: a report from the American Society of Echocardiography's Guidelines and Standards Committee and the Chamber Quantification Writing Group, developed in conjunction with the European Association of Echocardiography, a branch of the European Society of Cardiology. J Am Soc Echocardiogr. 2005;18:1440–63.
32. Vasan RS, Levy D. Defining diastolic heart failure: a call for standardized diagnostic criteria. Circulation. 2000;101:2118–21.

33. Kitzman DW, Little WC, Brubaker PH, et al. Pathophysiological characterization of isolated diastolic heart failure in comparison to systolic heart failure. JAMA. 2002;288:2144–50.
34. Bursi F, Weston SA, Redfield MM, et al. Systolic and diastolic heart failure in the community. JAMA. 2006;296:2209–16.
35. Roger VL. The heart failure epidemic. Int J Environ Res Public Health. 2010;7:1807–30.
36. Chugh SS, Reinier K, Teodorescu C, et al. Epidemiology of sudden cardiac death: clinical and research implications. Prog Cardiovasc Dis. 2008;51:213–28.
37. Owan TE, Hodge DO, Herges RM, et al. Trends in prevalence and outcome of heart failure with preserved ejection fraction. N Engl J Med. 2006;355:251–9.
38. Mokdad AH, Ford ES, Bowman BA, et al. Prevalence of obesity, diabetes, and obesity-related health risk factors, 2001. JAMA. 2003;289:76–9.
39. Jouven X, Empana JP, Schwartz PJ, et al. Heart-rate profile during exercise as a predictor of sudden death. N Engl J Med. 2005;352:1951–8.
40. Visser M, Kritchevsky SB, Newman AB, et al. Lower serum albumin concentration and change in muscle mass: the Health, Aging and Body Composition Study. Am J Clin Nutr. 2005;82: 531–7.
41. Levey AS, Bosch JP, Lewis JB, et al. A more accurate method to estimate glomerular filtration rate from serum creatinine: a new prediction equation. Modification of Diet in Renal Disease Study Group. Ann Intern Med. 1999;130:461–70.
42. Barzilay JI, Kronmal RA, Gottdiener JS, et al. The association of fasting glucose levels with congestive heart failure in diabetic adults > or =65 years: the Cardiovascular Health Study. J Am Coll Cardiol. 2004;43:2236–41.
43. Arques S, Ambrosi P, Gelisse R, et al. Hypoalbuminemia in elderly patients with acute diastolic heart failure. J Am Coll Cardiol. 2003;42:712–6.
44. Kannel WB, Belanger AJ. Epidemiology of heart failure. Am Heart J. 1991;121:951–7.

Chapter 7
Pathophysiology of Acute Decompensated Heart Failure

Ezra A. Amsterdam, Kathleen L. Tong, and Richard Summers

Introduction

Acute decompensated heart failure (ADHF) is a state of circulatory dysfunction that develops rapidly to fulfill the classic definition of cardiac failure: inability of the heart to provide adequate cardiac output for the needs of the body's tissues. Current refinement of this definition recognizes that the basis of this syndrome is impairment of the integrated function of the heart, peripheral vasculature, and related neurohormonal (NH) systems [1]. ADHF is an increasingly common and potentially lethal cause of acute respiratory insufficiency. It is the primary diagnosis in almost one million hospital admissions in this country and the secondary diagnosis in close to two million [2, 3]. ADHF is usually superimposed on a background of chronic heart failure (HF) but it may occur de novo. The clinical presentation is typically characterized by acute dyspnea resulting from pulmonary congestion due to rapid fluid accumulation in the pulmonary interstitial spaces and alveoli. Transudation of fluid into the alveoli is the basis of pulmonary edema, the extreme form of ADHF, which has been referred to as "flash" pulmonary edema. The pathophysiology of flash pulmonary edema is similar to that of less severe ADHF, but the physiologic derangements are more marked and the therapeutic urgency greater.

E.A. Amsterdam, MD (✉) • K.L. Tong, MD
Division of Cardiovascular Medicine, Department of Internal Medicine, Davis Medical Center,
University of California, 4860 Y Street, Sacramento, CA 95817, USA
e-mail: eaamsterdam@ucdavis.edu

R. Summers, MD
Division of Cardiovascular Medicine, Department of Internal Medicine, University of Mississippi
Medical Center, Jackson, Mississippi

W. Frank Peacock (ed.), *Short Stay Management of Acute Heart Failure*,
Contemporary Cardiology, DOI 10.1007/978-1-61779-627-2_7,
© Springer Science+Business Media, LLC 2012

Hemodynamic Dysfunction

There is normally a modest amount of transudation of protein-poor fluid from the pulmonary microcirculation into the interstitium of the lungs. The balance of this flux is determined by the interplay of the hydrostatic and oncotic forces in the pulmonary microvessels, as described by the Starling relationship [4]. These forces are normally in approximate equilibrium at pressures of ~25 mmHg. Acute pulmonary congestion, the clinical hallmark of ADHF, is due to a complex sequence of pathophysiologic events that increase the rate of fluid transudation into the pulmonary interstitium and alveoli. The immediate cause of congestion is a marked elevation of pulmonary capillary hydrostatic pressure that exceeds the oncotic pressure in these vessels. These events are initiated by a downward spiral of left ventricular (LV) systolic function resulting in reduced stroke volume and increased LV pressure. Whereas dilation of the right ventricle may be associated with acute, pressure or volume, LV dilation is not characteristic of ADHF.

Rapidly progressive LV diastolic dysfunction may also initiate markedly elevated left atrial pressure with resultant ADHF. When this occurs, neurohormonal and renal compensatory mechanisms are evoked to augment fluid retention and maintain systemic perfusion pressure and blood flow [5, 6]. The resulting increase in intravascular volume and pressure further elevates LV diastolic pressure which is transmitted to the left atrium and retrogrades to the pulmonary veins and capillaries, exacerbating the initial pulmonary congestion.

Irrespective of their origin, these physiologic derangements impair gas exchange between the alveoli and pulmonary capillaries, causing hypoxemia, acidosis, and dyspnea. Additionally, the increase in lung water reduces pulmonary compliance, thereby increasing the work of breathing and worsening the clinical state. Hypoxemia and acidosis can further reduce LV contractility and thereby exacerbate circulatory dysfunction. Thus, a vicious cycle of progressive circulatory decompensation can ensue (Fig. 7.1).

The pulmonary lymphatics have an essential role in the removal of excess lung water, and their function is a key determinant of the rate of fluid accumulation in the pulmonary vasculature [7]. Removal of fluid by the lymphatics is slower during acute accumulation than in the basal state. Therefore, pulmonary edema can occur at lower pulmonary pressures that are reached acutely than at higher pressures maintained chronically. This phenomenon is important in the pathogenesis of ADHF and especially of flash pulmonary edema.

Pathophysiology of Neurohormonal Compensatory Mechanisms

Neurohormonal controls play an essential role in the integration of normal circulatory physiology through the activity of the sympathetic nervous system, renin–angiotensin–aldosterone system, arginine vasopressin, and natriuretic peptides [1, 5, 6]. Endothelium-derived vasoactive factors and other mediators also contribute to this

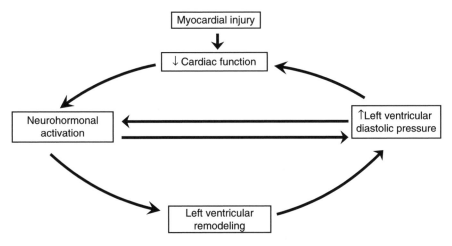

Fig. 7.1 Cardiac dysfunction and neurohormonal activation can promote a cycle of deleterious consequences that contribute to the pathophysiology of heart failure. See text for details

homeostatic organization. Several of these systems augment cardiac contractility, blood volume, sodium retention, and blood pressure, while others provide a counterbalance by promoting opposite cardiocirculatory effects. Under normal physiologic conditions, these mechanisms act in concert to modulate cardiac, renal, and vascular functions to maintain appropriate blood volume, perfusion pressure, cardiac output, and its distribution. However, when impairment of myocardial function results in reduced systemic perfusion, neurohormonal activity is augmented as a compensatory response to maintain cardiac output and blood pressure. Whereas this activation may be helpful for limited periods, the deleterious effects of excessive and persistent neurohormonal activity are central to the pathophysiology of chronic HF [1, 5, 6] (Fig 7.1).

There is less information regarding the role of maladaptive neurohormonal mechanisms in ADHF, but it appears that they are also prominent in this syndrome. In patients with ADHF, evidence of augmented neurohormonal activation and inflammatory mediator function is reflected by increases in circulating norepinephrine, renin and angiotensin II, aldosterone, arginine vasopressin, endothelin 1, and other cytokines [8–14]. In addition, it has recently been reported that ST-2, a member of the interleukin family, is associated with increased cardiac structural abnormalities and is a powerful prognostic indicator in patients with ADHF [15]. Excessive levels of these mediators have extensive pathophysiologic effects, including direct myocardial and vascular toxicity, decreased contractility, arrhythmias, vasoconstriction, increased cardiac afterload, renal sodium and water retention, and pulmonary congestion [6]. In addition, augmented activity of these mediators correlates with prognosis in patients with ADHF [15, 16]. These findings support the role of neurohormonal activation and increased cytokine activity in the pathogenesis of ADHF and have important implications for diagnosis, prognosis, and treatment.

The natriuretic peptides, of which B-type natriuretic peptide (BNP) is the most important, normally provide a counterbalance to the foregoing neurohormonal systems. BNP promotes natriuresis, reduces activity of the sympathetic nervous and rennin–angiotensin–aldosterone systems, inhibits vasopressin and endothelin, decreases systemic vascular resistance, and induces venodilation [17]. Thus far, the endogenous natriuretic peptides appear to have a relatively small role in the amelioration of ADHF. The clinical importance of BNP is in its use as a diagnostic tool and its therapeutic potential when applied in pharmacologic doses. BNP has assumed important diagnostic, therapeutic, and prognostic roles for managing patients with ADHF [18, 19]. In this regard, delayed measurement of BNP in patients with ADHF, which was accompanied by delayed treatment, was associated with increased mortality [20]. Further, it was recently reported that in patients admitted with ADHF, addition of NT-proBNP-guided therapy to multidisciplinary care improved clinical outcomes compared to multidisciplinary care alone, including mortality and rehospitalization [21].

As is clear from the foregoing, activation of the sympathetic nervous system, renin–angiotensin–aldosterone systems, vasopressin, and inflammatory markers in patients with HF has a profound and adverse effect on cardiac and renal function. The combination of this dual organ malfunction, which has been termed the cardiorenal syndrome [22], is associated with diuretic resistance and is common in ADHF. The pathophysiology of the syndrome appears to be related to a complex interplay of neurohormonal and hemodynamic mechanisms. It has important therapeutic and prognostic implications because conventional therapy is limited and clinical outcomes are poor. Whether worsening renal function specifically contributes to the progression of circulatory derangement or is a marker of advanced cardiac and kidney impairment is unclear [23].

Clinical Presentation

The demarcation between ADHF and chronic HF is not always clear. Three types of presentations of ADHF have been described [2] (1) progressive worsening of chronic HF into decompensation, which comprises a majority of admissions, (2) de novo ADHF, comprising ~20% of patients, and (3) acute ADHF superimposed on the stable chronic HF state. The usual sequence of events, as previously described, is acute LV failure causing abrupt increase in LV pressure and pulmonary congestion/edema. These are followed by the compensatory mechanisms that can produce further deterioration, which, if they persist, can progress to chronic HF. The ultimate clinical outcome is determined by the reversibility of ADHF, the underlying chronic pathophysiology, the triggers of ADHF, and the interplay of these variables.

In a typical clinical scenario, a patient with chronic HF will maintain stability unless there is a circulatory disruption that requires physiologic adjustment. Activation of the latter mechanisms to restore stable cardiac output and filling pressures can ultimately overwhelm homeostatic controls and result in the development of ADHF. When a patient arrives in the ED with ADHF, the critical efforts in the therapeutic process are rapid relief of pulmonary edema and improvement in oxygenation. This goal requires prompt relief of hemodynamic dysfunction to reduce left atrial pressure and alleviate pulmonary congestion [15]. Although it is common to observe rapid resolution of the acutely decompensated state by rapid reduction of preload and/or afterload, the hemodynamic adjustments initiated by most conventional acute therapies do not provide long-term circulatory stability [15, 16]. The derangements in the neurohormonal axis and other chronic control mechanisms that led to the decompensated state usually persist after the primary therapeutic interventions. Therefore, it is essential to immediately address these factors in the secondary phase of management.

Precipitating Factors and Clinical Outcome

Numerous clinical factors can provoke ADHF, and one or more precipitating factors or comorbidities have been identified in a majority of patients presenting with ADHF [2, 3, 24, 25]. Among the most frequent are myocardial ischemia, respiratory pathology, arrhythmias, uncontrolled hypertension, and dietary and medication noncompliance. Any of these factors singly or in combination can initiate the pathophysiologic processes resulting in acute circulatory decompensation when superimposed on chronic HF, or this may occur in the absence of the latter if the provocation is severe enough. Although average left ventricular ejection fraction is moderately reduced (35–40%) in patients with ADHF, it is preserved in a large minority of this population. Mortality in patients with ADHF has been reported to be 3–4% in hospitalized patients and 8–10% at 60–90-day follow-up, which is higher than for patients presenting with acute myocardial infarction without HF [2, 26]. Unfavorable clinical outcome in ADHF is associated with advanced age, acute coronary syndrome, renal insufficiency, respiratory processes, and hyponatremia.

Therapeutic Implications of Excessive Neurohormonal Activation

Based on the neurohormonal model of heart failure and the pharmacologic actions of current therapeutic modalities, the limitations and potentially deleterious role of some of these approaches can be appreciated. Thus, although diuretics, vasodilators, and positive inotropic agents may afford symptomatic relief and important therapeutic benefits acutely, their excessive use can exacerbate underlying detrimental neurohormonal overactivity on the myocardium, vasculature, kidney, and fluid and electrolyte balance (Fig. 7.1). Diuretics and vasodilators stimulate further activation of the sympathetic nervous system, renin–angiotensin–aldosterone system, vasopressin, and endothelin, as do direct vasodilators [6]. Additionally, the unfavorable myocardial effects of positive inotropic agents are similar to those of the endogenous catecholamines described previously [25]. These considerations have stimulated concern for judicious and physiologically rational application of these therapeutic approaches based on underlying pathophysiology to mitigate their undesirable effects.

Summary

ADHF is an increasingly common and potentially lethal form of heart failure. It is usually superimposed on a background of chronic HF, but it may occur de novo. Numerous provoking factors have been identified, and most patients with ADHF have important comorbidities. Early repeat hospitalizations are common in this patient population which has a high short-term posthospital mortality. The maladaptive compensatory neurohormonal mechanisms that contribute to chronic HF are also operative in ADHF. Although conventional therapy with diuretics and positive inotropic agents may yield early salutary clinical results, caution must be exercised with these methods because they have the potential to further augment adverse neurohormonal activation. The cardiorenal syndrome is a particularly challenging complication, the precise mechanisms of which have not been clarified. It is anticipated that current investigation of ADHF will afford enhanced approaches to its management.

References

1. Braunwald E, Bristow MR. Congestive heart failure: fifty years of progress. Circulation. 2000;102:14–23.
2. Yancy CW, Lopatin M, Stevenson LW, De Marco T, Fonarow GC. Clinical presentation, management, and in-hospital outcomes of patients admitted with acute decompensated heart failure with preserved systolic function: a report from the Acute Decompensated Heart Failure National Registry (ADHERE) Database. Circulation. 2005;112:3958–68.
3. Gheorghiade M, Zannad F, Sopko G, Klein L, Piña IL, Konstam MA, Massie BM, Roland E, Targum S, Collins SP, Filippatos G, Tavazzi L. Acute heart failure syndromes: current state and framework for future research. Circulation. 2005;112:3958–68.
4. Staub NC, Nagano H, Pearce ML. Pulmonary edema in dogs, especially the sequence of fluid accumulation in lungs. J Appl Physiol. 1967;22:227–40.
5. Francis GS, Benedict C, Johnstone DE, et al. Comparison of neuroendocrine activation in patients with left ventricular dysfunction with and without congestive heart failure. A substudy of the studies of left ventricular dysfunction SOLVD. Circulation. 1990;82:1724–9.
6. Summers R, Amsterdam E. Pathophysiology of acute decompensated heart failure. J Am Coll Cardiol. 2005;46:65–7.
7. Sampson JJ, Leeds SE, Uhley HN, Friedman M. The lymphatic system in pulmonary disease. In: Mayerson HS, editor. Lymph and the lymphatic system. Springfield, IL: Charles C. Thomas; 1968. p. 200.
8. Aukrust P, Ueland T, Lien E, et al. Cytokine network in congestive heart failure secondary to ischemic or idiopathic dilated cardiomyopathy. Am J Cardiol. 1999;83:376–82.

9. Aronson D, Burger AJ. Neurohormonal prediction of mortality following admission for decompensated heart failure. Am J Cardiol. 2003;91:245–8.
10. Aronson D, Burger AJ. Neurohumoral activation and ventricular arrhythmias in patients with decompensated congestive heart failure: role of endothelin. Pacing Clin Electrophysiol. 2003;26:703–10.
11. Milo O, Cotter G, Kaluski E, et al. Comparison of inflammatory and neurohormonal activation in cardiogenic pulmonary edema secondary to ischemic versus nonischemic causes. Am J Cardiol. 2003;92:222–6.
12. Chin BS, Conway DS, Chung NA, Blann AD, Gibbs CR, Lip GY. Interleukin-6, tissue factor and von Willebrand factor in acute decompensated heart failure: relationship to treatment and prognosis. Blood Coagul Fibrinolysis. 2003;14:515–21.
13. Mueller C, Laule-Kilian K, Christ A, et al. Inflammation and long-term mortality in acute congestive heart failure. Am Heart J. 2006;151:845–50.
14. Peschel T, Schonauer M, Thiele H, et al. Invasive assessment of bacterial endotoxin and inflammatory cytokines in patients with acute heart failure. Eur J Heart Fail. 2003;5:609–14.
15. Peacock WF, Allegra J, Ander D, et al. Management of acute decompensated heart failure in the emergency department. Congest Heart Fail. 2003;9 Suppl 1:S3–18.
16. Rame JE, Sheffield MA, Dries DL, et al. Outcomes after emergency department discharge with a primary diagnosis of heart failure. Am Heart J. 2001;142:714–9.
17. Hall C. Essential biochemistry and physiology of (NT-pro)BNP. Eur J Heart Fail. 2004;15(6):257–60.
18. Colucci WS, Elkayam U, Horton DP, et al. Intravenous nesiritide, a natriuretic peptide, in the treatment of decompensated congestive heart failure. N Engl J Med. 2000;343:246–53.
19. Maisel AS, McCord J, Nowak RM, et al. Bedside B-Type natriuretic peptide in the emergency diagnosis of heart failure with reduced or preserved ejection fraction: Results from the Breathing Not Properly Multinational Study. J Am Coll Cardiol. 2003;41:2010–7.
20. Maisel AS, Peacock WF, McMullin N, Jessie R, Fonarow GC, Wynne J, Mills RM. Timing of immunoreactive B-type natriuretic peptide levels and treatment delay in acute decompensated heart failure: an ADHERE (Acute decompensated heart failure national registry analysis). J Am Coll Cardiol. 2008;52:534–40.
21. Lainchbury JG, Troughton RW, Strangman KM, Frampton CM, Pilbrow A, Yandle TG, Hamid AK, Nicholls MG, Richards AM. N-terminal pro-B-type natriuretic peptide-guided treatment for chronic heart failure: results from the BATTLESCARRED (NT-proBNP-Assisted Treatment To Lessen Serial Cardiac Readmissions and Death) trial. J Am Coll Cardiol. 2009;55:53–60.
22. Bongartz LG, Cramer MJ, Doevendans PA, et al. The severe cardiorenal syndrome: Guyton revisited. Eur Heart J. 2005;26:11–7.
23. Liang K, Williams A, Greene E. Acute decompensated heart failure and the cardiorenal syndrome. Crit Care Med. 2008;36 Suppl 1:S75–88.
24. Fonarow GC, Abraham WT, Albert NM, Stough WG, Gheorghiade M, Greenberg BH, O'Connor CM, Pieper K, Sun JL, Yancy CW, Young JB. Factors identified as precipitating hospital admissions for heart failure and clinical outcomes: findings from OPTIMIZE-HF. Arch Intern Med. 2008;168:847–54.
25. Flaherty JD, Bax JJ, De Luca L, Rossi JS, Davidson CJ, Filippatos G, Liu PP, Konstam MA, Greenberg B, Mehra MR, Breithardt G, Pang PS, Young JB, Fonarow GC, Bonow RO, Gheorghiade M. Acute heart failure syndromes in patients with coronary artery disease early assessment and treatment. J Am Coll Cardiol. 2009;53:254–63.
26. Abraham WT, Adams KF, Fonarow GC, Costanzo MR, Berkowitz RL, LeJemtel TH, Cheng ML, Wynne J. In-hospital mortality in patients with acute decompensated heart failure requiring intravenous vasoactive medications: an analysis from the Acute Decompensated Heart Failure National Registry (ADHERE). J Am Coll Cardiol. 2005;46:57–64.

Part III
Emergency Medical Services and Emergency Department Assessment and Treatment

Chapter 8
The Out-of-Hospital Management of Acute Heart Failure

Marvin A. Wayne, Vincent N. Mosesso Jr., and A. Keith Wesley

Introduction

Emergency medical services (EMS) personnel frequently encounter patients with acute heart failure (AHF). Nearly one million hospitalizations annually are for AHF [1], and many of these patients are first cared for by EMS in the prehospital setting. AHF is one of only two cardiovascular diseases with an increasing prevalence; the other is atrial fibrillation. Five million Americans have the disease, and more than 500,000 are newly diagnosed each year. AHF is a major disease of our aging population [2] because most hospitalizations for AHF are of patients older than 65 years [3]. AHF is not only very prevalent, but also very deadly. The mortality rate for AHF has been reported to range from 8% to 25% [4]. Favorable outcome for AHF is dependent on rapid assessment and treatment initiated in the out-of-hospital setting [5–10].

Acute heart failure is defined as the abrupt onset or the rapidly progressive development of significant symptoms related to inadequate myocardial pumping function. Most commonly AHF presents as respiratory distress due to pulmonary congestion but can also present as poor systemic perfusion with or without pulmonary

M.A. Wayne, MD (✉)
University of Washington, Seattle, WA, USA

EMS Medical Program Director, Whatcom County, WA, USA

Emergency Department, Peacehealth St. Joseph Medical Center, Bellingham, WA, USA
e-mail: mwayne@cob.org

V.N. Mosesso Jr., MD
Emergency Medicine, University of Pittsburgh School of Medicine, Pittsburgh, PA, USA

Prehospital Care, University of Pittsburgh Medical Center, Pittsburgh, PA, USA

A.K. Wesley, MD
Medical Director, HealthEast Medical Transportation, St. Paul, MN, USA

W. Frank Peacock (ed.), *Short Stay Management of Acute Heart Failure*,
Contemporary Cardiology, DOI 10.1007/978-1-61779-627-2_8,
© Springer Science+Business Media, LLC 2012

congestion. Some cardiology organizations have classified the variety of AHF presentations into these syndromes: acute decompensated heart failure (new or acute on chronic), hypertensive AHF, acute pulmonary edema, cardiogenic shock, high-output failure, and right heart failure [11].

However, these are not distinct categories clinically, and during initial assessment and management, it is often difficult to clearly distinguish. Therefore, we prefer classifying AHF patients more in the manner of Mebazaa and colleagues [12], who suggested the following clinical scenarios:

1. Dyspnea with high SBP >140 mmHg
2. Dyspnea with normal SBP 100–140 mmHg
3. Dyspnea with low SBP <100 mmHg
4. Dyspnea with sign of acute coronary syndrome
5. Isolated right ventricular failure

Pathogenesis of Acute Heart Failure

Understanding the pathophysiology of AHF is helpful for appreciating the clinical presentation and for classifying patients into the above categories. This will lead to more specific and patient-tailored therapy.

AHF has a number of underlying etiologies as listed in Table 8.1. Nearly half of these cases are due to acute coronary syndrome, and another quarter are related to acute worsening of myocardial function (either systolic or diastolic). Please refer to Chap. 7 for full discussion of the pathophysiology of AHF.

It is important to appreciate that the pulmonary congestion is a reflection of increased volume and pressures in the left ventricle and left atrium and that often these patients are not volume overloaded. Rather the insufficient pumping of the heart leads to a redistribution of body water [13]. Over time and left untreated, most

Table 8.1 Precipitating causes of acute cardiogenic pulmonary Edema (APE)

Cause	Incidence (%)
Worsening heart failure	26
Coronary insufficiency	21
Subendocardial infarction	16
Transmural infarction	10
Acute dysrhythmia	9
Medication noncompliance	7
Dietary indiscretion	3
Valvular insufficiency	3
Other	5

From Marx J, Hockberger R, Walls R. Rosen's emergency medicine: concepts and clinical practice, 5th ed. Saint Louis: Mosby, 2002, with permission

patients will also develop excess total body water, but this is not typically the case with acute exacerbations, particularly new onset heart failure (e.g., due to large myocardial infarction or acute value dysfunction) or exacerbations of heart failure under effective long-term therapy.

Field Assessment

Assessment begins with a rapid, focused history and physical examination of the patient. This includes acute symptoms, recent illness, past history and prescribed medications, medication compliance, and diet. Together, this constitutes an important first step in the field diagnosis of AHF (Table 8.2). Critical elements of the physical examination include accurate determination of vital signs. Prehospital providers, even in the absence of peripheral edema, should strongly consider cardiogenic pulmonary edema in patients presenting with acute respiratory distress, hypoxemia, tachypnea, rales or wheezing, and marked hypertension. Such patients often have histories of poorly controlled hypertension and/or prior cardiac disease. Blood pressure of greater than 180/120 mmHg is common in this setting and is a good sign of reversibility. In these patients, a rapid reduction in blood pressure often produces prompt relief of respiratory distress. Marked hypertension associated with acute respiratory distress and wheezing, particularly in elderly patients without a history of asthma or pulmonary infection, is strongly suggestive of AHF. Such a presumptive diagnosis may be supported by the presence of cardiovascular medications

Table 8.2 Diagnosis of congestive heart failure

Prior history and comorbid states
- Chronic heart failure
- Hypertension
- Ischemic heart disease
- Valvular heart disease
- Anemia
- Dysrhythmias
- Thyroid disease

Current situation
- Medications (prescribed regimen and current compliance, other drug use)
- Symptoms of acute coronary syndromes
- Diet or exercise indiscretions in patients with known heart failure
- Signs of pulmonary edema such as tachypnea, low oxygen saturation, rales, and peripheral edema
- Lack of signs of chronic obstructive pulmonary disease, asthma, or airway obstruction
- Lack of signs of pneumonia or sepsis, such as fever and purulent sputum

Tools
- Pulse oximetry
- End-tidal carbon dioxide waveform morphology and trending
- 12-lead ECG and continuous rhythm monitoring

and the absence of respiratory medications, such as metered-dose inhalers. Even when these facts are present, out-of-hospital personnel should always consider alternate etiologies such as pulmonary embolism, pneumonia, COPD and asthma, and drug overdose before diagnosing patients as having APE. Cardiac rhythm monitoring and 12-lead electrocardiograms (ECGs) are essential in patients suspected of AHF, particularly for identifying arrhythmia and/or acute coronary syndrome that may be the inciting event, and should be placed on the patient shortly after arrival on the scene.

Electrocardiogram

Standard 12-lead ECG should be obtained on all patients to ascertain the presence of acute and/or chronic cardiac changes that may be creating or contributing to the current episode.

In addition to the ECG, a number of other diagnostic aids have been developed to improve accuracy in the evaluation and diagnosis of AHF. Although not currently used in the prehospital environment, a rapid bedside assay of blood levels of B-type natriuretic peptide (BNP) is now available. BNP is a neurohormone secreted mainly by the cardiac ventricles in response to volume expansion and pressure over-load which rises in the setting of acute heart failure [14–19]. Application of such testing in the out-of-hospital environment may be a logical extension and further aid in diagnosis. Noninvasive cardiac output (NICO) devices, such as impedance cardiography [20, 21], have also been suggested as diagnostic tools, but their complexities and cost have to date precluded their out-of-hospital use.

APE is often difficult to distinguish clinically from an exacerbation of chronic obstructive pulmonary disease (COPD) or other acute pulmonary disorders. The misdiagnosis of AHF in the out-of-hospital setting has been documented to be 23% in one study [22] and 32% in another [23]. The need for the correct identification of precipitating events, and the rapid initiation of appropriate treatment, is critical to achieve a positive outcome. Inappropriate therapy, as a result of misdiagnosis, may result in harm to the patient. Hoffman and Reynolds reported that adverse effects were more common in misdiagnosed patients. Untoward effects included (a) respiratory depression in patients receiving morphine, (b) hypotension and bradycardia in patients receiving both morphine and nitroglycerin, and (c) hypotension and arrhythmias associated with hypokalemia in patients receiving furosemide.

Emergency Medical Services Scope of Practice

Before one can make recommendations on the out-of-hospital care of AHF, it is vital to understand the scope of practice of the EMS health-care provider. While some countries, primarily European, staff their EMS with physicians and nurses, the majority of countries use individuals with limited and specific training in out-of-hospital care of the acutely ill and injured.

Although there is some degree of variability in differentiation, most of the western hemisphere and Australia utilize a tiered level of providers who at entry have the training and equipment to provide basic life support care for cardiac arrest and provide first aid care to victims of trauma and those complaining of chest pain and respiratory distress. The highest qualification of training includes the ability to administer drug therapy and utilize advanced airway techniques. For purposes of illustration, the US EMS scope of practice will be presented.

The United States recently adopted the National Scope of Practice for EMS providers, a document created by the National Highway and Traffic Safety Administration in 2007. This describes four levels of prehospital providers. The first level, the emergency medical responder (EMR), was previously titled the first responder. This provider is trained in CPR and the use of the automatic external defibrillator (AED), as well as basic first aid, including oxygen administration and care of simple trauma. They are not associated with transportation of the patient by ambulance.

The following are the minimum psychomotor skills of the EMR:

- Airway and breathing

  - Insertion of airway adjuncts intended to go into the oropharynx
  - Use of positive pressure ventilation devices such as the bag valve mask (BVM)
  - Suction of the upper airway
  - Supplemental oxygen therapy

- Pharmacological interventions

  - Use of unit-dose auto-injectors for the administration of life-saving medications intended for self or peer rescue in hazardous materials situations (e.g., MARK I, etc.)

- Medical/cardiac care

  - Use of an automated external defibrillator

The next level is the emergency medical technician (EMT). This provider has the capabilities of the EMR, in addition to noninvasive monitoring and assisting the patient with the administration of their own medications. This level of provider is given minimal education in pathophysiology, and their treatments are primarily driven by patient complaint and symptoms. As for airway management, most states currently allow this level to place nonvisualized airways such as the King LT or Combitube. This level of provider is the minimum allowed to transport the patient in an ambulance.

The following are the minimum psychomotor skills of the EMT:

- Airway and breathing

  - Insertion of airway adjuncts intended to go into the oropharynx or nasopharynx
  - Use of positive pressure ventilation devices such as manually triggered ventilators and automatic transport ventilators

- Pharmacological interventions

    - Assist patients in taking their own prescribed medications, such as inhaled bronchodilators
    - Administration of the following medications with appropriate medical oversight:

        - Oral glucose for suspected hypoglycemia
        - Aspirin for chest pain of suspected ischemic origin

The next level, the advanced EMT (AEMT), is able to establish an intravenous line and administer a limited list of medications. Many states currently allow the EMT to administer many of the medications listed only for the advanced EMT.

The following are the minimum psychomotor skills of the AEMT:

- Airway and breathing

    - Insertion of airways that are NOT intended to be placed into the trachea
    - Tracheobronchial suctioning of an already intubated patient

- Assessment
- Pharmacological interventions

    - Establish and maintain peripheral intravenous access
    - Establish and maintain intraosseous access in a pediatric patient
    - Administer (nonmedicated) intravenous fluid therapy
    - Administer sublingual nitroglycerin to a patient experiencing chest pain of suspected ischemic origin
    - Administer subcutaneous or intramuscular epinephrine to a patient in anaphylaxis
    - Administer glucagon to a hypoglycemic patient
    - Administer intravenous dextrose to a hypoglycemic patient
    - Administer inhaled beta-agonists to a patient experiencing difficulty breathing and wheezing
    - Administer an opioid antagonist to a patient suspected of opioid overdose
    - Administer nitrous oxide for pain relief

The highest defined prehospital provider level is the paramedic. This level is permitted to administer the widest range of medications and procedures which are usually limited only by medical director authorization and in some instances state rule.

The following are the minimum psychomotor skills of the paramedic:

- Airway and breathing

    - Perform endotracheal intubation (ETI)
    - Perform percutaneous cricothyrotomy
    - Decompress the pleural space
    - Perform gastric decompression

- Pharmacological interventions
  - Insert an intraosseous cannula
  - Enteral and parenteral administration of approved prescription medications
  - Access indwelling catheters and implanted central IV ports for fluid and medication administration
  - Administer medications by IV infusion
  - Maintain an infusion of blood or blood products

- Medical/cardiac care
  - Perform cardioversion, manual defibrillation, and transcutaneous pacing

The Emergency Medical Services Challenge

Due to the significant variability in scope of practice by the four EMS levels of training, the ability to provide care for the patient with AHF is limited by each state's implementation of this scope of practice model and the willingness of an EMS medical director to authorize various treatment modalities.

At first blush, the National Scope of Practice model would appear to limit the administration of nitroglycerin for AHF only to paramedics. This would limit care for many persons living in areas with only basic life support EMS response, which is often the case outside urban areas. However, since the EMT may assist the patient with administration of their own medications, and it is reasonable to assume that a large number of AHF patients would have NTG prescribed by their physician, EMS personnel will be able to help assure properly aggressive treatment with NTG.

CPAP involves the administration of oxygen via a positive pressure device for spontaneously breathing patients. The EMT is allowed to assist a patient's ventilations with a BVM and to provide positive pressure ventilation to the cardiac arrest victim. The application of CPAP has proven clinical benefit, is arguably easier than ventilating with a BVM, and has a similar or lower risk of adverse effects, so many areas do allow EMTS to utilize this modality.

For the medical director of a paramedic service, the greatest challenge has been to adopt treatment protocols based on the current understanding of the pathophysiology of AHF. Traditionally, the use of diuretics by EMS has been commonplace, and the role of nitroglycerin has not been well accepted. Many service protocols include the administration of morphine for AHF despite no data to support its use. Further, some services that include NTG in their protocols are extremely conservative, allowing paramedics to administer NTG in a manner more appropriate for angina than the high adrenergic state of AHF. Some also rely too heavily on the transdermal route of NTG despite the poor pharmacodynamic properties of this route.

Table 8.3 Management of acute congestive heart failure: Overview

- Identify CHF
- Identify and treat specific etiology when possible
- Provide oxygen and ventilatory support when needed
- Reduce LV preload
- Reduce LV afterload
- Provide inotropic support when needed
- Select receiving facility based on needed resources

Prehospital Management of Acute Pulmonary Edema

The prehospital management of AHF must be tempered by the inherent limitations of assessment modalities, diagnostic testing, and personnel expertise in this setting. The focus should be on therapies that will most likely lead to immediate benefit with low risk of harm should the working diagnosis of AHF be incorrect. Even in the emergency department, the primary condition causing the patient's dyspnea and other symptoms may not be clear. Primary objectives for the treatment of AHF are to reduce pulmonary capillary hydrostatic pressure, to redistribute pulmonary fluid, and to improve forward blood flow. These goals may be achieved by reducing LV preload and afterload, providing ventilatory and inotropic supports, and identifying and treating the underlying etiology of the syndrome (Table 8.3).

Notwithstanding the inherent limitations of blood pressure as a reflection of perfusion, from a practical standpoint, it is perhaps the best initial gauge for directing therapy of AHF. Table 8.4 presents an approach to therapy based on blood pressure. As blood pressure changes, then therapies should change accordingly. While clinical judgment and consideration of patient specific factors must impact treatment decisions, this table should provide a useful conceptual guide to serve as a starting point.

General therapy in addition to above specific measures:

1. IV access
2. 12-lead ECG and monitor cardiac rhythm (rate and rhythm management as indicated)
3. ASA (chewed) and transport to PCI-capable facility, if concern for ACS
4. Bronchodilator (nebulized) if wheezing
5. Waveform capnography if available to monitor ETCO2; waveform may help in diagnosis

Reduction of Left Ventricular Preload

The initial effort to reduce the pulmonary congestion in patients presenting with APE should be to reduce the pressure and volume of blood flow to the pulmonary vasculature. This may be accomplished by dilating the venous capacitance system.

Table 8.4 Hemodynamic approach to AHF treatment

	Hemodynamic management	Oxygenation and ventilation	Volume management
Systolic blood pressure	Goal is normalizing systemic perfusion and cardiac preload/afterload	Goals are O2 sat 94–99%, adequate air exchange and relief of dyspnea	Goal is appropriate amount of intravascular and total body water
>150	Aggressive use of vasodilators (high-dose nitrates, consider ACE inhibitors)	High-flow oxygen, strongly consider CPAP	Diuresis if evidence of peripheral edema
90–150	Careful use of vasodilators (low-dose nitrates)	Oxygen as needed to maintain sat, consider CPAP if significant respiratory distress	Diuresis if evidence of peripheral edema
70–89	Inotropic agents (dobutamine)	Oxygen to maintain sat, CPAP with extreme caution (hypotension, AMS)	Avoid diuresis and consider need for careful IV fluid administration
< 70	Dual inotropes/vasopressors (dopamine, norepineph-rine), mechanical assist (aortic balloon pump)	Oxygen to maintain sat, consider intubation and mechanical ventilation	Avoid diuresis Administer IV fluids unless clear pulmonary congestion, especially if using PPV

CPAP continuous positive airway pressure, *AMS* altered mental status, *IV* intravenous, *PPV* positive pressure ventilation

This will result in decreased blood return to the right ventricle (preload), hence reducing blood flow to the pulmonary vascular bed. The net result is a reduction in LV preload, which then allows the LV output to more closely match inflow from the pulmonary system. Pharmacologic therapy to reduce LV preload includes the use of nitrates primarily. Loop diuretics such as furosemide should only be used in the prehospital setting when there is clear evidence of total volume overload, such as worsening peripheral edema or known acute weight gain. If antianxiety medication is needed, small doses of benzodiazepines, such as midazolam or lorazepam, are preferred over morphine and other opioids due to the higher adverse effect profile of the latter.

Nitrates

Nitroglycerin and related drugs at low dosages are primarily venodilators but also cause arterial vasodilation at higher doses. Intracellularly, they react with and convert sulfhydryl groups to S-nitrosothiols and nitric oxide. These reactive groups then activate the enzyme guanylate cyclase which catalyzes the formation of cyclic guanosine monophosphate (cGMP). This nucleotide induces the reentry of calcium back into the sarcoplasmic reticulum of vascular smooth muscle thereby causing its relaxation.

Nitroglycerin is currently the vasodilator agent of choice for the reduction of LV preload in the field setting. It is fast acting, efficient, and easy to administer [24]. Nitroglycerin's effectiveness in reducing mortality in patients with APE in the prehospital setting has been demonstrated by Bertini [25]. In this study, even hypotensive patients (systolic blood pressure <100 mmHg) were found to respond positively to nitroglycerin. Likewise, Hoffman and Reynolds compared a number of prehospital management protocols for APE and concluded that nitroglycerin was beneficial, whereas morphine and furosemide had no additive effect when combined with nitroglycerin and were occasionally deleterious. The beneficial vasodilation effect of nitroglycerin must be closely monitored to avoid excessive reduction in blood pressure, which may occur from both the decrease in venous return and arterial vasodilation. Thus, a potential disadvantage of nitroglycerin is that it can lead to excessive hypotension, particularly in patients without adequate preload (e.g., hypovolemia and inferior wall myocardial infarction (MI) with significant right ventricular (RV) involvement). Note that nitrates should be avoided in patients who recently took a phosphodiesterase inhibitor [these are drugs used for pulmonary hypertension and erectile dysfunction, such as Viagra (sildenafil), Levitra (vardenafil), and Cialis (tadalafil)].

Morphine

Although morphine has been used for decades to treat acute MI, unstable angina, and AHF, few clinical trials have demonstrated its effectiveness for these conditions. Its popularity in treating pulmonary edema arose because of its vasodilatory and antianxiety effects. However, morphine's vasodilatory effects are transient and are the result of histamine release. Recently, concerns have been raised over the use of morphine in treating AHF in the ED. A retrospective study of the ED management of APE and intensive care unit (ICU) admissions showed that morphine administered in the ED was associated with significant increases in ICU admissions and the need for ETIs when compared with treatment with sublingual captopril [26].

A prospective study of morphine use in prehospital APE treatment showed that the drug was minimally effective as single therapy or in combination with nitrates [22]. Furthermore, the effects of morphine in depressing respiration and the central nervous system may be particularly deleterious in misdiagnosed patients. The authors strongly recommended against using morphine for routine treatment of acute heart failure.

Furosemide

Furosemide has been a mainstay of treatment for APE since the 1960s although its effectiveness has been examined in only a few studies. Its primary mechanism of action involves the inhibition of sodium reabsorption in the ascending limb of

Henle's loop in the renal medulla. This results in an increased excretion of salt and water in urine. The net effect of this action is a lowering of plasma volume, a decrease in LV preload, and a decrease in pulmonary congestion. These effects are beneficial in patients presenting with cardiovascular volume overload. In addition to its diuretic effects, furosemide also induces neurohumoral changes. These include both vasodilatation (by promoting renal prostaglandin E2 and atrial natriuretic peptide secretion) and vasoconstricting effects. The latter, via the feedback loop, can result in peripheral elevation of mean arterial pressure, LV pressure, heart rate, and systemic vascular resistance through enhancement of the renin–angiotensin system (RAS). Stroke volume index and pulmonary capillary wedge pressure initially decrease but subsequently increase after the RAS enhancement (usually within 15 min). The latter effects are not beneficial in the treatment of AHF particularly in the absence of volume overload [27]. Furthermore, misdiagnosis of AHF and subsequent inducement of inappropriate diuresis can lead to increased morbidity and mortality in patients with other conditions such as pneumonia, sepsis, or COPD. Thus, while furosemide is still an important and beneficial component of medical therapy for chronic heart failure, it should be used very judiciously for the initial treatment of AHF. Because of the limited patient information and evaluation capabilities in the prehospital environment, furosemide should be reserved for selected cases when it will be clearly safe to administer [28].

Combined Drug Therapies with Nitroglycerin, Furosemide, and Morphine

Nitrates are frequently combined with loop diuretics in treating pulmonary edema. A complex, randomized, prospective clinical study from Israel investigated the efficacy and safety of these drugs in treating patients presenting with severe pulmonary edema in the prehospital setting [29]. This study concluded that intravenous (IV) nitrates administered as repeated high-dose boluses (3 mg every 5 min) after a low dose (40 mg) of furosemide were associated with lower ETI and MI rates than the administration of low-dose nitrates (1 mg/h, increased by 1 mg/h every 10 min) and high-dose furosemide (80 mg every 15 min). A prospective observational study on the use of sublingual nitroglycerin in the prehospital setting in 300 patients with presumed MI or CHF analyzed treatment-related adverse events. Only four patients experienced adverse events, most of which were bradycardic-hypotensive reactions, and all recovered subsequently [30].

A retrospective case review evaluated outcomes of 57 patients presumed to have prehospital APE who were treated in the field with combinations of nitroglycerin, furosemide, and/or morphine [11]. Although only a small study, any combination treatment including nitroglycerin was associated with both subjective and objective (respiratory and heart rates, blood pressure, respiratory distress, mental status) improvement. Combination treatment with furosemide and morphine without nitroglycerin, on the other hand, resulted in a substantial number of patients not responding to treatment and some actually deteriorating. Ultimately, 23 of 57 (47%) patients in this study were found not to have pulmonary edema. A larger retrospective case series evaluated outcomes in 493 patients receiving prehospital nitroglycerin, furosemide, and/or morphine versus no treatment for CHF. Mortality was significantly reduced in those receiving any prehospital drug treatment but especially in the subset of critical patients (5% vs. 33%, $p < 0.01$) [31].

Reduction of Left Ventricular Afterload

A variety of pharmacologic agents, including nitroglycerin at higher doses, angiotensin-converting enzyme (ACE) inhibitors, nitroprusside, dobutamine, and dopamine, may be useful in the reduction of LV afterload.

Nitrates at Higher Doses

High-dose nitrates can reduce both preload and afterload.

CHF patients present with very elevated arterial and venous pressures; frequent doses of nitrates may be required to control blood pressure and afterload. Some patients develop tolerance to nitroglycerin, but this is not of concern in the prehospital environment. Another concern with high dose nitrates is that certain patients are very sensitive to even normal doses and may experience marked hypotension. These are typically patients with tenuous preload status (e.g., preexisting hypovolemia or significant RV infarction in the setting of inferior wall MI). It is therefore critical to monitor blood pressure during high-dose nitrate therapy.

Angiotensin Converting Enzyme Inhibitors

ACE inhibitors play a primary role in chronic CHF therapy and have therapeutic advantages for treating APE. These include reducing both preload and afterload, increasing splanchnic flow, decreasing LV diastolic dysfunction, reducing sodium retention, and reducing sympathetic stimulation. Captopril (Capoten) is an ACE inhibitor that has been studied in the prehospital setting [11]. When a standard tablet is administered sublingually, it rapidly dissolves and has an onset of action of less than 10 min. Clinical effects are seen within 15 min, with peak effects within 30 min [31, 32]. A retrospective study of 181 patients with APE treated in the ED examined the relationship between pharmacologic treatments and rates of ICU admissions [24]. Patients in this study were treated with captopril (26%), nitroglycerin (81%), morphine (49%), and/or loop diuretics (73%). Patients receiving captopril had decreased rates of ICU admissions and ETIs, as well as shorter ICU stays.

A prospective, placebo-controlled, randomized study evaluated the addition of sublingual captopril to the standard treatment regimen (oxygen, nitrates, morphine, and furosemide) in patients brought to the ED with APE [32]. Using a clinical APE distress score for assessment, the addition of captopril was found to significantly reduce distress scores over the first 40 min compared with placebo. This study indicated that certain features of ACE inhibitors make them attractive for field use, including ease of sublingual administration, fast onset of action, and low cost. However, captopril use may be associated with potential concerns, which include occasional hypotension and a variable duration of effect in comparison to nitrates [33].

In addition to the sublingual route, ACE inhibitors may also be administered intravenously. Enalapril maleate (Vasotec IV) is the only IV ACE inhibitor currently available in the United States. Enalapril also has a somewhat variable effect on blood pressure and a much longer duration of action than NTG, so caution is appropriate. Generally, it is reasonable to consider in patients with extremely high blood pressure and those not responding to or with contraindication to nitrates and CPAP alone. Lower dosing, such as 1.25 mg, should be considered in the prehospital setting especially for elderly patients. Enalapril may be useful in patients on CPAP since it is difficult to administer NTG sublingually in these patients; NitroPaste has suboptimal absorption, and most ground EMS agencies do not use IV NTG.

Nitroprusside

APE patients presenting with severe hypertension and those refractory to nitrate and ACE inhibitor treatments may be candidates for treatment with nitroprusside sodium. However, the need to continuously monitor blood pressure, with a carefully titrated continuous infusion, and the requirement of glass containers shielded from light typically preclude its utility in the field environment. When used out of hospital, it is usually by air medical services or critical care transport teams performing interfacility transfers.

Ventilatory Support

Patients with acute CHF may be treated with a spectrum of ventilatory support modalities based on the patient's clinical condition and comorbid factors. Initial treatment includes oxygen therapy to maintain oxygen saturation of at least 93–94%. Current guidelines recommend oxygen administration only as needed and to the extent needed to maintain this level of saturation. Inhaled bronchodilators should be administered when bronchospasm is evident. True bronchospasm may be triggered by interstitial edema, especially in patients with underlying reactive airway disease. Initial concerns that the beta-agonist effect of bronchodilators such as albuterol could result in injury to the myocardium were dispelled by a study that found no rise in cardiac necrosis markers in AHF patients receiving broncho-dilators [34].

In cases of severe respiratory distress or impending respiratory failure (ineffective respiratory effort, hypoxemia, hypercarbia), assisted ventilation is needed. Traditionally, this has been accomplished in tandem with ETI. However, ETI is a challenge to accomplish effectively in noncomatose, nonparalyzed patients with the limited resources and personnel usually available in the field setting. Further, ETI is associated with various infectious (e.g., nosocomial pneumonia, sinusitis) and noninfectious complications (e.g., barotrauma; oral, nasal, or laryngeal trauma; respiratory muscle weakness; prolonged weaning). To avoid these complications and lengthy ICU stays, noninvasive ventilatory support is being increasingly used. ETI remains necessary when altered mental status requires airway protection or when other patient characteristics prevent the successful application of noninvasive positive pressure ventilation.

Noninvasive Positive Pressure Ventilation

Noninvasive positive pressure ventilation (NIPPV) is now considered an effective adjunctive treatment of AHF/APE [35–37]. NIPPV improves ventilation and oxygenation in the patient with APE by several mechanisms. Its ability to increase intra-alveolar air pressure shifts the flow of fluid back into the pulmonary capillaries and thereby reduces pulmonary congestion and opens more alveolar for effective gas exchange. NIPPV decreases the mechanical work of breathing and thereby decreases myocardial demand. Two different methods of providing NIPPV are used: continuous positive airway pressure (CPAP), which provides a constant level of positive pressure applied throughout inspiration and exhalation, and bi-level positive airway pressure (BiPAP), which allows provision of higher pressure during inspiration than expiration.

The concept of prehospital CPAP administration was examined by Kosowsky and found safe and practical [23]. In this study, trained paramedics applied CPAP in 19 patients with cardiogenic pulmonary edema and showed that none required field intubation and that hemoglobin oxygen saturation increased from a mean of 83.3% to 95.4% after CPAP administration via a face mask. Two patients intolerant of CPAP required ETI on ED arrival, and an additional five patients required ETI within 24 h. There were no adverse events related to CPAP therapy. Since then, there have been several prehospital studies to examine the value of prehospital CPAP.

Hubble and Richards [4] examined the impact of CPAP by EMS when they implemented it in one of two adjoining counties. Care in both county systems was the same except for the addition of CPAP by one. In the county without CPAP, 25% of the AHF patients required intubation, while in those receiving CPAP, only 9% required intubation. Those without CPAP were also more likely to die (odds ratio 7.4).

Another prehospital study [38] found a 30% reduction in the need for intubation and a 21% absolute reduction in mortality following application of CPAP by paramedics.

BiPAP has been investigated as an alternative to CPAP in a number of conditions but has shown a significant advantage over CPAP only in patients whose respiratory failure is due to COPD exacerbation [39]. A number of individual studies reported some success with BiPAP, and some problems, including increased rates of MI [40], associated with its use in treating acute CHF.

In an out-of-hospital study of patients with presumed CHF, EMS personnel considered the use of BiPAP to be safe and judged this method to improve dyspnea and respiratory distress in their patients [40]. Although oxygen saturation was significantly greater for the BiPAP plus conventional treatment group, compared with the conventional treatment group, treatment times, length of hospital stay, intubation rate, and death rates were not significantly different between the groups. Of the two types of noninvasive ventilatory support, there is good supporting evidence for the effectiveness of CPAP. The technology is reasonable for field implementation, but there is room for further refinement, especially regarding the volume of oxygen required. Greater experience of field providers should also lead to better outcomes because this therapy is not only patient dependent but operator dependent as well. In the case of BiPAP, the risk–benefit ratio is conflicting in the literature. In addition, the existing technology for BiPAP is suboptimal for out-of-hospital use. However, this too may show greater field use in the future.

This review focuses on the importance of understanding that the pathogenesis of AHF is usually related to intravascular fluid redistribution rather than to primary volume overload. Management of suspected AHF begins with correct assessment and management of underlying causes of elevated ventricular filling pressures and continues by improving oxygenation with the application of ventilatory support, reduction of LV preload and afterload with nitroglycerin, and inotropic support in the setting of symptomatic hypotension.

The EMS scope of practice places both limitations as well as unique opportunities for the implementation of appropriate prehospital treatment of AHF. The EMS medical director must understand the national, state, and local scope of EMS practice to determine the best method to implement the following therapies.

Finally, EMS personnel should choose an appropriate receiving facility for the patient with moderate or severe AHF. In particular, this decision should be guided by concern for ACS, particularly STEMI, and by the potential needed for advanced invasive therapies such as aortic balloon pump. Transport time and distance considerations and the level of providers are also important considerations.

Conclusion

AHF is a common and often life-threatening condition encountered by prehospital emergency medical personnel. Patients with this condition must receive rapid, accurate assessment and aggressive treatment. For patients with elevated blood pressure, high-dose nitrates represent the out-of-hospital treatment of choice, whereas diuretics and morphine should be reserved for select patient groups. More data are needed on the efficacy and safety of ACE inhibitors to justify their use in the field. CPAP has been shown to be effective, and the growing clinical experience in the prehospital setting has been strongly positive. Emerging diagnostic assays and tools offer promise of fast and accurate diagnosis of CHF. Finally, transport of APE patients should be matched with the cardiovascular care resources of receiving facilities to optimize chances of survival.

Acknowledgment Portions of this chapter are reprinted with the permission of the National Association of EMS Physicians from Mosesso VN Jr, Dunford J, Blackwell T, and Griswell JK. Prehospital therapy for acute congestive heart failure: state of the art. Prehosp Emerg Care 2003;7:13–23.

References

1. Roger VL, Go AS, Llyod-Jones DM, et al. Heart Disease and Stroke Statistics—2011 Update: Chapter 9. Circulation. 2011;123(4):e18–209.
2. Nohria A, Lewis E, Stevenson LW. Medical management of advanced heart failure. JAMA. 2002;287:628–40.
3. Croft JB, Giles WH, Pollard RA, et al. Heart failure survival among older adults in the United States: a poor prognosis for an emerging epidemic in the Medicare population. Arch Intern Med. 1999;159:505–10.
4. Hubble MW, Richards ME, Jarvis R, Millikan T, Young D. Effectiveness of Prehospital continuous positive airway pressure in the management of acute pulmonary edema. Prehosp Emerg. 2006;10:430–9.
5. Emerman CL. Treatment of the acute decompensation of heart failure: Efficacy and pharmacoeconomics of early initiation of therapy in the emergency department. Rev Cardiovasc Med. 2003;4 Suppl 7:S13–20.
6. Peacock WF, Emerman CL. Emergency department management of patients with acute decompensated heart failure. Heart Fail Rev. 2004;9:187–93.
7. Nguyen HB, Rivers EP, Havstad S, et al. Critical care in the emergency department: a physiologic assessment and outcome evaluation. Acad Emerg Med. 2000;7:1354–61.
8. Rivers E, Nguyen B, Havstad S, et al. Early goal-directed therapy in the treatment of severe sepsis and septic shock. N Engl J Med. 2001;345:1368–77.
9. Sebat F, Johnson D, Musthafa AA, et al. A multidisciplinary community hospital program for early and rapid resuscitation of shock in nontrauma patients. Chest. 2005;127:1729–43.
10. Hunt SA, Baker DW, Chin MH, et al. ACC/AHA guidelines for the evaluation and management of chronic heart failure in the adult: executive summary. A report of the American College of Cardiology/American Heart Association Task Force on Practice Guidelines (Committee to revise the 1995 Guidelines for the Evaluation and Management of Heart Failure). J Am Coll Cardiol. 2001;38:2101–13.
11. Cotter G, Moshkovitz Y, Milovanov O, et al. Acute heart failure: a novel approach to its pathogenesis and treatment. Eur J Heart Failure. 2002;4:227–34.
12. Mebazaa A, Gheorghiade M, et al. Practical recommendations for prehospital and early in-hospital management of patients presenting with acute heart failure syndromes. Crit Care Med. 2008;36(Suppl):S129–39.
13. Cotter G, Kaluski E, Moshkovitz Y, et al. Pulmonary edema: new insight on pathogenesis and treatment. Curr Opin Cardiol. 2001;16:159–63.

14. Maisel AS, Krishnaswamy P, Nowak RM, et al. Rapid measurement of B-type natriuretic peptide in the emergency diagnosis of heart failure. N Engl J Med. 2002;347:161–7.
15. Maisel A. B-type natriuretic peptide in the diagnosis and management of congestive heart failure. Cardiol Clin. 2001;19:557–71.
16. Dao Q, Krishnaswamy P, Kazanegra R, et al. Utility of B-type natriuretic peptide in the diagnosis of congestive heart failure in an urgent-care setting. J Am Coll Cardiol. 2001;37:379–85.
17. Morrison LK, Harrison A, Krishnaswamy P, et al. Utility of a rapid B-natriuretic peptide assay in differentiating congestive heart failure from lung disease in patients presenting with dyspnea. J Am Coll Cardiol. 2002;39:202–9.
18. Tabbibizar R, Maisel A. The impact of B-type natriuretic peptide levels on the diagnoses and management of congestive heart failure. Curr Opin Cardiol. 2002;17:340–5.
19. Teboul A, Gaffinel A, Meune C, et al. Management of acute dyspnea: use and feasibility of brain natriuretic peptide (BNP) assay in the prehospital setting. Resuscitation. 2004;12:25.
20. Ventura HO, Pranulis MF, Young C, Smart FW. Impedance cardiography: a bridge between research and clinical practice in the treatment of heart failure. Congest Heart Fail. 2000;6: 94–102.
21. Tang WH, Tong W. Measuring impedance in congestive heart failure: current options and clinical applications. Am Heart J. 2009;157(3):402–11.
22. Hoffman JR, Reynolds S. Comparison of nitroglycerin, morphine and furosemide in treatment of presumed prehospital pulmonary edema. Chest. 1987;92:586–93.
23. Kosowsky JM, Stephanides SL, Branson RD, Sayre MR. Prehospital use of continuous positive airway pressure (CPAP) for presumed pulmonary edema: a preliminary case series. Prehosp Emerg Care. 2001;5:190–6.
24. Kukovetz WR, Holzmann S. Mechanisms of nitrate-induced vasodilation and tolerance. Eur J Clin Pharmacol. 1990;38:9.
25. Bertini G, Giglioli C, Biggeri A, et al. Intravenous nitrates in the prehospital management of acute pulmonary edema. Ann Emerg Med. 1997;30:493–9.
26. Sacchetti A, Ramoska E, Moakes ME, et al. Effect of ED management on ICU use in acute pulmonary edema. Am J Emerg Med. 1999;7:571–4.
27. Hill JA, Yancy CW, Abraham WT. Beyond diuretics: management of volume overload in acute heart failure syndromes. Am J Med. 2006;119(12A):S37–44.
28. Cleland JGF, Coletta A, Witte K. Practical applications of intravenous diuretic therapy in decompensated heart failure. Am J Med. 2006;119(12A):S26–36.
29. Cotter G, Metzkor E, Kaluski E, et al. Randomised trial of high-dose isosorbide dinitrate plus low-dose furosemide versus high-dose furosemide plus low-dose isosorbide dinitrate in severe pulmonary oedema. Lancet. 1998;351:389–93.
30. Wuerz R, Swope G, Meador S, et al. Safety of prehospital nitroglycerin. Ann Emerg Med. 1994;23:31–6.
31. Dorthridge D. Frusemide or nitrates for acute heart failure? Lancet. 1996;347:667–8.
32. Leeman M, Deguate JP. Invasive hemodynamic evaluation of sublingual captopril and nifedipine in patients with arterial hypertension after abdominal aortic surgery. Crit Care Med. 1995;23:847.
33. Ahmed A. Interaction between aspirin and angiotensin-converting enzyme inhibitors: should they be used together in older adults with heart failure? J Am Geriatr Soc. 2002;50: 1293–6.
34. Singer AJ, et al. Bronchodilator therapy in acute decompensated heart failure patients without a history of chronic obstructive pulmonary disease. Ann Emerg Med. 2008;51:25–34.
35. Meduri GU, Turner RE, Abou-Shala N. Noninvasive positive pressure ventilation via face mask: first-line intervention in patients with acute hypercapnic and hypoxemic respiratory failure. Chest. 1996;109:179–93.
36. Brochard L, Mancebo J, Wysocki M, et al. Noninvasive ventilation for acute exacerbations of chronic obstructive pulmonary disease. N Engl J Med. 1995;333:817–22.

37. Masip J, Roque M, Sa'nchez B. Noninvasive ventilation in acute cardiogenic pulmonary edema systematic review and meta-analysis. JAMA. 2005;294:3124–30.
38. Thompson J, Petrie DA. Out-of-hospital continuous positive airway pressure ventilation versus usual care in acute respiratory failure: a randomized controlled trial. Ann Emerg Med. 2008;52:232–41.
39. Mehta S, Jay GD, Woolard RH, et al. Randomized, prospective trial of bilevel versus continuous positive airway pressure in acute pulmonary edema. Crit Care Med. 1997;25:620–8.
40. Masip J, Betbese AJ, Paez J, et al. Non-invasive pressure support ventilation versus conventional oxygen therapy in acute cardiogenic pulmonary oedema: a randomised trial. Lancet. 2000;356:2126–32.

Chapter 9
Dyspnea Assessment and Airway Management in Acute Heart Failure Syndromes Patients

Masood Zaman and Peter S. Pang

Dyspnea is the most common presenting symptom in patients with acute heart failure syndromes (AHFS) [1–4]. Alleviating this sensation of breathlessness is a critical goal of early AHFS management. For the vast majority of patients, traditional AHFS therapies such as intravenous (IV) loop diuretics, nitrovasodilators, and oxygen are able to improve dyspnea [5]. For other patients, the severity of their respiratory distress requires use of additional treatment modalities, such as noninvasive positive pressure ventilation, or rarely endotracheal intubation, to ensure adequate oxygenation and ventilation. In this chapter, we review the assessment of dyspnea followed by airway management in AHFS.

Assessment of Dyspnea

Despite the importance of dyspnea relief to patients and caregivers, as well as its use as an endpoint in clinical trials, no validated dyspnea assessment tool currently exists [6]. Measurement scales such as Likert or visual analog scales are commonly used instruments to assess dyspnea in clinical trials [6–8]. From a clinical perspective however, the severity of dyspnea is rarely quantitatively assessed; rather its presence or absence combined with a clinical impression regarding its severity guides initial management. Furthermore, the exact pathophysiologic mechanisms by which AHFS patients experience the sensation of dyspnea is not fully known [9]. Thus, targeting another parameter, for

M. Zaman, MD • P.S. Pang, MD (✉)
Department of Emergency Medicine, Center for Cardiovascular Innovation -
Department of Medicine, Northwestern University Feinberg School of Medicine,
Chicago, IL, USA
e-mail: ppang@northwestern.edu

W. Frank Peacock (ed.), *Short Stay Management of Acute Heart Failure*,
Contemporary Cardiology, DOI 10.1007/978-1-61779-627-2_9,
© Springer Science+Business Media, LLC 2012

Table 9.1 The New York Heart Association functional classification [14]

Class I	Patients with cardiac disease but without resulting limitation of physical activity. Ordinary physical activity does not cause undue fatigue, palpitation, dyspnea, or anginal pain
Class II	Patients with cardiac disease resulting in slight limitation of physical activity. They are comfortable at rest. Ordinary physical activity results in fatigue, palpitation, dyspnea, or anginal pain
Class III	Patients with cardiac disease resulting in marked limitation of physical activity. They are comfortable at rest. Less than ordinary activity causes fatigue, palpitation, dyspnea, or anginal pain
Class IV	Patients with cardiac disease resulting in inability to carry on any physical activity without discomfort. Symptoms of heart failure or the anginal syndrome may be present even at rest. If any physical activity is undertaken, discomfort increases

Adapted from: The Criteria Committee of the New York Heart Association. *Nomenclature and Criteria for Diagnosis of the Heart and Great Vessels*, 9th ed. Boston, MA: Little Brown & Co; 1994:253–256

example, high blood pressure, with the goal of alleviating dyspnea has been proposed, but this relationship has yet to be conclusively defined [10–12]. The association of dyspnea with hard outcomes, such as mortality and/or re-hospitalization, has been shown by retrospective analysis, but still requires prospective confirmation [13].

Guidelines on assessment of dyspnea in AHFS or dyspnea-guided therapy do not exist, alluding to the lack of evidence in this area, or the fact that current therapy appears to improve, but not completely resolve, dyspnea in many patients. A commonly used classification scheme used in chronic HF is the NYHA classification: where the presence or absence of dyspnea is a dominant classification characteristic (see Table 9.1). As patients commonly complain of dyspnea at time of arrival to the hospital, however, this is not as useful in AHFS as most patients would be categorized as class III or IV.

At the present time, we suggest the following: (1) All AHFS patients should be asked if they feel short of breath, or have a sensation of breathlessness. Determining the impact of breathlessness on a patient's daily living may also provide a reference point for severity. For example, a patient who normally walks three blocks without dyspnea can now walk only five steps minimal activity. In addition, whether the patient experiences orthopnea or paroxysmal nocturnal dyspnea should also be determined. If a change from baseline is noted, the suspicion for worsening volume overload is increased (2). After treatment, patients should be reassessed to determine response to therapy. Caution is warranted for patients with minimal improvement. While undertreatment is one possibility, other causes of dyspnea (e.g., pulmonary embolism, emphysema) should be considered (Fig. 9.1).

Airway Management

While most AHFS patients do not require definitive airway control, those with severe respiratory distress require emergent and decisive management. Even those with only mild to moderate respiratory distress should be carefully assessed to determine the need for supplemental oxygen. This includes a thorough history, as clinical conditions permit, to assess for other causes contributing to dyspnea (e.g., fever and cough suggesting pneumonia, history of chronic obstructive pulmonary disease). In addition, careful assessment vital signs, including oxygen saturation, as well as of volume status is important.

For patients who require supplemental oxygen, the method of delivery (i.e. nasal cannula, varying oxygen-delivering masks, or a ventilator after endotracheal intubation) depends on the condition in which the patient presents as well as response to initial therapy. Moribund patients require definitive airway control with endotracheal intubation, whereas those whose clinical condition can be stabilized or rapidly reversed may be managed with alternative methods such as noninvasive ventilation with bi-level positive airway pressure (BPAP) or continuous positive airway pressure (CPAP). Unfortunately, no quick, simple, and universal method exists to determine which patients will rapidly improve with NIV from those who require definitive airway control. At the present time, this continues to be a clinical decision—with experience demonstrating that even patients who appear in the greatest distress often recover without intubation if initial therapy is begun rapidly (e.g., flash pulmonary edema).

For those who require definitive airway management, rapid sequence intubation (RSI) is the preferred method. This involves the simultaneous administration of a sedative along with a paralytic. A key step in RSI is preoxygenation to minimize the risk of hypoxia after the patient is paralyzed. Patients who present with pulmonary edema will not be able to tolerate prolonged periods of apnea compared to healthy adults and will experience oxygen desaturation more rapidly [15]. The risk of aspiration versus hypoxia needs to be carefully considered for these patients as preoxygenation with BVM may be necessary. RSI is the preferred mode of intubation in the emergency department and is both safe and effective [15].

Rapid Sequence Intubation

In RSI, unconsciousness is achieved using a fast-acting sedative agent. Etomidate is one of the most common induction agents used in RSI and is preferred because of its rapid onset and offset of action [15]. The induction dose of etomidate is 0.3 mg/kg IV. The most commonly used benzodiazepine in RSI is Midazolam at a dose of 0.3 mg/kg IV. Midazolam has some negative inotropic effects, however, and should generally be avoided to prevent further cardiovascular decompensation in patients requiring intubation due to AHFS [15].

Paralysis during RSI completely relaxes the patient's musculature facilitating first-pass success [15]. Succinylcholine is the most commonly used paralytic agent owing to its rapid onset of action and relatively brief half-life. Succinylcholine is a depolarizing neuromuscular blocking agent and binds to acetylcholine receptors systemically, but the desired effect of paralysis occurs through its action at the motor end plates. Succinylcholine also stimulates muscarinic receptors in the myocardium and can be a negative chronotrope [15]. This is important to recognize as sinus bradycardia may occur, but is uncommon with a single dose. If clinically indicated, atropine rapidly reverses bradycardia. When succinylcholine is contraindicated, other alternatives available such as vecuronium and rocuronium (both of which are non-depolarizing paralytics) have been used successfully in RSI.

Endotracheal intubation generally has few immediate side effects for otherwise healthy individuals but may pose substantial risk for those with underlying cardiovascular disease. Intubation induces catecholamine release that can lead to an increase in heart rate and blood pressure resulting in an overall increase in myocardial oxygen demand. Fentanyl, a synthetic opioid, can be used to potentially attenuate this reaction. The dose of fentanyl is 3 µg/kg and is given over 60 s prior to intubation [15].

Noninvasive Ventilation

Noninvasive ventilation is an important maneuver for both symptomatic and therapeutic management. The benefits of noninvasive ventilation include a decrease in some of the risks associated with endotracheal intubation, preservation of speech and swallowing along with patient comfort [16]. Appropriate patient selection is key to implementing noninvasive ventilation. Those unable to protect their airway (e.g., patient's with altered mental status) are not candidates for noninvasive ventilation.

There are two primary NIV modalities, continuous positive airway pressure (CPAP) and bi-level positive airway pressure (BPAP). CPAP differs from BPAP in that it provides a fixed level of positive pressure throughout the respiratory cycle whereas BPAP, as the name implies, provides two levels of support during the respiratory cycle, once during the inspiratory phase and then again during expiration. CPAP is similar to positive end expiratory pressure (PEEP), which is used in traditional mechanical ventilation. The purpose of CPAP (and PEEP) is to increase the functional residual capacity of the lungs by prevention of alveolar collapse that would occur secondary to injury or pulmonary edema [16]. In addition to end expiratory pressure, BPAP provides inspiratory pressure and may be preferred in patient with hypercarbia and increased work of breathing [16].

A systematic review published by Masip et al. looked at the role of noninvasive ventilation for acute cardiogenic pulmonary edema [17]. This meta-analysis described outcome differences in patients treated with conventional oxygen therapy versus noninvasive ventilation and also analyzed studies that compared the outcome differences between the two different methods of noninvasive ventilation. For this meta-analysis, treatment failure was defined as the need for intubation or in-hospital mortality.

When comparing conventional therapy with noninvasive ventilation, the results significantly favored CPAP. CPAP decreased the need for intubation by 60% with a decrease in mortality by 40%. The results for BPAP did not reach statistical significance; however, BPAP compared to conventional therapy showed ~50% reduction in the need for intubation and a trend towards decreased mortality. The meta-analysis of studies comparing BPAP and CPAP found no significant differences between the two modalities [17]. The authors strongly encouraged the use of noninvasive ventilation for the management of cardiogenic pulmonary edema although they did not recommend one method over another.

More recently, a multicenter randomized controlled trial called 3CPO (Cardiogenic Pulmonary Oedema trialists group) compared conventional oxygen therapy, BPAP, and CPAP in patients presenting to emergency departments in the United Kingdom with acute cardiogenic pulmonary edema [18]. For the 1,069 subjects enrolled, no significant mortality differences were found at 7 days between patients treated with conventional therapy and those treated with noninvasive ventilation. Additionally, no significant difference was found between BPAP or CPAP for intubation and mortality rates at 7 days. The study did demonstrate an improvement in patient reported dyspnea, acidosis, and hypercapnia with noninvasive ventilation versus conventional oxygen therapy [18].

The American College of Emergency Physicians' clinical policy guideline on the management of AHFS gives a level B recommendation for the use of CPAP and level C recommendation for the use of BPAP [19]. The level C recommendation for BPAP was a result of a single study suggesting a higher incidence of myocardial infarction, although follow-up studies have not shown such an association [18].

Although the 3CPO study did not show any difference in the need for intubation or short-term mortality between NIV and conventional oxygen therapy, we continue to recommend the use of noninvasive ventilation, specifically CPAP, for patients presenting to the emergency department with dyspnea from cardiogenic pulmonary edema who are at low risk for aspiration and do not require immediate endotracheal intubation. Importantly, the 3CPO study did not show any harm from NIV. CPAP should be initiated at 10–15 cm H20 and titrated in 2 cm H20 increments based on the patient's clinical status and degree of hypoxemia [16]. Close interval assessments are needed to ensure compliance and to assess improvement or worsening in clinical status. Although arterial blood gases are rarely performed in the ED setting, patients who are failing to improve with CPAP may be retaining CO_2, which is an indication to switch to BPAP, to improve ventilatory support. Some patients may find the tight-fitting mask to be claustrophobic or painful, and low doses of morphine, used with caution, may be utilized to ensure compliance.

Conclusion

Assessing breathlessness and ensuring its relief is a major goal of initial AHFS management. For patients who present moribund or with altered mental status and respiratory distress, immediate endotracheal intubation with RSI is recommended, recognizing that hypoxia may worsen rapidly secondary to paralysis in patients with cardiogenic pulmonary edema. For patients with moderate to severe respiratory distress, immediate use of NIV may rapidly improve patient's signs and symptoms.

Appendix 1: Assessment of Supplemental Oxygen Needs for Dyspneic AHFS Patients

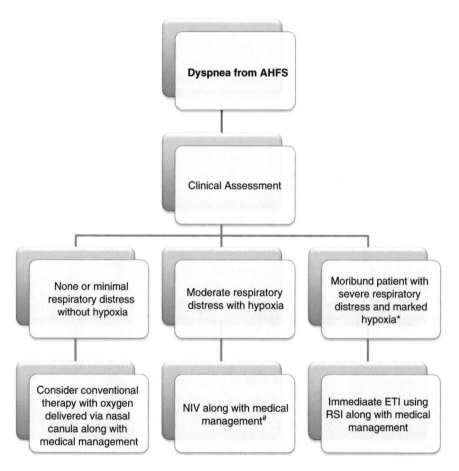

Fig. 9.1 Assessment of Supplemental Oxygen Needs for Dyspneic AHFS Patients
*If the clinical situation permits, a brief trial of NIV along with medical management may rapidly turn these patients around #In patients who are not at risk for aspiration. Although we recommend NIV, conventional oxygen therapy may be used instead
AHFS acute heart failure syndrome, *NIV* non-invasive ventilation, *ETI* endotracheal intubation, *RSI* rapid sequence intubation

References

1. Adams JKF, Fonarow GC, Emerman CL, LeJemtel TH, Costanzo MR, Abraham WT, et al. Characteristics and outcomes of patients hospitalized for heart failure in the United States: Rationale, design, and preliminary observations from the first 100,000 cases in the Acute Decompensated Heart Failure National Registry (ADHERE). Am Heart J. 2005;149(2):209–16.
2. VMAC Investigators. Intravenous nesiritide vs. nitroglycerin for treatment of decompensated congestive heart failure: a randomized controlled trial. JAMA. 2002;287(12):1531–40.
3. Hernandez AF. Acute study of clinical effectiveness of nesiritide in decompensated heart failure trial (ASCEND-HF)—Nesiritide or placebo for improved symptoms and outcomes in acute decompensated HF. American Heart Association Scientific Sessions. Chicago, IL: AHA; 2010.
4. Massie BM, Metra M, Ponikowski P, Teerlink J, Cotter G, et al. Rolofylline, an adenosine A1-receptor antagonist, in acute heart failure. N Engl J Med. 2010;363(15):1419–28.
5. Mebazaa A, Pang PS, Tavares M, Collins SP, Storrow AB, Laribi S, et al. The impact of early standard therapy on dyspnoea in patients with acute heart failure: the URGENT-dyspnoea study. Eur Heart J. 2010;31(7):832–41.
6. Pang PS, Cleland JG, Teerlink JR, Collins SP, Lindsell CJ, Sopko G, et al. A proposal to standardize dyspnoea measurement in clinical trials of acute heart failure syndromes: the need for a uniform approach. Eur Heart J. 2008;29(6):816–24.
7. McMurray JJ, Teerlink JR, Cotter G, Bourge RC, Cleland JG, Jondeau G, et al. Effects of tezosentan on symptoms and clinical outcomes in patients with acute heart failure: the VERITAS randomized controlled trials. JAMA. 2007;298(17):2009–19.
8. Gheorghiade M, Konstam MA, Burnett Jr JC, Grinfeld L, Maggioni AP, Swedberg K, et al. Short-term clinical effects of tolvaptan, an oral vasopressin antagonist, in patients hospitalized for heart failure: the EVEREST Clinical Status Trials. JAMA. 2007;297(12):1332–43.
9. Teerlink JR. Dyspnea as an end point in clinical trials of therapies for acute decompensated heart failure. Am Heart J. 2003;145(2 Suppl):S26–33.
10. Teerlink JR, Metra M, Felker GM, Ponikowski P, Voors AA, Weatherley BD, et al. Relaxin for the treatment of patients with acute heart failure (Pre-RELAX-AHF): a multicentre, randomised, placebo-controlled, parallel-group, dose-finding phase IIb study. Lancet. 2009;373(9673):1429–39.
11. Shah MR, Hasselblad V, Stinnett SS, Gheorghiade M, Swedberg K, Califf RM, et al. Hemodynamic profiles of advanced heart failure: association with clinical characteristics and long-term outcomes. J Card Fail. 2001;7(2):105–13.
12. Shah MR, Hasselblad V, Stinnett SS, Kramer JM, Grossman S, Gheorghiade M, et al. Dissociation between hemodynamic changes and symptom improvement in patients with advanced congestive heart failure. Eur J Heart Fail. 2002;4(3):297–304.
13. Metra M, Cleland JG, Davison Weatherley B, Dittrich HC, Givertz MM, Massie BM, et al. Dyspnoea in patients with acute heart failure: an analysis of its clinical course, determinants, and relationship to 60-day outcomes in the PROTECT pilot study. Eur J Heart Fail. 2010;12(5):499–507.
14. The Criteria Committee of the New York Heart Association, editor. Nomenclature and criteria for diagnosis of diseases of the heart and great vessels. 9th ed. Boston: Little Brown; 1994.
15. Walls RM. Airway. In: John A, Marx M, Robert S, Hockberger M, Ron M, Walls M, James G, Adams M, William G, Barsan M, Michelle H, Biros M, et al., editors. Marx: Rosen's emergency medicine: concepts and clinical practice. 7th ed. Philadelphia: Mosby Elsevier; 2009.
16. Anderson ML, Younger JG. Mechanical ventilation and noninvasive ventilatory support. In: John A, Marx M, Robert S, Hockberger M, Ron M, Walls M, James G, Adams M, William G, Barsan M, Michelle H, Biros M, et al., editors. Marx: Rosen's emergency medicine: concepts and clinical practice. 7th ed. Philadelphia: Mosby Elsevier; 2009.

17. Masip J, Roque M, Sanchez B, Fernandez R, Subirana M, Exposito JA. Noninvasive ventilation in acute cardiogenic pulmonary edema: systematic review and meta-analysis. JAMA. 2005;294(24):3124–30.
18. Gray A, Goodacre S, Newby DE, Masson M, Sampson F, Nicholl J. Noninvasive ventilation in acute cardiogenic pulmonary edema. N Engl J Med. 2008;359(2):142–51.
19. Jagoda A, Decker W, Edlow J, Fesmire F, Godwin S, Howell J, et al. Clinical policy: critical issues in the evaluation and management of adult patients presenting to the emergency department with acute heart failure syndromes. Ann Emerg Med. 2007;49(5):627–69.

Chapter 10
Volume Assessment in the Emergency Department

Anna Marie Chang and Judd E. Hollander

In the emergency department (ED), a myriad of diagnoses may present similarly. For example, heart failure (HF), chronic obstructive pulmonary disease (COPD), and pulmonary embolism may all present as shortness of breath. To further cloud the picture, acute decompensated heart failure (ADHF) represents a heterogeneous group of disorders with various etiologies, and the optimal treatments for each disorder may be different, based on volume and perfusion status. Accurate volume assessment is paramount in the ED for the diagnosis of heart failure.

Background

In the out-of-hospital (or prehospital) realm, it has been shown that early treatment of patients suspected of suffering from ADHF improved mortality [1]. However, patients that did not have heart failure but received empiric treatment with medications targeting heart failure (furosemide, nitroglycerin, and morphine) had a higher mortality than patients who remained untreated. Those patients ultimately found to not have heart failure who received bronchodilators had a mortality rate of 3.6%. Patients ultimately found not to have heart failure but who received heart failure therapy had an increased mortality to 13.6%. The non-HF group that received no

A.M. Chang, MD (✉)
Emergency Cardiac Care Fellow, Department of Emergency Medicine,
University of Pennsylvania, Philadelphia, PA, USA
e-mail: changam@uphs.upenn.edu

J.E. Hollander, MD
Department of Emergency Medicine, University of Pennsylvania,
Philadelphia, PA, USA

W. Frank Peacock (ed.), *Short Stay Management of Acute Heart Failure*,
Contemporary Cardiology, DOI 10.1007/978-1-61779-627-2_10,
© Springer Science+Business Media, LLC 2012

therapy had a mortality of only 8.2%, highlighting the importance of having a correct diagnosis and volume assessment prior to treatment [1].

Hemodynamic profiles have been used to stratify patients presenting with acute heart failure. In 1978, Forrester et al. demonstrated four patient profiles after acute myocardial infarction that predicted outcomes [2, 3]. These profiles were based on the presence or absence of congestion (pulmonary capillary wedge pressure (PCWP) > or ≤18 mm Hg) and adequacy of perfusion (cardiac index >2.2 l/min/m [2]) which could be ascertained by Swan-Ganz catheter readings. The findings were extended to patients with acute heart failure by Stevenson [4]. For example, indications of congestion included a recent history of orthopnea and/or physical examination with evidence of jugular venous distention, rales, hepatojugular reflux, ascites, peripheral edema, leftward radiation of the pulmonic heart sound, or a square wave blood pressure response to the Valsalva maneuver. Compromised perfusion was defined by presence of a narrow proportional pulse pressure pulsus alternans, symptomatic hypotension (without orthostasis), cool extremities, or impaired mentation. Physicians synthesized the presence or absence of any or all of these signs to make a subjective assessment of the patients' volume and perfusion status when wedge pressures or cardiac index measures were not available. Profile I represents no congestion or hypoperfusion (dry-warm); profile II, congestion without hypoperfusion (wet-warm); profile III, hypoperfusion without congestion (dry-cold); and profile IV, both congestion and hypoperfusion (wet-cold) [5]. These clinical profiles predict short-term survival, with patients fitting profile II and IV having twice the mortality rate compared to profile I. It appears that increased volume and congestion (wet) predict a worse prognosis, and perhaps these patients need to be more aggressively treated. The rest of this chapter will discuss methods to help assess volume overload.

The Gold Standard

The gold standard for determining blood volume is radioisotopic measurement. It is generally held that a reliable blood volume analysis can be provided by the dual-labeling radioisotope technique, which includes red cell volume measurement using 51-Cr or 99-mTc as a label and a separate plasma volume assessment using 125-I- or 131-I-tagged human serum albumin (International Committee for Standardization in Hematology). More recently, it has been suggested that blood volumes can be estimated from a single 125-I- or 131-I-HSA assessment effectively, rapidly, and at a lower cost [6]. However, the definition of rapid from these studies is 1.5 h. Although radioisotope blood volume analysis may be useful in ideal conditions, there are no ED-based clinical studies that show effectiveness. In the ED, we need to rely on tools that are faster and more widely available.

History and Physical Examination

The 2009 American College of Cardiology/American Heart Association Revised Guidelines recommend volume assessment for all patients with heart failure during the initial evaluation and with follow-up examinations [7]. Physicians should begin their evaluation of a patient with a history and physical examination. The guidelines recommend measurement of body weight, sitting and standing blood pressures, jugular venous distension, and hepatojugular reflux, as well as edema in the legs and abdomen. It also recommends evaluation for pulmonary rales and hepatomegaly [7]. These are the factors that have been the standards of hemodynamic profiling. However, Stevenson and Perloff demonstrated that physical signs have limited accuracy in estimating hemodynamics in chronic HF [8]. Furthermore, the inter-rater reliability for hemodynamic profiling among emergency physicians was poor to fair at best, with observers agreeing on the hemodynamic profile only 64% of the time [9]. Despite the lack of data on the reliability of physical examination findings, practice guidelines emphasize their importance in the evaluation of patients with HF, and they should be determined [7].

In nondifferentiated dyspneic patients in the ED, the diagnosis is even more difficult. In a meta-analysis of 18 studies by Wang et al., a history of congestive heart failure or myocardial infarction were the most helpful features to identify patients with potential heart failure [10]. Risk factors for HF that were also helpful included hypertension, diabetes, valvular heart disease, older age, male sex, and obesity. Those who reported symptoms of paroxysmal nocturnal dyspnea, ortho-pnea, or dyspnea on exertion were also more likely to have HF; however, these were less reliable than past medical history. This is true in many patients with chronic HF, who have elevated intravascular volume without overt peripheral edema or rales. However, depending on the study, signs and symptoms have varying sensitivity and specificity. Butman et al. reported that JVD was both specific and sensitive for an increased PCWP [11], while another study, defining volume overload as a PCWP > 18 mm Hg, concluded that JVD and HJR had a predictive accuracy of only 81% [12]. The presence of rales has a sensitivity and specificity as low as the 50% range [8]. Further information about sensitivity and specificity of history and physical exami-nation findings can be found in Table 10.1.

In physical examination teachings, the S3 is highly specific for ventricular dys-function and elevated left ventricular filling pressures. In fact, the presence of an S3 has the highest positive likelihood ratio (LR 11.0) for volume overload [10]. However, the inter-rater reliability of this physical exam finding is very low [13], and it is often difficult to auscultate in patients with confounding diseases (e.g., COPD and obesity) and in noisy environments such as the emergency department. In fact, the 2009 updated guidelines do not list heart sounds as a method to assess volume status or the diagnosis of heart failure [7].

Another confounding factor to the diagnosis of volume overload may be the presence of hypoperfusion. Although the majority of patients with HF do not present

Table 10.1 History and physical examination findings and their association with volume overload and heart failure diagnosis

Finding	Sensitivity	Specificity	Summary LR (95% CI)	
			Positive	Negative
Initial clinical judgment	0.61	0.86	4.4 (1.8–10.0)	0.45 (0.28–0.73)
History				
Heart failure	0.60	0.90	5.8 (4.1–8.0)	0.45 (0.38–0.53)
Myocardial infarction	0.40	0.87	3.1 (2.0–4.9)	0.69 (0.58–0.82)
Coronary artery disease	0.52	0.70	1.8 (1.1–2.8)	0.68 (0.48–0.96)
Diabetes mellitus	0.28	0.83	1.7 (1.0–2.7)	0.86 (0.73–1.0)
Hypertension	0.60	0.56	1.4 (1.1–1.7)	0.71 (0.55–0.93)
Smoking	0.62	0.27	0.84 (0.58–1.2)	1.4 (0.58–3.8)
COPD	0.34	0.57	0.81 (0.60–1.1)	1.1 (0.95–1.4)
Symptoms				
PND	0.41	0.84	2.6 (1.5–4.5)	0.70 (0.54–0.91)
Orthopnea	0.50	0.77	2.2 (1.2–3.9)	0.65 (0.45–0.92)
Edema	0.51	0.76	2.1 (0.92–5.0)	0.64 (0.39–1.1)
Dyspnea on exertion	0.84	0.34	1.3 (1.2–1.4)	0.48 (0.35–0.67)
Cough	0.36	0.61	0.93 (0.70–1.2)	1.0 (0.87–1.3)
Physical examination				
Third heart sound	0.13	0.99	11 (4.9–25.0)	0.88 (0.83–0.94)
Abdominojugular reflux	0.24	0.96	6.4 (0.81–51.0)	0.79 (0.62–1.0)
Jugular venous distension	0.39	0.92	5.1 (3.2–7.9)	0.66 (0.57–0.77)
Rales	0.60	0.78	2.8 (1.9–4.1)	0.51 (0.37–0.70)
Any murmur	0.27	0.90	2.6 (1.7–4.1)	0.81 (0.73–0.90)
Lower extremity edema	0.50	0.78	2.3 (1.5–3.7)	0.64 (0.47–0.87)
Valsalva maneuver	0.73	0.65	2.1 (1.0–4.2)	0.41 (0.17–1.0)
SBP < 100 mm Hg	0.06	0.97	2.0 (0.60–6.6)	0.97 (0.91–1.0)
Fourth heart sound	0.05	0.97	1.6 (0.47–5.5)	0.98 (0.93–1.0)
SBP > 150 mm Hg	0.28	0.73	1.0 (0.69–1.6)	0.99 (0.84–1.2)
Wheezing	0.22	0.58	0.52 (0.38–0.71)	1.3 (1.1–1.7)
Ascites	0.01	0.97	0.33 (0.04–2.9)	1.0 (0.99–1.1)

Abbreviations: LR likelihood ratio, *CI* confidence interval, *PND* paroxysmal nocturnal dyspnea, *SBP* systolic blood pressure, *COPD* chronic obstructive pulmonary disease

with hypoperfusion, their cardiac function may be severely depressed. Conversely, patients with hypoperfusion may have a concurrent illness, or be suffering from hypovolemia rather than pump failure, or have excessive vasodilation from their heart failure; this must be considered when taking the history. When patients present with more severe volume deficits, orthostatic symptoms and hypotension may suggest hypovolemia and not necessarily hypoperfusion. Orthostatic symptoms may include dizziness upon standing, shortness of breath with exertion or at rest, weakness, malaise, and syncope if the deficit is severe. However, the utility of orthostatic vital signs in the emergency department has been questioned. In a sample of 132 presumed euvolemic patients, 43% had "positive" orthostatic vital signs [14]. In a comparison of over 200 ill patients and 20 control patients, orthostatic changes in systolic blood pressure and diastolic blood pressure demonstrated no statistically significant association with level of dehydration, and it was impossible to define a group of patients who had a "positive" tilt-table test [15].

The combination of history and physical examination findings may aid the physician in diagnosing volume overload. However, diagnostic imaging, natriuretic peptides, and other noninvasive techniques are also available to address the issue.

Chest Radiography

Chest radiographs may aid in the diagnosis of volume overload, or may help guide the differential diagnosis of the acutely dyspneic patient in the emergency department. In the presence of heart failure, one may find pulmonary venous congestion, cardiomegaly, and interstitial edema. However, the absence of radiography findings does not exclude heart failure [7]. Collins et al. found that up to 20% of patients who were eventually diagnosed with heart failure had negative chest radiographs at the time of evaluation in the emergency department [16]. Furthermore, in late-stage heart failure patients, chest radiography has unreliable sensitivity, specificity, and predictive value for identifying individuals with high PCWP.

Natriuretic Peptides

The natriuretic peptides (NP) are hemodynamically active neurohormones that are released into the bloodstream when there is increased myocardial pressure and stretching, so that they can enable vasodilation and natriuresis. It is released as a prohormone and cleaved into the biologically active BNP and NT-proBNP. Assays for BNP and its synthetic by-product NT-proBNP are commercially available.

Compared with BNP, NT-proBNP has a longer plasma half-life [17]. There is ample evidence that both BNP and NT-proBNP are useful in diagnosing and predicting prognosis in heart failure, including the Breathing Not Properly Multinational Trial (BNP Trial) [18], the Rapid Emergency Department Heart Failure Outpatient Trial (REDHOT) [19], PRIDE (pro-BNP Investigation of Dyspnea in the Emergency Department) [17], and the ESCAPE (Evaluation Study of Congestive Heart Failure and Pulmonary Artery Catheterization Effectiveness) Trial [20]. These molecules behave similarly and are elevated in the setting of heart failure. These studies demonstrated that BNP and NT-proBNP are useful in the diagnosis and risk stratification of patients with heart failure.

Furthermore, the natriuretic peptides also provide an overall assessment of volume status. In studies of patients on hemodialysis, plasma BNP levels before and after hemodialysis correlate with the degree of body fluid and volume retention [21, 22] and with inferior vena cava diameter measurements that are reflective of hydration status.

However, because the NPs can be elevated with any type of myocardial stress, independent of volume status (e.g., myocardial infarction, pulmonary embolus), physician judgment must also be used. Both BNP and NT-proBNP interpretation must be used carefully in obese individuals [23], older patients, and those with renal disease or on hemodialysis [22]; all these factors affect the sensitivity and specificity of the test. Knowledge of the patient's baseline levels and any associated change may also be useful.

For more detailed information regarding the diagnostic and prognostic utility of natriuretic peptides, please refer to Chap. 5.

Phonocardiography

Auscultation of an S3 heart sound is difficult in the emergency department setting, and as mentioned previously, interobserver concordance is low [13]. Phonoelectrocardiographic devices have been developed in order to improve detection of abnormal heart sounds, specifically an S3 or S4. The Audicor system is an acoustic cardiogram that collects both sound and electrical data. Earlier studies showed that it has increased the likelihood of the diagnosis of HF and left ventricular dysfunction [24, 25]. However, in a multinational study of over 990 patients, although the system was specific for the diagnosis of acute decompensated heart failure and affected physician confidence, its lack of sensitivity did not improve diagnostic rates [26]. Furthermore, the test did not have any independent prognostic information.

Ultrasonography

Ultrasound has become increasingly available at the bedside. It has been shown to be useful in a myriad of conditions and has been helpful in the assessment of volume status in the critically ill patient [27] including septic shock and trauma [28].

The inferior vena cava diameter (IVCd) has been shown to indicate volume status and blood loss. In a study of 31 healthy male volunteers who were donating 450 ml of blood, IVCd measured both during inspiration (IVCi) and during expiration (IVCe) showed a decrease of 5 mm after blood loss [29]. The wide variation between individuals of IVC diameter makes isolated measurements difficult to interpret for volume status (Fig. 10.1).

Studies have addressed using respiratory variation in IVCd as a marker for the diagnosis of HF. IVCd is dynamic and changes with changes in intrathoracic pressure. During inspiration, intrathoracic pressure decreases thereby increasing venous return and causing distention of the IVC. During expiration, an increase in intrathoracic pressure causes a collapse of the IVC [27, 30]. A measurement for this variation in IVC diameter is the IVC collapse index (IVC-CI). The IVC-CI is equal to the difference between the IVCDe and the IVC diameter in inspiration (IVCi) divided

Fig. 10.1 (**a, b**) 100% collapse of IVC secondary to volume depletion and over 75% collapse of IVC. The *white arrow* indicates IVC seen on short axis view. Image reproduced with permission of Drs. Alfred Cheng and Anthony Dean, Hospital of the University of Pennsylvania

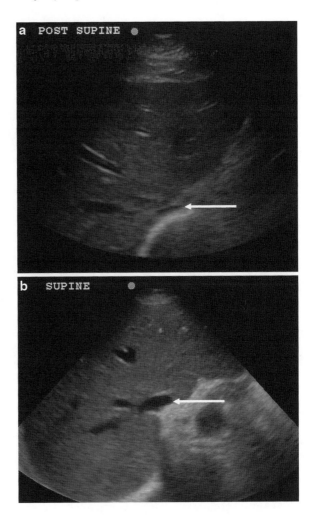

by the IVCe. Absolute values for a normal IVC-CI do not exist; however, the IVC-CI in normal healthy subjects is typically between 0.25 and 0.75 (see Fig. 10.1b). In HF, volume overload dilates the IVC to the point that decreased intrathoracic pressure does not change the resulting diameter and thus the IVC-CI remains close to 1 (Fig. 10.2).

Another diagnostic use of thoracic ultrasound is the assessment of pulmonary water by the identification of the presence of sonographic artifacts, known as B-lines, lung comets, or comet tails. These imply thickened interstitial or fluid-filled alveoli. B-lines occur most commonly in patients with HF and correlate with elevated PCWP and extravascular pulmonary water [31]. Clinical studies using these ultrasound findings have shown good sensitivity and specificity for distinguishing between congestive heart failure and COPD (sensitivity range, 85.7–100%; specificity range, 92–97.7%) [32]. In a study of 94 patients presenting to the ED with

Fig. 10.2 Plethoric IVC, a sign of volume overload. The *white arrow* indicates IVC seen on short axis view. Image reproduced with permission of Drs. Alfred Cheng and Anthony Dean, Hospital of the University of Pennsylvania

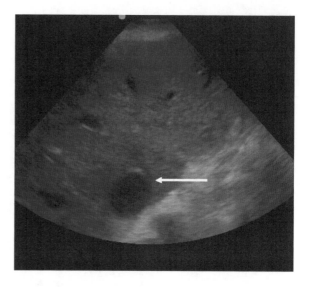

acute shortness of breath, an US that showed comet tails had a positive likelihood ratio (LR+) of 3.88 and a negative likelihood ratio (LR−) of 0.5 [33]. However, as with any ultrasound technology, there is room for much user heterogeneity. Many of these studies require multiple lung fields and zones to assess total volume status as well. This makes it a potentially time-consuming and not the most user-friendly modality.

Impedance Monitors

Impedance cardiography (ICG) is a noninvasive measurement of cardiac output, cardiac index, and thoracic fluid content. Electrical impedance is the resistance to flow of an electrical alternating current, and the human thorax is an inhomogeneous electrical conductor. Bone and tissue are poor conductors while blood and fluids are good conductors and decrease impedance. When a high frequency electrical current is injected across the thorax, paired electrodes can be used to measure impedance reflected as voltage changes. The changes in thoracic voltage result from changes that occur from blood volumetric and velocity alterations related to the cardiac cycle. By analyzing these changes and their relation with ECG-derived timing measures, variations in blood flow through the great vessels result in estimates of stroke volume [34].

ICG directly measures certain parameters including heart rate, thoracic fluid content (1/baseline impedance [per k ohm]), velocity index (first time derivative/baseline impedance [per 1,000 s]), acceleration index (second time derivative/baseline impedance [per 100 s]), and pre-ejection period (time from EKG Q wave to aortic valve opening [ms]) [35]. It would make sense that by measuring the thoracic fluid content, one can estimate the hemodynamics and fluid profile of a patient.

In the outpatient setting, Packer et al. [35] followed 212 stable HF patients who underwent serial clinical and ICG evaluation every 2 weeks for 26 weeks and who were followed up for the occurrence of death or worsening of HF requiring hospitalization or emergent care. Those with a higher thoracic fluid content (TFC) were at an increased risk for hospitalization and emergent care [35].

The bioimpedance cardiography in advanced heart failure (BIG) substudy was conducted within the ESCAPE Trial and was designed to determine the utility of bioimpedance cardiography as an adjunct tool for HF monitoring in hospitalized patients with advanced HF [34]. TFC was not predictive of poor outcomes, as it had been in the outpatient setting. In patients with systolic HF, TFC was poorly correlated with invasively measured RAP and PCWP. It can be inferred from the poor correlation between the pulmonary artery catheter (PAC)-derived and ICG-derived clinical profiles that in general that ICG is a poor surrogate for PAC-derived data in chronic heart failure patients who are readmitted to the hospital and should not be used as an alternative.

Bioimpedance Vector Analysis

A further use of bioimpedance is known is BIVA, or bioelectrical impedance vector analysis, which is a noninvasive technique to estimate body mass and water composition by bioelectrical impedance measurements, resistance, and reactance [36]. To measure BIVA, the patient lies supine on a nonconductive surface, without metal contacts, with straddle inferior limbs at 45° and superior limbs abducted at 30° to avoid skin contacts with the trunk. Two skin electrodes are applied, one on the right hand and the other on the right foot. These measures are then compared to the normal distribution adjusted by patient's height and weight, age, and sex. This is plotted within ellipses, as well as measurements of vectors measured in degrees of elevation from the x-axis is termed the phase angle (PA), and has prognostic value in many clinical situations. Short vectors are associated with edema, whereas long vectors indicate dehydration [37].

In disease entities where volume assessment is crucial, there appears to be a correlation between BIVA values and hydration status. BIVA was useful in predicting fluid overload in critically ill patients. In a cohort of 121 patients in an intensive care unit, central venous pressure values >12 mm Hg were associated with shorter impedance vectors in 93% of patients, indicating fluid overload [38]. In 22 HF patients, using deuterium dilution as the standard for total body water evaluation, BIVA measurements had excellent correlation with total body water content ($r = 0.93$, $p = 0.01$) [39]. Di Somma et al. enrolled 51 patients in an ED, half of whom were ultimately diagnosed with ADHF based on clinical and laboratory findings. BIVA of ADHF patients was compared with BIVA of controls, and the difference was statistically significant ($P < 0007$); the numbers reported in ADHF patients had greater hydration (76.7±4.0%) compared with controls (73.1±1.9%). In patients with average hydration values >80.5%, there was a correlation with events at 3 months (death or rehospitalization for cardiogenic event) with a sensitivity of 22% and specificity of 94.2% (positive likelihood ratio 4.6, positive predictive value 66.7, negative predictive value 74.1) [36]. However, there are many limitations to this type of procedure in the ED. It is still a new technology that has not gained widespread use; the utility of the tool above and beyond what are already available has not been proven in an undifferentiated ED population, and it cannot be used on uncooperative patients.

Conclusion

It is difficult to accurately assess volume status on patients in the ED. Only through careful history taking, physical examination, and the assortment of the tools and diagnostic tests that are available in the ED can physicians put together a profile of the patient. Ultrasound skills such as measurement of IVC show promise; more training is needed for most practitioners to make it useful. New technologies such as BIVA show promise; however, future studies need to address its utility in the diverse patient population seen in the ED.

References

1. Wuerz RC, Meador SA. Effects of prehospital medications on mortality and length of stay in congestive heart failure. Ann Emerg Med. 1992;21(6):669–74.
2. Forrester J, Diamond G, Chatterjee K, Swan H. Medical therapy of acute myocardial infarction by application of hemodynamic subsets. N Eng J Med. 1976;295:1356–413.
3. Forrester JS, Diamond G, Chatterjee K, Swan HJ. Medical therapy of acute myocardial infarction by application of hemodynamic subsets (first of two parts). N Engl J Med. 1976;295(24): 1356–62.
4. Stevenson LW. Tailored therapy to hemodynamic goals for advanced heart failure. Eur J Heart Fail. 1999;1(3):251–7.
5. Nohria A. Clinical assessment identifies hemodynamic profiles that predict outcomes in patients admitted with heart failure. J Am Coll Cardiol. 2003;41(10):1797–804.
6. Moralidis E, Papanastassiou E, Arsos G, et al. A single measurement with (51)Cr-tagged red cells or (125)I-labeled human serum albumin in the prediction of fractional and whole blood volumes: an assessment of the limitations. Physiol Meas. 2009;30(7):559–71.
7. Hunt SA, Abraham WT, Chin MH, et al. 2009 Focused update incorporated into the ACC/AHA 2005 Guidelines for the Diagnosis and Management of Heart Failure in Adults A Report of the American College of Cardiology Foundation/American Heart Association Task Force on Practice Guidelines Developed in Collaboration With the International Society for Heart and Lung Transplantation. J Am Coll Cardiol. 2009;53(15):e1–90.
8. Stevenson L, Perloff J. The limited reliability of physical signs for estimating hemodynamics in chronic heart failure. JAMA. 1989;261:884–8.
9. Chaudhry A, Singer AJ, Chohan J, Russo V, Lee C. Inter-rater reliability of hemodynamic profiling of patients with heart failure in the ED. Am J Emerg Med. 2008;26(2):196–201.

10. Wang CS, FitzGerald JM, Schulzer M, Mak E, Ayas NT. Does this dyspneic patient in the emergency department have congestive heart failure? JAMA. 2005;294(15):1944–56.

11. Butman SM, Ewy GA, Standen JR, Kern KB, Hahn E. Bedside cardiovascular examination in patients with severe chronic heart failure: importance of rest or inducible jugular venous distension. J Am Coll Cardiol. 1993;22(4):968–74.

12. Marantz PR, Kaplan MC, Alderman MH. Clinical diagnosis of congestive heart failure in patients with acute dyspnea. Chest. 1990;97(4):776–81.

13. Marcus GM, Marcus G, Vessey J, et al. Relationship between accurate auscultation of a clinically useful third heart sound and level of experience. Arch Intern Med. 2006;166(6):617–22.

14. Koziol-McLain J, Lowenstein SR, Fuller B. Orthostatic vital signs in emergency department patients. Ann Emerg Med. 1991;20(6):606–10.

15. Levitt MA, Lopez B, Lieberman ME, Sutton M. Evaluation of the tilt test in an adult emergency medicine population. Ann Emerg Med. 1992;21(6):713–8.

16. Collins SP, Lindsell CJ, Storrow AB, Abraham WT. Prevalence of negative chest radiography results in the emergency department patient with decompensated heart failure. Ann Emerg Med. 2006;47(1):13–8.

17. Januzzi J, Camargo CA, Anwaruddin S, et al. The N-terminal Pro-BNP Investigation of Dyspnea in the Emergency department (PRIDE) study. Am J Cardiol. 2005;95(8):948–54.

18. Maisel AS, Krishnaswamy P, Nowak RM, et al. Rapid measurement of B-type natriuretic peptide in the emergency diagnosis of heart failure. N Engl J Med. 2002;347(3):161–7.

19. Maisel A, Hollander JE, Guss D, et al. Primary results of the Rapid Emergency Department Heart Failure Outpatient Trial (REDHOT): a multicenter study of B-type natriuretic peptide levels, emergency department decision making, and outcomes in patients presenting with shortness of breath. J Am Coll Cardiol. 2004;44(6):1328–33.

20. The ESCAPE Investigators and ESCAPE Study Coordinators. Evaluation study of congestive heart failure and pulmonary artery catheterization effectiveness: the ESCAPE trial. JAMA. 2005;294(13):1625–33.

21. Lee SW, Song JH, Kim GA, Lim HJ, Kim M. Plasma brain natriuretic peptide concentration on assessment of hydration status in hemodialysis patient. Am J Kidney Dis. 2003;41(6):1257–66.

22. Garg R, Singh A, Khaja A, Martin A, Aggarwal K. How does volume status affect bnp and troponin levels as markers of cardiovascular status in peritoneal dialysis? Congest Heart Fail. 2009;15(5):240–4.

23. Krauser DG, Lloyd-Jones DM, Chae CU, et al. Effect of body mass index on natriuretic peptide levels in patients with acute congestive heart failure: a ProBNP Investigation of Dyspnea in the Emergency Department (PRIDE) substudy. Am Heart J. 2005;149(4):744–50.

24. Collins SP, Lindsell CJ, Peacock WF, et al. The combined utility of an S3 heart sound and B-type natriuretic peptide levels in emergency department patients with dyspnea. J Card Fail. 2006;12(4):286–92.

25. Collins S, Peacock W, Clopton P, et al. 152: Audicor S3 outperforms emergency physicians' ability to diagnose acute heart failure at the bedside. Ann Emerg Med. 2007;50(3):S49.

26. Collins SP, Peacock WF, Lindsell CJ, et al. S3 detection as a diagnostic and prognostic aid in emergency department patients with acute dyspnea. Ann Emerg Med. 2009;53(6):748–57.

27. Carr BG, Dean AJ, Everett WW, et al. Intensivist bedside ultrasound (INBU) for volume assessment in the intensive care unit: a pilot study. J Trauma. 2007;63(3):495–500. Discussion 500–502.

28. Yanagawa Y, Sakamoto T, Okada Y. Hypovolemic shock evaluated by sonographic measurement of the inferior vena cava during resuscitation in trauma patients. J Trauma. 2007;63(6):1245–8. discussion 1248.

29. Lyon M, Blaivas M, Brannam L. Sonographic measurement of the inferior vena cava as a marker of blood loss. Am J Emerg Med. 2005;23(1):45–50.

30. Kimura BJ, Dalugdugan R, Gilcrease GW, et al. The effect of breathing manner on inferior vena caval diameter. Eur J Echocardiogr. 2010;12(2):120–3.

31. Agricola E, Bove T, Oppizzi M, et al. "Ultrasound comet-tail images": a marker of pulmonary edema: a comparative study with wedge pressure and extravascular lung water. Chest. 2005;127(5):1690–5.

32. Noble VE, Murray AF, Capp R, et al. Ultrasound assessment for extravascular lung water in patients undergoing hemodialysis. Chest. 2009;135(6):1433–9.
33. Liteplo AS, Marill KA, Villen T, et al. Emergency thoracic ultrasound in the differentiation of the etiology of shortness of breath (ETUDES): sonographic B-lines and N-terminal pro-brain-type natriuretic peptide in diagnosing congestive heart failure. Acad Emerg Med. 2009;16(3): 201–10.
34. Kamath SA, Drazner MH, Tasissa G, et al. Correlation of impedance cardiography with invasive hemodynamic measurements in patients with advanced heart failure: the BioImpedance CardioGraphy (BIG) Substudy of the ESCAPE Trial. Am Heart J. 2009;158(2):217–23.
35. Packer M, Abraham WT, Mehra MR. Utility of impedance cardiography for the identification of short-term risk of clinical decompensation in stable patients with chronic heart failure. J Am Coll Cardiol. 2006;47(11):2245–52.
36. Di Somma S, De Berardinis B, Bongiovanni C, et al. Use of BNP and bioimpedance to drive therapy in heart failure patients. Congest Heart Fail. 2010;16 Suppl 1:S56–61.
37. Piccoli A. Bioelectric impedance vector distribution in peritoneal dialysis patients with different hydration status. Kidney Int. 2004;65(3):1050–63.
38. Piccoli A, Pittoni G, Facco E, Favaro E, Pillon L. Relationship between central venous pressure and bioimpedance vector analysis in critically ill patients. Crit Care Med. 2000;28(1): 132–7.
39. Uszko-Lencer NHMK, Bothmer F, van Pol PEJ, Schols AMWJ. Measuring body composition in chronic heart failure: a comparison of methods. Eur J Heart Fail. 2006;8(2):208–14.

Chapter 11
Diagnostic and Prognostic Biomarkers in Emergency Department Heart Failure

Yang Xue, Arrash Fard, Navaid Iqbal, and Alan Maisel

Introduction

In the USA, there are three million heart failure admissions per year, with 35% of cases progressing to death or readmissions within 60 days. In spite of major advances in therapy, prognosis for heart failure remains poor. Challenges still remain in timely diagnosis of acute heart failure and accurate risk stratification of patients with heart failure. Biomarkers, with their objectivity and widespread availability, have an indispensible role in improving heart failure management. Among the biomarkers available today, natriuretic peptides are the most validated and accepted for acute heart failure diagnosis. For prognostic evaluation of heart failure, natriuretic peptides, troponin, creatinine, blood urea nitrogen (BUN), serum sodium, and novel biomarkers such as mid-region proadrenomedullin (MR-proADM) and C-terminal pre-pro-vasopressin (copeptin) have all been shown to be effective in identifying high-risk patients who are more likely to have adverse clinical outcomes.

It is important to note that heart failure is a complicated disease, involving dysfunctions in multiple physiological processes. A biomarker representing a single pathophysiological process is unlikely to be sufficient for the evaluation of heart failure patients. A multimarker approach utilizing biomarkers representing different pathophysiological processes is required to adequately assess the risk profile of a given heart failure patient. As a result, significant effort has been placed on biomarker research, leading to the emergence of several promising novel biomarkers for heart failure diagnosis and risk stratification.

Y. Xue, MD (✉) • A. Fard, MD • N. Iqbal, MD • A. Maisel, MD
VA San Diego Healthcare System, San Diego, CA, USA
e-mail: yxue100@yahoo.com

W. Frank Peacock (ed.), *Short Stay Management of Acute Heart Failure*,
Contemporary Cardiology, DOI 10.1007/978-1-61779-627-2_11,
© Springer Science+Business Media, LLC 2012

Natriuretic Peptides

Natriuretic peptides have become a staple in assisting the clinical diagnosis of acute heart failure. The most relevant biomarkers in this peptide family are B-type natriuretic peptide (BNP), N-terminal prohormone BNP (NT-proBNP), and atrial natriuretic peptide (ANP). BNP was originally isolated from the porcine brain, leading to its original name "brain natriuretic peptide," although it is made predominantly in the cardiac ventricles in humans. BNP is a 32-amino-acid peptide hormone with an in vivo half-life of 20 min. BNP is a cleavage product of NT-proBNP, which itself is a cleavage product of prohormone BNP, a 134-amino-acid peptide. NT-proBNP is a 76-amino-acid peptide with an in vivo half-life of 120 min. ANP is a 28-amino-acid peptide hormone first isolated from the atrial tissue of rats. Among the three, BNP and NT-proBNP are more validated by clinical trials and more widely used in today's clinical practice (Table 11.1). Natriuretic peptides are released by the cardiac ventricles in response to increased wall stress caused by the volume expansion and pressure overload that accompanies heart failure. They are protective hormones that serve to counteract the physiological abnormalities of heart failure. Their functions include increasing glomerular filtration rate (GFR), increasing sodium and water excretion, increasing vasodilation by relaxing arterioles and venules, inhibiting cardiac hypertrophy, and inhibiting renin and aldosterone secretion [1].

The need for biomarkers in diagnosing acute heart failure stemmed from the fact that differentiating between pulmonary and cardiac causes of acute dyspnea has traditionally been a challenge as the physical exam, laboratory, and radiographical finding between the two conditions have significant overlap. Delayed diagnosis and therapy for acute heart failure not only increase morbidity and cost but also lead to increased mortality, making accurate diagnosis of heart failure in the emergency department imperative. A quick, simple, and objective test can greatly aid in the diagnostic workup of patients with acute dyspnea. BNP and NT-proBNP have emerged to fill in the role of this much-needed supplement to history and physical exam. Over the years, the use of natriuretic peptides has expanded into prognostic evaluation of heart failure patients.

Table 11.1 Characteristics of BNP and NT-proBNP

	BNP	NT-proBNP
Components	BNP molecule	NT fragments (1–76) NT-proBNP (1–108)
Molecular weight	4 kDa	8.5 kDa
Genesis	Cleavage from NT-proBNP	Release from ventricular myocytes
Half-life	20 min	120 min
Clearance mechanism	Neutral endopeptidase clearance receptors	Renal clearance
Increase with normal aging	+	++++
Correlation with estimated glomerular filtration rate	−0.20	−0.60
Approved cutoff(s) for CHF diagnosis	100 pg/mL	Age < 75: 125 pg/mL Age > 75: 450 pg/mL
Studies completed	1,370	39
Entry on US market	Nov 2000	Dec 2002

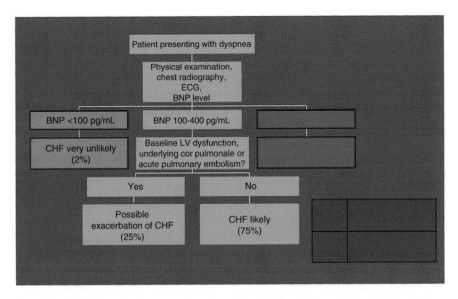

Fig. 11.1 Algorithm using B-type natriuretic peptide (BNP) and N-terminal prohormone B-type natriuretic peptide (NT-proBNP) levels to rule in and rule out congestive heart failure (CHF). ECG indicates electrocardiography; *LV* left ventricular (Copyright MedReviews, LLC. Reprinted with permission of MedReviews, LLC. Maisel A. B-Type natriuretic peptide measurements in diagnosing congestive heart failure in the dyspneic emergency department patient. Rev Cardiovas Med. 2002; 3(suppl 4):S10–S17. Reviews in Cardiovascular Medicine is a copyrighted publication of MedReviews, LLC. All rights reserved)

Natriuretic Peptides in the Diagnosis of Acute Heart Failure

Although BNP was first isolated by Sudoh et al. in 1988, its role as a biomarker in acute heart failure was not established until 2002. The multicenter Breathing Not Properly trial, by Maisel et al., was the first study to validate the effectiveness of BNP in the diagnostic workup of patients presenting to the emergency department (ED) with acute dyspnea. In this study, a BNP > 100 pg/mL was shown to be 73% specific and 90% sensitive for the diagnosis of acute heart failure with a diagnostic accuracy of 83.4%. The negative predictive value of BNP < 50 pg/mL for acute heart failure was 96% [2]. Besides BNP, NT-proBNP has also been studied extensively for the diagnostic evaluation of patients with acute dyspnea. In a study by Januzzi et al., NT-proBNP was shown to have comparable sensitivity and slightly higher specificity (90% sensitive and 85% specificity) for the diagnosis of acute heart failure [3]. Natriuretic peptide levels are highly reproducible and can be checked with ease in a typical clinical laboratory. Adding natriuretic peptide levels to the standard diagnostic evaluation of acutely dyspneic patients can significantly reduce clinical indecision and diagnostic lag time, leading to their widespread acceptance (Fig. 11.1). ANP, although discovered around the same time as BNP, suffers from in vitro instability, which has limited its use in routine clinical practice. Recently, biochemical assays targeting a stable fragment of the ANP prohormone, mid-region proANP (MR-proANP) became available, leading to the emergence of ANP as

Table 11.2 MR-proANP vs. BNP for diagnosis of acute heart failure

Measure	Sensitivity	Specificity	Accuracy
MR-proANP 120 pmol/L	95.56	59.85	72.64
BNP 100 pg/mL	96.98	61.90	73.50
Difference	1.42	2.05	0.86
Upper 95% limit	2.82	3.84	2.10
Noninferiority p	<0.0001	<0.0001	<0.0001

MR-pro ANP mid-regional pro atrial natriuretic peptide, *BNP* B-type natriuretic peptide

a diagnostic in acute heart failure. The diagnostic utility of MR-proANP was examined in a large-scale multinational study, Biomarker in Acute Heart Failure (BACH) trial by Maisel et al. in 2008. In the BACH trial, 1,641 patients with acute dyspnea were studied for the diagnostic accuracy of MR-proANP for acute heart failure. This study demonstrated that MR-proANP ≥ 120 pmol/L was noninferior to BNP > 100 pg/L for the diagnosis of acute heart failure (Table 11.2). Requiring both BNP and MR-proANP to be elevated increased the diagnostic accuracy of acute heart failure to 76.6% comparing 73.6% for BNP elevation alone. In addition, MR-proANP measurements added to the diagnostic accuracy of BNP in patients with intermediate BNP value and obesity, but not in renal insufficiency, elderly patients, and patients with edema. MR-proANP added to the diagnostic utility of NT-proBNP in patients with intermediate values, obesity, renal insufficiency, elderly patients, and patients with edema [4].

Natriuretic Peptides in the Prognostic Evaluation of Heart Failure

Another important function of natriuretic peptides is their use in the risk stratification of heart failure patients. The ability to accurately risk stratify patients can allow clinicians to tailor therapy to fit each patient's needs. These individualized treatments will not only decrease morbidity and mortality but also reduce cost to the overall health system. Both BNP and NT-proBNP have been studied with promising results in the prognostic evaluation of heart failure patients.

Multiple natriuretic peptide studies have been performed in the ED setting, mostly in patients presenting with acute dyspnea. While the majority of these studies focused on the diagnostic utility of natriuretic peptides, major prognostic evidence had arisen as well. For example, the ADHERE (Acute Decompensated Heart Failure National Registry) database of 65,275 acute heart failure patients showed that BNP level at the time of admission had a nearly linear relationship with the risk for in-hospital mortality. The adjusted odds ratio for mortality between BNP quartile 4 (BNP > 1,730 pg/mL) and BNP quartile 1 (BNP < 430 pg/mL) was 2.23 with $p < 0.0001$. In addition, initial ED BNP levels can identify patients at high risk for 30-day mortality or readmission [5]. NT-proBNP is also highly prognostic in patients with acute heart failure. Januzzi et al. demonstrated that an ED NT-proBNP level greater than 1,000 pg/mL is indicative of severe heart failure and is associated with adverse prognosis. Furthermore, the IMPROVE-CHF (Canadian Multicenter

Improved Management of Patients with Congestive Heart Failure) study showed that knowing a patient's NT-proBNP level during ED evaluation can decrease the duration of the ED visit by 21% and reduce 60-day rehospitalization rate by 35% in addition to reducing overall medical costs [6].

The prognostic value of natriuretic peptides can play an important role in guiding treatment strategies. Having a baseline natriuretic peptide level when a patient's heart failure is stable can go a long way to assist with prognostic evaluation when he/she goes into acute heart failure. Acute heart failure patients whose natriuretic peptide levels remain elevated despite appropriate inpatient therapy often have a poorer prognosis and require closer follow-up in the outpatient setting. For example, Bettencourt et al. showed that among 182 patients admitted to the hospital for acute heart failure, discharge NT-proBNP above median (>4,137 pg/mL) was associated with increased postdischarge adverse outcomes. He also showed that the change in NT-proBNP values with treatment is highly prognostic. Patients with NT-proBNP increase greater than 30% from admission to discharge had the worse outcome, followed by patients with less than 30% change in NT-proBNP levels. Patients with more than 30% decrease in NT-proBNP levels had the best outcome. The single best predictor of mortality and readmission in this study was the change in NT-proBNP levels from admission to discharge [7]. Within the hospital setting, the current general consensus is to obtain a natriuretic peptide value with admission and again prior to discharge when the patient is deemed to be clinically optivolemic. Repeat natriuretic peptide levels are suggested if there is clinical deterioration. While some trials have shown that the lower the natriuretic peptide level at discharge, the lower the risk of death and readmission, overall, the literature has been inconsistent. Still, an as-low-as-possible natriuretic peptide level is a reasonable goal for clinicians to aim for while treating a patient for acute heart failure. In fact, a BNP level of <350 pg/mL or NT-proBNP level < 4,000 pg/mL at discharge is generally linked to a stable posthospital course, which is especially true if the patient is clinically optivolemic.

As to why a patient's natriuretic peptide levels can remain elevated despite recommended in-hospital treatment, the answer may be multifactorial. First, the high natriuretic peptide levels could reflect the severity of patient's baseline heart failure, which may result in persistently elevated ventricular wall stress. Second, excessive treatment with diuretics may cause the patient to enter a prerenal state leading to a decreased GFR. Because natriuretic peptides are partly cleared by the kidneys, a decreased GFR can lead to inappropriately elevated natriuretic peptide levels due to poor clearance. In patients with concurrent right heart failure leading to edema and ascites, significant diuresis can occur prior to any effects on ventricular preload, resulting in persistent elevation of ventricular wall stress despite diuresis. Finally, there is the possibility that the treatment was inadequate and ventricular wall stress remains elevated despite treatment [3].

Perhaps the most exciting and rapidly expanding use of natriuretic peptides is in the outpatient setting, where natriuretic peptides can help to identify patients who are at high risk for future adverse events. For example, the Framingham Offspring Study, which evaluated 3,346 asymptomatic outpatients, demonstrated that elevated natriuretic peptide levels were predictive of future adverse cardiovascular events and mortality. In this particular cohort, BNP values above the 80th percentile were associated with increased risk for death (hazard ratio = 1.62, $p = 0.02$), first major cardiovascular event (hazard ratio = 1.76, $p = 0.03$), atrial fibrillation (hazard ratio = 1.91, $p = 0.02$), stroke or transient ischemic attack (hazard ratio = 1.99, $p = 0.02$), and heart failure (hazard ratio = 3.07, $p = 0.002$) [8]. These natriuretic peptide elevations in asymptomatic patients may reflect a change in cardiac or renal function that has not yet manifested as clinical deterioration. Measuring natriuretic peptides in these patients can help to identify clinical deteriorations early on and assist with therapeutic interventions to prevent the development of significant symptoms.

In outpatient management of heart failure, it is very important to know each patient's optivolemic natriuretic peptide level, which can serve as a baseline for comparison during subsequent evaluations. This is especially true in cases where symptoms have not yet appeared. A greater than 50% rise of natriuretic peptide levels from baseline is associated with high risk for impending heart failure decompensation. The clinician must also keep in mind that small changes in natriuretic peptide levels (<50% of baseline levels) could reflect biological variability in some patients and may not represent a forthcoming clinical event. Therefore, a detailed history, physical exam, and standard laboratory values are still very important in heart failure management.

Natriuretic Peptide-Guided Heart Failure Therapy

With increasing data supporting the prognostic utility of natriuretic peptide, there have been several attempts to use natriuretic peptides to guide outpatient heart failure therapy with relative success. The first large-scale natriuretic peptide-guided therapy study was the STAR-BNP study by Troughton et al. STAR-BNP was a multicenter study comparing the outcomes of BNP-guided therapy against standard clinical therapy according to current guidelines. A total of 220 NYHA class II and III patients optimally managed with ACE inhibitors, beta-blockers, and diuretics were involved in the study. These patients were randomized to receive either BNP-guided therapy with a goal BNP of <100 pg/mL or standard clinical therapy according to guidelines at the time. The patients were followed for up to 15 months for a primary endpoint of heart failure-related death or admission. By the end of the study, the BNP-guided arm had significantly fewer patients reaching primary endpoint than the standard clinical therapy arm (24% vs. 52%, $p < 0.001$) [9]. The STAR-BNP study was followed by the BATTLESCARRED study, which was a large-scale study comparing NT-proBNP-guided therapy, intensive clinical management (treatment by a heart failure management team led by heart failure specialists), and usual care (treatment at the discretion of a primary care physician). A total of 366 patients were enrolled and followed for up to 3 years. The study found that 1-year mortality was significantly less in both the NT-proBNP-guided therapy arm (9.1%) and the intensive clinical management arm (9.1%) when compared to the usual care arm (18.%; $p = 0.03$). In addition, the study found that in patients less than 75 years of age, the

3-year mortality is significantly lower in the NT-proBNP-guided arm (15.5%) when compared to both the intensive clinical management arm (30.9%, $p = 0.048$) and the usual care arm (31.3% and $p = 0.021$), highlighting the long-term benefit of natriuretic peptide-guided therapy [10]. The largest natriuretic peptide-guided heart failure therapy trial was the TIME-CHF trial, which was a prospective randomized study evaluating the effectiveness of NT-proBNP-guided therapy versus symptom-guided therapy with a total of 499 chronic heart failure patients followed for up to 18 months. This study found similar rates of survival free of all-cause hospitalizations between the NT-proBNP-guided therapy arm and symptom-guided therapy arm (41% vs. 40%, respectively; $p = 0.39$). Additionally, NT-proBNP-guided heart failure therapy led to higher rates of survival free of all-cause hospitalizations in patients aged 60–75 years ($p < 0.02$) [11]. These studies have consistently shown the long-term effectiveness of natriuretic peptide-guided heart failure therapy, highlighting the potential benefit of adding natriuretic peptides to future heart failure treatment algorithms.

Natriuretic Peptides for Heart Failure Screening

Finally, using natriuretic peptides in screening for asymptomatic heart failure patients is also a possibility in the future, as many patients with left ventricular dysfunction would have elevations in natriuretic peptide levels prior to developing symptoms of heart failure. This would be a far more convenient and cost-effective method than the current gold standard for left ventricular dysfunction detection, the echocardiogram. There are many reasons why screening with natriuretic peptides would be beneficial. First of all, cardiac disorders are common and are a source of considerable morbidity and mortality. Additionally, natriuretic peptides are elevated early in the disease process, often before symptoms develop and thus can allow for early treatment. Finally, early treatment in heart failure is associated with better outcomes and is more cost-effective than delayed action. The future of natriuretic peptide use in the outpatient setting, whether it be managing chronic heart failure or screening for new cases, is bright, and the utility of natriuretic peptides is only going to increase with time.

Caveats of Natriuretic Peptide Use

In order to optimally use natriuretic peptides in clinical practice, the clinician must be aware of important caveats and limitations of their use:

- Obesity: Natriuretic peptide levels are generally lower in obese patients both with and without heart failure. The reason for this is currently not completely understood. It may have to do with increased natriuretic peptide receptor-C clearance receptors on adipocytes. This is supported by the fact that obese patients still have elevated levels of precursor hormones despite having low BNP and

NT-proBNP levels. Measured natriuretic peptide levels in obese patients should be multiplied by a factor of two to three to account for this discrepancy.

• Gray zone: In relation to diagnosis, moderate increases in natriuretic peptides fall into the "gray zone" where the evidence is not as strong in supporting an acute heart failure diagnosis. In these cases, clinical acumen is especially important, and other causes of myocardial stress should to be considered, such as pulmonary hypertension, pulmonary embolism, arrhythmias, acute coronary syndrome, pneumonia, or COPD with cor pulmonale.

• Renal disease: As mentioned above, renal disease can influence natriuretic peptide levels through several mechanisms including decreased clearance of natriuretic peptides and counter-regulatory responses from cardiorenal syndrome. It has been suggested that natriuretic peptide cutoffs for patients with a GFR <60 mL/min may need to be raised. Detailed knowledge of a patient's renal function is important when natriuretic peptides are used for clinical assessment.

• Shock: Natriuretic peptide values have been shown to be unreliable in cases of shock and therefore should be avoided in hemodynamically unstable patients.

Blood Urea Nitrogen

BUN is a serum by-product of protein metabolism. It is probably one of the oldest prognostic biomarkers in heart failure. Urea is formed by the liver and carried by the blood to the kidneys for excretion. Diseased or damaged kidneys cause BUN to accumulate in the blood as the GFR goes down. Conditions such as hypovolemic shock, congestive heart failure, high protein diet, and bleeding into the gastrointestinal tract will also cause BUN elevations. BUN plays a unique role as a short-term as well as long-term prognostic marker in patients with heart failure. In 2005, Fonarrow et al. analyzed the ADHERE database for predictors of in-hospital mortality among 65,275 acute heart failure admissions. Of the 39 variables evaluated in this database, BUN≥43 mg/dL was the single best predictor of mortality, followed by admission systolic blood pressure <115 mmHg and serum creatinine ≥2.75 mg/dL (243.1 μmol/L) [12]. Another study done by Aronson et al. in 2004, which involved 541 patients with acute heart failure, examined the prognostic utility of BUN, serum creatinine, BUN/creatinine ratio, and estimated creatinine clearance. There were 177 mortalities in this cohort, and the mean follow-up period was 343 ± 185 days. The risk of all-cause mortality increased significantly with each quartile of BUN, with an adjusted relative risk of 2.3 in patients in the upper quartiles ($p = 0.005$). Creatinine and estimated creatinine clearance were not statistically significant predictors of mortality after adjustment for other covariates. BUN/creatinine ratio yielded similar prognostic information as BUN (adjusted relative risk = 2.3; $p = 0.0007$ for patients in the upper quartiles) [13]. As seen in these studies, elevated BUN levels are strongly associated with adverse outcomes in patients hospitalized for acute heart failure. Therefore, BUN levels should be considered in the routine prognostic evaluation of patients with acute heart failure.

Creatinine

Creatinine is a breakdown product of creatine phosphate in muscle tissue. It is usually produced at a fairly constant rate. Creatinine is cleared by the kidneys with little-to-no tubular reabsorption. Creatinine accumulates in the blood when GFR decreases in the setting of renal dysfunction. As a result, serum creatinine levels are commonly used to calculate the creatinine clearance, which is a surrogate for GFR and renal function. Since renal dysfunction is a negative prognostic factor in patients with heart failure, elevations of creatinine are associated with poor outcomes in heart failure patients. This was shown in a study by Vaz Perez et al. in 2009, involving 128 patients who were hospitalized for acute heart failure. In this study, elevated admission creatinine level was a strong predictor of both 1-year and 5-year mortality. For 1-year mortality, creatinine and ejection fracture were both independent predictors of mortality in multivariable analysis ($p < 0.001$), whereas body mass index and NYHA class did not reach statistical significance. In the multivariate analysis for 5-year mortality, creatinine and NYHA class were independent predictors of all-cause mortality ($p < 0.001$), whereas body mass index and age did not reach statistical significance [14]. In another study by Aronson et al. involving 467 patients with acute heart failure, persistent creatinine elevation above baseline was associated with significantly worse outcomes. Persistent creatinine elevation in this study was defined as ≥0.5 mg/dL increase in serum creatinine above baseline for more than 30 days. Transient creatinine elevation was defined as creatinine elevation ≥0.5 mg/dL above baseline that subsequently decreased to <0.5 mg/dL above baseline within 30 days. Persistent creatinine elevation was seen in 115 patients and transient creatinine elevation was seen in 39 patients. The 6-month mortality rates were 17.3% in patients without creatinine elevation, 20.5% in patients with transient creatinine elevation, and 46.1% in patients with persistent creatinine elevation. Compared to patients stable creatinine (<0.5 mg/dL increase from baseline), the adjusted hazard ratio for mortality was 3.2 ($p < 0.0001$) in patients with persistent creatinine elevation [15]. These studies highlighted the fact that elevated creatinine level is a strong predictor of medium- and long-term mortality in patients with heart failure and can serve as a fast and inexpensive biomarker to help identify patients at high risk for mortality.

Troponin

Troponin, a biomarker widely used for the diagnosis of myocardial infarction, is increasingly being recognized as a valuable biomarker for risk stratification of heart failure patients. Elevated troponin levels have long been associated with increased in-hospital and long-term mortality, as shown by Peacock et al. in an analysis of the ADHERE database. In this analysis, patients admitted for acute heart failure were risk stratified by admission troponin levels. Positive troponin was defined as troponin I greater than 1,000 ng/L and troponin T greater than 100 ng/L. From this database,

4,240 patients had positive troponin by this definition. Patients with positive troponin had significantly increased risk for in-hospital mortality when compared to patients with negative troponin (odds ratio=2.55; $p<0.001$) [16]. These findings have also been shown in the recently published BACH trial where acute heart failure patients with elevated troponin had significantly increased mortality [6]. Recently, the availability of new high-sensitivity troponin assays capable of measuring troponin I in the ng/L range made it possible to detect troponin levels in virtually all patients with heart failure. In a study by our group, we examined 144 patients hospitalized for acute heart failure with serial measurements of troponin I. Using a high-sensitivity troponin I assay, troponin levels were detectable in every patient in the study. We found that patients with small troponin elevations at discharge (troponin I > 23.25 ng/L) have significantly higher risk for 90-day mortality and readmission than patients with troponin I less than 23.25 ng/L (hazard ratio=3.547; $p=0.003$). Patients with small troponin elevations and BNP elevations are at even higher risk for mortality and readmission comparing to patients without elevations in troponin and BNP (hazard ratio=15.972; $p=0.007$). In addition, we found that patients with increasing troponin levels during hospitalization have significantly increased risk for 90-day mortality than those with stable or decreasing troponin levels (hazard ratio=4.520; $p=0.047$) [17]. The significance of our findings lies in the fact that every patient included in the analysis had measurable troponin levels, thus extending the prognostic value of troponin to the entire acute heart failure population. Furthermore, since the trend of troponin levels during acute heart failure treatment is prognostic of adverse events, serial measurements of troponin levels should be considered during hospitalization for acute heart failure. Once validated by larger trials, high-sensitivity troponin measurements are likely to become a routine part of the evaluation and treatment of acute heart failure patients.

Sodium

It is well known that hyponatremia is a common consequence of heart failure and is associated with worse outcomes. The cause of hyponatremia in heart failure is complex and involves several pathophysiological processes. Decreased cardiac output due to heart failure leads to activation of the renin–angiotensin–aldosterone system (RAAS), increased sympathetic discharge, and the release of vasopressin from the posterior pituitary gland. The RAAS decreases sodium and water delivery to the collecting duct by increasing tubular reabsorption while further stimulating the sympathetic nervous system and increasing vasopressin release. The sympathetic nervous system also stimulates RAAS and further potentiates sodium and water conservation via renal afferent vasoconstriction and direct action on the proximal tubules. Finally, vasopressin upregulates aquaporin channels in the collecting ducts, leading to increased water reabsorption. The combined effect of these pathophysiological pathways forms a vicious cycle of sodium and free water retention, leading to hyponatremia, worse heart failure symptoms, and increased mortality [18].

As a result, serum sodium measurements could help to give clinicians a glimpse of the prognosis of a patient. In a trial by Kearney et al. involving 553 outpatients, serum sodium was shown to be an independent predictor of all-cause mortality during their 5-year follow-up period. In fact, for a 2 mmol/L decrease in serum sodium, the calculated hazard ratio was 1.22 ($p<0.01$) [19]. Furthermore, in a retrospective study of 4,031 outpatients with heart failure by Lee et al., serum sodium <136 mmol/L was associated with a 50% increased risk of mortality at both 30 days and 1 year [20]. Finally, Klein et al. reported from the OPTIME-CHF study that serum sodium is a significant predictor of increased 60-day mortality with a hazard ratio of 1.18 per 3 mEq/dL decrease in serum sodium ($p=0.018$). Hyponatremic patients also had longer hospital stays and higher 60-day rehospitalization rates in this study [15]. Although hyponatremia is associated with worse outcomes in heart failure patients, one must keep in mind that multiple factors influence serum sodium levels, including both pathophysiological processes and medications, which must be taken into consideration when serum sodium is used for the prognostic evaluation of heart failure patients.

Emerging Biomarkers of Heart Failure

Over the past decade, significant progress has been made in the discovery of new biomarkers representing different physiological processes with the potential to improve the accuracy of diagnostic and prognostic evaluation of heart failure patients. The biomarkers worth mentioning are mid-region proadrenomedullin (MR-proADM), C-terminal pre-pro-vasopressin (copeptin), and ST2.

Mid-region Proadrenomedullin

Adrenomedullin (ADM) is a 52-amino-acid ringed peptide with C-terminal amidation. It was first isolated from human pheochromocytoma cells. Since its first report, studies examining the effects of ADM have increased exponentially, highlighting its important role in physiology. ADM is a peptide hormone with natriuretic, vasodilatory, and hypotensive effects mediated by cyclic adenosine monophosphate (cAMP), nitric oxide, and renal prostaglandin systems. ADM expression is seen in many tissues and organ systems, including cardiovascular, renal, pulmonary, cerebrovascular, gastrointestinal, and endocrine tissues. ADM acts as both a circulating hormone and a local autocrine and paracrine hormone. ADM plasma concentrations are increased in hypertension, chronic renal disease, and heart failure [21]. Despite its important role in many disease processes, for many years, the clinical application of ADM was limited by its in vitro instability. This problem has been solved by the emergence of the mid-region (MR) biomarkers, which are stable fragments of prohormones. One of these mid-region markers is MR-proADM, which is a stable fragment of proadrenomedullin. MR-proADM is released in a one-to-one fashion to the active ADM, and its serum levels mirror that of ADM [22].

The prognostic potential of MR-proADM was demonstrated in the recently published BACH trial. Among the 1,641 patients enrolled in the study, 568 patients were diagnosed with acute heart failure. In this acute heart failure population, MR-proADM not only carried independent prognostic value but was also found to be superior to both BNP and NT-proBNP in predicting mortality within 14 days. MR-proADM also provided significant additive incremental predictive value for 90-day mortality when added to BNP and NT-proBNP [6]. Despite the promising results shown above, MR-proADM is still a very nascent biomarker. Significant work is needed to fully define its role in clinical management of heart failure patients.

Copeptin

Copeptin is a powerful new mid-region biomarker discovered in recent years. It is a fragment of the vasopressin prohormone pre-pro-vasopressin. Pre-pro-vasopressin is cleaved into copeptin and vasopressin inside the posterior pituitary gland. Postcleavage, both copeptin and vasopressin are released in equimolar amounts into circulation and cleared by the kidneys. It is well known that vasopressin is a major contributor to hyponatremia. In addition, elevated vasopressin is consistently seen in patients with severe heart failure, highlighting vasopressin's potential as a prognostic biomarker. However, vasopressin has not been widely used in clinical practice due to its rapid clearance and in vitro instability. Unlike vasopressin, copeptin is very stable in vitro, making it an ideal surrogate biomarker for vasopressin. In the BACH trial, which is the largest trial examining copeptin in patients with acute heart failure, elevated copeptin levels were associated with increased 14-day mortality, heart failure-related readmissions, and heart failure-related emergency department visits. In addition, mortality is significantly increased in patients with elevated copeptin (above median) and low sodium (below median: <139 mEq/L) (data not yet published). These findings highlighted the prognostic utility of copeptin in patients with acute heart failure and opened the door to future copeptin-guided vasopressin antagonist therapy in acute heart failure patients.

ST2

ST2 is yet another up-and-coming cardiac biomarker that has recently gained increasing interest in heart failure. ST2 is a member of the interleukin-1 receptor family of proteins and acts as the receptor to IL-33. It was first identified in cultured cardiac myocytes [23]. The ST2 gene was found to be highly upregulated when mechanical strain was applied to myocytes. Mice with ST2 gene knockout can develop severe cardiac hypertrophy, fibrosis, and heart failure, suggesting that ST2 may have a cardioprotective effect in response to myocyte strain and injury. There are two transcripts of the ST2 gene, soluble and the membrane-bound IL-33 receptors. The interactions between IL-33 and the two ST2 forms are complex and currently incompletely understood, but some light has been shed on their functions. The IL-33/

ST2 complex is believed to be protective to the myocardium under strain by acting as an activated fibroblast-cardiomyocyte paracrine system that works to prevent hypertrophy and fibrosis. The soluble ST2 receptor is believed to play a modulating role in the interaction between IL-33 and the membrane-bound ST2 receptor. Over the long term, the IL-33/ST2 complex may have a role in the inflammatory and remodeling processes of the myocardium in heart failure patients [24].

Despite some of the lingering questions about the exact physiological functions of ST2, the fact that it is significantly upregulated during myocyte strain has spawned several studies to assess its role as a biomarker in heart failure. In a trial of 139 patients with severe (NYHA III–IV) heart failure, Weinberg et al. found that baseline ST2 levels correlated very well with baseline BNP and proANP levels. Furthermore, a change in ST2 value at 2 weeks (when compared to baseline values) was predictive of mortality or heart transplantation in both univariate and multivariate analyses [25]. Another trial by Bayes-Genis et al. found a similar benefit in using a change in ST2 to risk stratify heart failure patients. They found that if the ratio of ST2 at 14 days, compared to baseline ST2, was greater than 0.75, it had an AUC of 0.772 for predicting 1-year cardiac events [26]. When applied to patients presenting to the ED with dyspnea, ST2 also had promising results. A post hoc analysis of the PRIDE (Pro-Brain Natriuretic Peptide Investigation of Dyspnea in the Emergency Department) study found that ST2 levels were higher in patients with acute heart failure than those without, but ST2 was inferior to NT-proBNP for diagnosing acute heart failure. Additionally, a ST2 value of 0.20 ng/mL or higher predicted 1-year mortality with a hazard ratios of 5.6 ($p < 0.001$) for all patients with dyspnea and 9.3 ($p = 0.03$) for patients with acute heart failure. Furthermore, a ST2 value of 0.29 ng/mL or higher is predictive of 1-year mortality with an AUC of 0.80 ($p < 0.001$) [27]. Finally, there has also been work on ST2's abilities to predict sudden cardiac death. One small study involving 99 patients showed that the combination of ST2 and NT-proBNP can help to identify patients at high risk for sudden cardiac death [28]. ST2 has also been shown to be predictive of adverse outcomes in stable outpatients. In a study by Daniels et al., which examined 558 stable patients who were referred for outpatient echocardiogram, elevated ST2 levels were associated with increased right atrial size, right ventricular dysfunction, and increased 1-year mortality. In this study, patients with increased BNP and ST2 levels are at even higher risk for mortality when compared to patients with normal BNP and ST2 levels [29]. Although significant work is still required before it is ready for clinical use, ST2 as a marker of myocardial inflammation, remodeling, and strain is an exciting new addition to the biomarker arsenal for the evaluation of heart failure patients.

Conclusion

Although significant work is still needed to further define their role in the overall management of heart failure patients, biomarkers with their objectivity, reproducibility, and accessibility are excellent adjuncts to physical examination and imaging studies in heart failure diagnosis and risk stratification. With advances in basic science, new biomarkers representing different physiological processes continue to emerge. Along with traditional predictors of prognosis, biomarkers can help to identify high-risk patients who need closer monitoring and more aggressive therapy. By continually enhancing our understanding of the underlying pathophysiology and improving our ability to identify high-risk individuals, biomarkers will undoubtedly improve the effectiveness of heart failure diagnosis and risk stratification, leading to better patient outcomes.

References

1. Maisel A, Mueller C, Adams Jr K, et al. State of the art: using natriuretic peptide levels in clinical practice. Eur J Heart Fail. 2008;10(9):824–39.
2. Maisel AS, Krishnaswamy P, Nowak RM, et al. Rapid measurement of B-type natriuretic peptide in the emergency diagnosis of heart failure. N Engl J Med. 2002;347(3):161–7.
3. Januzzi Jr JL, Camargo CA, Anwaruddin S, et al. The N-terminal Pro-BNP investigation of dyspnea in the emergency department (PRIDE) study. Am J Cardiol. 2005;95(8):948–54.
4. Maisel A, Mueller C, Nowak R, et al. Mid-region pro-hormone markers for diagnosis and prognosis in acute dyspnea: results from the BACH (Biomarkers in Acute Heart Failure) trial. J Am Coll Cardiol. 2010;55(19):2062–76.
5. Fonarow GC, Peacock WF, Phillips CO, et al. Admission B-type natriuretic peptide levels and in-hospital mortality in acute decompensated heart failure. J Am Coll Cardiol. 2007;49(19): 1943–50.
6. Moe GW, Howlett J, Januzzi JL, et al. N-terminal pro-B-type natriuretic peptide testing improves the management of patients with suspected acute heart failure: primary results of the Canadian prospective randomized multicenter IMPROVE-CHF study. Circulation. 2007;115(24):3103–10.
7. Bettencourt P, Azevedo A, Pimenta J, et al. N-terminal-pro-brain natriuretic peptide predicts outcome after hospital discharge in heart failure patients. Circulation. 2004;110:2168–74.
8. Wang TJ, Larson MG, Levy D, et al. Plasma natriuretic peptide levels and the risk of cardio-vascular events and death. N Engl J Med. 2004;350(7):655–63.
9. Jourdain P, Jondeau G, Funck F, et al. Plasma brain natriuretic peptide-guided therapy to improve outcome in heart failure: the STARS-BNP Multicenter Study. J Am Coll Cardiol. 2007;49(16):1733–9.
10. Lainchbury JG, Troughton RW, Strangman KM. N-terminal pro-B-type natriuretic peptide-guided treatment for chronic heart failure: results from the BATTLESCARRED (NT-proBNP-Assisted Treatment To Lessen Serial Cardiac Readmissions and Death) trial. J Am Coll Cardiol. 2009;55(1):53–60.
11. Pfisterer M, Buser P, Rickli H. BNP-guided vs symptom-guided heart failure therapy: the Trial of Intensified vs Standard Medical Therapy in Elderly Patients With Congestive Heart Failure (TIME-CHF) randomized trial. JAMA. 2009;301(4):383–92.
12. Fonarow GC, Adams Jr KF, Abraham WT, et al. Risk stratification for in-hospital mortality in acutely decompensated heart failure: classification and regression tree analysis. JAMA. 2005;293:572–80.
13. Aronson D, Mittleman MA, Burger AJ. Elevated blood urea nitrogen level as a predictor of mortality in patients admitted for decompensated heart failure. Am J Med. 2004;116:466–73.
14. Vaz Pérez A, Otawa K, Zimmermann AV, et al. The impact of impaired renal function on mortality in patients with acutely decompensated chronic heart failure. Eur J Heart Fail. 2010; 12(2):122–8.
15. Aronson D, Burger AJ. The relationship between transient and persistent worsening renal function and mortality in patients with acute decompensated heart failure. J Card Fail. 2010; 16(7):541–7.

16. Peacock 4th WF, De Marco T, Fonarow GC, et al. Cardiac troponin and outcome in acute heart failure. N Engl J Med. 2008;358(20):2117–26.
17. Xue Y, Clopton P, Peacock WF, et al. Serial changes in high-sensitive troponin I predict outcome in patients with decompensated heart failure. Eur J Heart Fail. 2011;13(1):37–42.
18. Klein L, O'Connor CM, Leimberger JD, et al. OPTIME-CHF Investigators. Lower serum sodium is associated with increased short-term mortality in hospitalized patients with worsening heart failure: results from the Outcomes of a Prospective Trial of Intravenous Milrinone for Exacerbations of Chronic Heart Failure (OPTIME-CHF) study. Circulation. 2005;111(19): 2454–60.
19. Kearney MT, Fox KA, Lee AJ, et al. Predicting death due to progressive heart failure in patients with mild-to-moderate chronic heart failure. J Am Coll Cardiol. 2002;40(10):1801–8.
20. Lee DS, Austin PC, Rouleau JL, et al. Predicting mortality among patients hospitalized for heart failure: derivation and validation of a clinical model. JAMA. 2003;290(19):2581–7.
21. Jougasaki M, Burnett Jr JC. Adrenomedullin: potential in physiology and pathophysiology. Life Sci. 2000;66(10):855–72.
22. Morgenthaler NG, Struck J, Alonso C, et al. Measurement of midregional proadrenomedullin in plasma with an immunoluminometricassay. Clin Chem. 2005;51:1823–9.
23. Weinberg EO, Shimpo M, de Keulenaer GW, et al. Expression and regulation of ST2, an interleukin-1 receptor family member, in cardiomyocytes and myocardial infarction. Circulation. 2002;106(23):2961–6.
24. Shah RV, Januzzi Jr JL. ST2: a novel remodeling biomarker in acute and chronic heart failure. Curr Heart Fail Rep. 2010;7(1):9–14.
25. Weinberg EO, Shimpo M, Hurwitz S, et al. Identification of serum soluble ST2 receptor as a novel heart failure biomarker. Circulation. 2003;107(5):721–6.
26. Bayes-Genis A, Pascual-Figal D, Januzzi JL, et al. Soluble ST2 monitoring provides additional risk stratification for outpatients with decompensated heart failure. Rev Esp Cardiol. 2010;63(10):1171–8.
27. Januzzi Jr JL, Peacock WF, Maisel AS, et al. Measurement of the interleukin family member ST2 in patients with acute dyspnea: results from the PRIDE (Pro-Brain Natriuretic Peptide Investigation of Dyspnea in the Emergency Department) study. J Am Coll Cardiol. 2007;50(7):607–13.
28. Pascual-Figal DA, Ordoñez-Llanos J, Tornel PL, et al. Soluble ST2 for predicting sudden cardiac death in patients with chronic heart failure and left ventricular systolic dysfunction. J Am Coll Cardiol. 2009;54(23):2174–9.
29. Daniels LB, Clopton P, Iqbal N, et al. Association of ST2 levels with cardiac structure and function and mortality in outpatients. Am Heart J. 2010;160(4):721–8.

Chapter 12
Emergency Department Therapy
of Acute Heart Failure

Phillip D. Levy

Overview

Acute heart failure (HF) is as a disorder of heterogeneous etiology that is largely defined by a single, homogenous symptom: dyspnea [1]. Other findings, including signs of systemic venous congestion and/or hypoperfusion, fatigue, weakness, and chest pain, may accompany breathlessness, but the degree to which they are present can vary greatly between patients. Consequently, conventional therapy is most often directed toward alleviation of dyspnea with the need for additional intervention dependent on the presence of other clinical abnormalities [2].

While most instances (~80%) of acute HF occur in patients with a history of chronic disease, a de novo presentation is not uncommon. Acute heart failure syndromes (AHFS), therefore, are often more than simple exacerbations of underlying chronic disease, and effective management requires an approach that considers the complex nature of this disorder. Often presumed to be a direct consequence of volume overload, AHFS is more accurately depicted by a model that considers the superimposition of potentially divergent precipitants on underlying systolic, diastolic, or mixed cardiac dysfunction [1, 3]. Effective treatment of AHFS, therefore, requires an understanding of the interplay between basal cardiovascular pathophysiology and those factors which specifically contribute to the decompensated state.

P.D. Levy, MD, MPH (✉)
Department of Emergency Medicine, Wayne State University School of Medicine,
Detroit, MI, USA
e-mail: plevy@med.wayne.edu

W. Frank Peacock (ed.), *Short Stay Management of Acute Heart Failure*,
Contemporary Cardiology, DOI 10.1007/978-1-61779-627-2_12,
© Springer Science+Business Media, LLC 2012

General Approach to Treatment

Treatment of AHFS can be broadly divided into a *stabilization phase*, where initial intervention directed toward immediate life-threatening conditions is followed by subsequent efforts to alleviate symptoms through targeted management of acute precipitants and an *in-hospital phase*, which involves continued remediation of residual signs and symptoms and ongoing surveillance for interval development of renal or cardiac injury [1]. The latter also includes initiation or up-titration of chronic therapy that is in accordance with existing, evidence-based guidelines such as those put forth by the Heart Failure Society of America [2] or the American College of Cardiology/American Heart Association [4] and predischarge planning with an eye on transition to the early postdischarge period.

The focus of this chapter will be on the stabilization phase of AHFS treatment, which generally occurs within the first 24–48 h of care. Initiation of this phase usually takes place (~80% of the time) in the emergency department (ED) and continues for most, depending on severity, in an inpatient (~85%) or observation unit (OU) setting. The primary goal of treatment during this early phase is symptom reduction which is often achieved by rebalancing hemodynamics and volume status [1]. The need to prevent myocardial or renal injury during this phase has gained increasing prominence with evolving data that show worse outcomes when these develop in hospital [5]. Cognizance of this is especially important because, in some cases, such myocardial and renal injury may be iatrogenically mediated through inappropriate or excessive medication administration (especially diuretics) [6], underscoring the need to deliver patient appropriate, targeted therapy.

Precipitants and Targeted Therapy

The goal of targeted therapy is to deliver the right medication to the right patient at the right time [7]. Doing so enables, at least in the acute phase of management, mitigation of the physiological perturbation which is most directly causing or contributing to cardiac decompensation. Common precipitants of AHFS (and their resulting consequences) include:

- *Acute hypertension*—an abrupt rise in blood pressure which causes impedance to forward flow by a structurally and/or functionally compromised left ventricle; net effect is a mismatch between necessary and achievable stroke volume resulting in a backflow of fluid from systemic to pulmonary vasculature ("vascular failure"); typically occurs in a patient with chronic hypertension.
- *Excess fluid accumulation*—neurohormonal activation (principally aldosterone and arginine vasopressin), worsening renal function, high dietary sodium consumption, excess fluid intake (or intravenous administration if AHFS develops in hospital), or medication noncompliance, either singularly or in combination, leads to fluid accumulation and increased preload; net effect is the presentation

of excess volume to a left ventricle which is incapable of responding by the Frank–Starling mechanism; consequence is a buildup of fluid in the lungs and onset of clinical pulmonary congestion ("congestive failure").

- *Acute or subacute myocardial dysfunction*—onset of ischemic, inflammatory (from infectious and noninfectious causes), or idiopathic myocardial damage that results in rapid development of cardiac dysfunction (either regionally or globally); net effect is to limit the heart's pumping ability which produces a precipitous decline in cardiac output ("pump failure").
- *Deterioration of advanced chronic heart failure*—overexertion, medication-related (under, over, or inappropriate use), worsening renal function, or indolent (i.e., "smoldering") myocardial necrosis; net effect is a progression of underlying advanced disease and an intolerable acute or subacute increase in baseline symptoms.
- *Dysrhythmia*—development of tachycardia (often atrial fibrillation) or, less commonly, bradycardia (often medication-related), which reduces the time spent in systole and/or diastole; net effect is to limit cardiac output through a decrease in ventricular filling and stroke volume.
- *Aortic or mitral valve dysfunction*—stenotic, regurgitant, or mechanical valve abnormality which develops acutely (often from infection or, in the case of mitral regurgitation, from ischemic complications such as left ventricular dilation with leaflet tethering or papillary muscle rupture) or subacutely (typically from worsening of underlying chronic valve disease); net effect is an increase in end-diastolic volume with consequent backflow into the pulmonary vasculature.

Identifying the specific precipitant (and hence, the acute pathophysiology to be targeted) can be facilitated by consideration of clinical variables. To make rapid but precise treatment decisions during the stabilization phase, such variables should be readily identifiable on presentation or available shortly after arrival. These variables can then be combined to yield clinical profiles that are more (or less) amenable to certain therapies.

Clinical Profiles

Clinical profiles in acute HF are defined by the presence (or absence) of relatively consistent features within important variable categories including presenting signs and symptoms (pulmonary congestion with or without systemic edema and evidence of hypoperfusion), hemodynamic parameters (primarily blood pressure and heart rate), and rapidly available diagnostic test results (electrocardiographic changes consistent with ischemia or infarct, biomarker indicators of acute renal and myocardial stress or injury, and findings consistent with heart failure on chest radiography) [1, 3, 8]. This approach differs from prior conceptual models of AHFS that incorporated pulmonary capillary wedge pressure and cardiac index (i.e., the "quadrants" of HF [9]), resulting in a framework that is more broadly applicable and user-friendly, without need for invasive hemodynamic assessment (which, with the exception of patients with advanced chronic heart failure or refractory cardiogenic shock, is associated with an unacceptable risk/benefit ratio).

In deriving clinical profiles (Table 12.1), blood pressure serves as a critical branch point [1, 3, 8]. Reasons for this relate to its clear importance as a precipitating factor (more than 50% of all AHFS episodes are associated with a systolic blood pressure >140 mm Hg) [10] and its role as the principal determinant of in-hospital morbidity and mortality [11]. While interpretation of these profiles within the context of echocardiograhically determined cardiac function may be useful for de novo cases where the underlying physiology is not known or in patients with refractory symptoms, in most circumstances, such information will not dramatically impact intervention during the stabilization phase. Moreover, for some patients with decompensated chronic disease, the presenting clinical profile may be more dependent on acute, precipitating factors than previously established echocardiographic abnormalities or underlying etiology (i.e., ischemic or nonischemic), and overreliance on the latter information may preclude application of situation-appropriate therapeutic intervention. An example of this would be the administration of aggressive diuresis to an established HF patient with reduced ejection fraction and systemic edema when in fact their acute decompensation was triggered by an episode of atrial fibrillation with rapid ventricular rate.

Specific Targets of Therapy

The importance of appropriate ED treatment of acute HF cannot be sufficiently underscored. Data from ADHERE (Acute Decompensated Heart Failure Registry) show that when intravenous (IV) vasoactive medications are started early by ED physicians rather than waiting for the inpatient service, outcomes such as mortality rate (4.3% vs. 10.9%), intensive care unit admission rate (4% vs. 20%), and total hospital length of stay (3 days vs. 7 days) are dramatically improved [12]. Therefore, knowing which agents to administer and the correct circumstance in which to administer them is critical. An overview of therapeutic targets within the context of clinical profiles can be found in Fig. 12.1. These targets are discussed in greater detail in the following sections with increased emphasis placed on those that are particularly relevant to management of the short-stay HF patient. While each is presented in isolation, there may be some overlap of targets in an individual patient, and as shown in Fig. 12.1, use of a combined approach to therapy may be warranted.

Acute Hypertension (Afterload)

As noted, elevated BP (systolic BP > 140 mm Hg) is present in more than half of all patients with AHFS, and for those with substantial dyspnea, appropriate, early vasodilatation can lead to substantial improvement in symptoms [13]. A number of

Table 12.1 Clinical profiles of acute heart failure

Profile	Common precipitants	Signs and symptoms	Hemodynamics on presentation
Profoundly hypertensive	Abrupt rise in BP	Rapid onset of dyspnea ("flash pulmonary edema"); systemic edema may be absent; diaphoresis with adequate perfusion typical	Systolic BP>160 mm Hg; sinus tachycardia and hypoxia common
Normal to moderately hypertensive	Progressive fluid accumulation	Gradual or subacute worsening of dyspnea; moderate to severe systemic edema; minimal distress with adequate perfusion	Systolic BP>100 mm Hg but <160 mm Hg; tachycardia and hypoxia uncommon
Hypotensive	Deterioration of advanced, chronic disease; excessive diuresis	Mild dyspnea; often with cool, edematous extremities	Systolic BP<90 mm Hg; HR often normal but may be <60 beats per min if on baseline medications with rate control effects
Cardiogenic shock	Myocardial injury, valve dysfunction	Rapid onset of dyspnea with evidence of profound hypoperfusion	Systolic BP<90 mm Hg; tachycardia common (unless on rate control agents)—may be ventricular in origin
Arrhythmogenic	Ventricular or supraventricular dysrhythmia	"Palpitations" and "dizziness"; mild to moderate dyspnea (often secondary feature); systemic edema may be present or absent	Systolic BP variable; HR <60 or >120 beats per min; hypoxia
Acute coronary syndrome	Acute myocardial ischemia or infarct	Chest pain with dyspnea	Systolic BP>100 mm Hg; HR variable; hypoxia less common
Isolated right heart failure	Right ventricular ischemia or infarct (right coronary or left circumflex); pulmonary hypertension; tricuspid or pulmonary valve dysfunction; pulmonary artery obstruction (embolism)	Dyspnea without rales; systemic edema if subacute or long standing	BP variable; tachycardia and hypoxia often present

BP blood pressure, *HR* heart rate

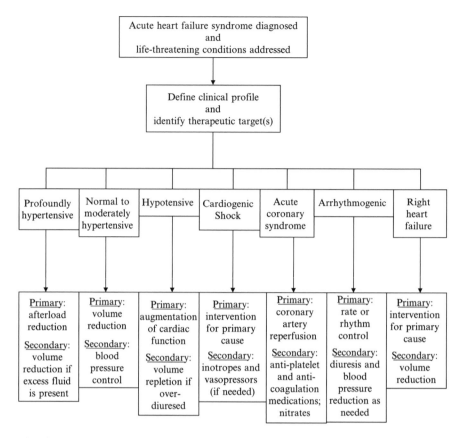

Fig. 12.1 Therapeutic targets for specific acute heart failure clinical profiles

agents can produce afterload reduction, yet only a handful have been rigorously tested in the management of AHFS, and head-to-head comparison trials are sorely lacking. Regardless, it has been postulated that in patients with acute hypertensive HF, the decision to implement therapy focused primarily on BP control (rather than volume reduction) may be more important than actual agent used [7]. Though such a hypothesis has not been tested in clinical trials, as shown in STAT (Studying the Treatment of Acute Hypertension), the degree of BP reduction has critical bearing on outcomes, with an increase in adverse event rates when the systolic BP declines to less than 120 mm Hg [14]. Thus, when managing acute hypertension with any agent, close monitoring and frequent BP measurement is essential.

Nitrovasodilators

Nitrates have long been considered the first-line agents for AHFS associated with acute hypertension. As a class, nitrates work by providing an exogenous source of nitric oxide which is then available to bind to soluble guanylate cyclase, thereby producing vascular smooth muscle relaxation [15]. At modest doses, this effect occurs predominantly in the venous circulation, resulting in increased capacitance and a marked reduction in preload. This produces ventricular unloading with diminished end-diastolic volume and consequently, a profound decrease in pulmonary capillary wedge pressure (PCWP) [16, 17]. At higher doses (i.e., ≥150–250 mcg/min), arteriolar dilation occurs, which helps to improve cardiac output through a reduction in afterload [18–20]. This effect may be more pronounced when systemic vascular resistance is severely elevated [21] and may be mediated through a dose-dependent, differential effect on the augmentation index—a measure of the amplified pressure wave that is reflected back to the central circulation from the periphery (i.e., a ratio of central/peripheral pulse pressure) [22]. Nitrate tolerance is a common but poorly understood phenomenon thought to involve O_2 free radical formation and nitric oxide (NO) synthase inhibition which can decrease the hemodynamic response to ongoing administration despite up-titration [23, 24].

Nitroglycerin (glyceryl trinitrate) is the most common nitrate used in the United States and is typically given as an initial sublingual tablet or spray (400 mcg/dose) to enable quick absorption and rapid onset of action. For persistent symptoms, transdermal application (1–2 in. of 2% ointment), or for more severe cases, IV administration may be required. Because the half-life of nitroglycerin (NTG) is short (<5 min), a continuous infusion (rate, 20–400 mcg/min) may be needed to maintain effect. Higher doses of IV NTG (or its relative, isosorbide dinitrate [ISDN]) may be particularly useful in patients with profound BP elevations and respiratory distress (i.e., hypertensive cardiogenic pulmonary edema). When delivered to such patients by repeat IV bolus (every 3–5 min), both high-dose NTG (2 mg) [25] and ISDN (4 mg) [26, 27] have been associated with a reduction in the need for mechanical ventilation and intensive care unit admission, a lower incidence of cardiac injury (as evidenced by biomarkers), and a shorter total hospital length of stay. In studies to date, substantial doses of NTG (mean [SD]=6.50 [±3.47 mg]) and ISDN (mean [SD]=11.4 mg [±6.8 mg]) have been given with a low incidence of hypotension (<4%) and no report of adverse neurologic, renal, or cardiac events. While sustained administration of such aggressive therapy may not be appropriate for the OU, most patients who respond do so quickly, often circumventing the need for continued IV nitrate therapy. Results of a topical high-dose nitrate strategy (two sublingual NTG tablets followed by application of ten NitroDerm TTS patches) have recently been reported with demonstration of a reduced intensive care unit admission rate and greater improvement in cardiac stress in the high-dose nitrate arm [28]. Importantly, this strategy was implemented in a nonmonitored setting (general medical ward), thus enabling possible extrapolation to the OU. Preload-dependent conditions, such as right heart ischemia, pericardial effusion/pericarditis, or restrictive cardiomyopathy, should be considered a contraindication to nitrate therapy (regardless of dose).

Sodium nitroprusside (NTP) is another nitric oxide donor which can be used in profoundly hypertensive and dyspneic patients. The administration of NTP results in both preload and afterload reduction even at lower doses and has been shown to be effective for patients with refractory elevations in systemic vascular resistance [29].

Controlled trials of NTP in acute HF are lacking with only one small ($n = 37$) study showing no difference in BP control or transmitral Doppler flow parameters in patients with hypertension and left ventricular filling abnormalities who received relatively low doses of NTG (max dose, 50 mcg/min) or NTP (max dose, 1 mcg/kg/min) [30]. Because NTP can cause significant and slightly prolonged reduction in blood pressure as well as reflex tachycardia, invasive arterial monitoring and close supervision are recommended [31]. Furthermore, NTP may increase the risk of "coronary steal syndrome" which results in focal decreased cardiac perfusion from generalized vasodilation in the setting of a fixed coronary constriction (e.g., atherosclerosis) and cyanide toxicity (though this risk can be minimized concurrent administration of thiosulfate). As such, NTP is not ideal for use in short-stay management of AHFS or in the OU setting.

Natriuretic Peptides

Since its approval by the Food and Drug Administration in 2001, nesiritide, a recombinant form of brain natriuretic peptide (BNP), has been promoted as an alternative to existing vasodilator therapy with potential advantages because of its combined neurohormonal and hemodynamic effects [32]. Published in 2002, the VMAC (Vasodilation in the Management of Acute Congestive Heart Failure) trial stood as the early "definitive" study of nesiritide, comparing it with NTG and placebo [33]. While nesiritide showed a more rapid and persistent effect on PCWP, there were limited differences in the degree of symptom improvement [33]. The subsequent PROACTION (Prospective Randomized Outcomes Study of Acutely Decompensated Congestive Heart Failure Treated Initially in Outpatients with Natrecor) study found that nesiritide use was safe in the OU and offered some improvement in the 30-day alive and out of hospital rate but no clinical advantage over standard therapy in the acute setting [34]. Shortly thereafter, the safety of nesiritide was called into question by two meta-analyzes which found an increased risk of renal dysfunction (relative risk [95% CI] = 1.54 [1.19–1.98]) and mortality (relative risk [95% CI] = 1.81 [1.02–3.27]) [35, 36]. Despite widespread adoption, utilization of nesiritide steadily decreased after these data were published [37], which, in part, prompted a large-scale (>7,000 patients) safety and efficacy study. This trial, ASCEND-HF (Acute Study of Clinical Effectiveness of Nesiritide in Decompensated Heart Failure), was completed in 2010 finding a statistical (but not clinically significant) difference in dyspnea and an increased risk of hypotension with use of nesiritide (vs. placebo) without evidence of additional harm or benefit [38]. Nesiritide thus appears to be a reasonable and safe option for management of AHFS, though it is unclear what are the specific indications for its implementation.

Other natriuretic peptide compounds, include ularitide (a synthetic analog of urodilatin, an atrial-NP derivative) and CD-NP (a chimer of c-type and d-type NP) [39], have been developed and are currently subject to preliminary investigation, but their clinical viability has yet to be determined.

Angiotensin Converting Enzyme Inhibitors

Angiotensin converting enzyme (ACE) inhibitors have been used in the setting of acute HF with hypertension. As a class, they are effective antihypertensives and provide antagonism of the renin–angiotensin–aldosterone system, making them ideal agents for HF treatment. Abundant data show substantial benefit from the use of oral ACE inhibitors in chronic HF (i.e., disease regression, symptom improvement, decreased mortality) [40–42], but few studies have been conducted in the acute setting. Notwithstanding, results from these limited trials are encouraging with demonstration of rapid symptom improvement and decreased intubation after a single dose of sublingual captopril (25 mg) and significant reduction in BP after IV administration of enalaprilat (1 mg) [43, 44]. While such signals suggest efficacy, there is potential for adverse events such as sustained hypotension due to their relatively longer half-lives, renal dysfunction, and hyperkalemia. Therefore, absent further safety data, ACE inhibitors should be used with caution during the stabilization phase of AHFS care.

Calcium Channel Blockers

Due to their negative inotropic effects, beta-blocking agents and nondihydropyridine calcium channel blockers (CCBs) are considered contraindicated in the initial management of AHFS [45]. It has also been recommended to avoid rapid-onset dihydropyridine CCBs, such as sublingual nifedipine, as they produce unpredictable effects on peripheral resistance and have been correlated with an increased risk of coronary and cerebral hypoperfusion [46]. In recent years, however, a new generation of short-acting IV dihydropyridine CCBs (i.e., nicardipine and clevidipine) has been developed, leading to renewed interest in their use for hypertensive emergencies including AHFS. A recent subanalysis of the VELOCITY (The Evaluation of the Effect of Ultra-Short-Acting Clevidipine in the Treatment of Patients With Severe Hypertension). trial found such agents to be safe in the setting of AHFS [47]. A phase III trial of clevidipine in AHFS (An Efficacy and Safety Study of Blood Pressure Control in Acute Heart Failure - A Pilot Study). is currently underway and should help define the role of short-acting CCBs in the management of acute hypertensive HF.

Other Agents

Relaxin is a peptide hormone released in pregnancy that helps regulate hemodynamic function and renovascular blood flow. Specific effects of relaxin include production of nitric oxide, vascular endothelial growth factor, and matrix metalloproteinases, as well as inhibition of endothelin and angiotensin II. Such effects result in a number of vascular changes (especially systemic and renal vasodilation) that may be beneficial in acute hypertensive HF [48]. Preliminary study (Pre-RELAX AHF—Phase II Multicenter, Randomized, Double-blind, Placebo-Controlled Study to Evaluate the

Efficacy and Safety of Relaxin in Subjects With Acute Heart Failure) suggests greater improvement of dyspnea at all time points and a reduction in the composite of cardiovascular death or readmission due to heart or renal failure at day 60 (2.6% [95% CI 0.4–16.8] vs. 17.2% [9.6–29.6]; $p=0.053$) with use of relaxin (compared to placebo) [49]. Definitive conclusions regarding the potential utility of relaxin in AHFS, however, await the results on an ongoing phase III trial.

Cinaciguat is a direct-acting soluble guanylate cyclase activator which produces a net effect similar to nitrate medications without the need for nitric oxide itself [50]. Cinaciguat offers the potential to overcome reductions in nitric oxide-mediated guanylate cyclase function (and hence nitrate bioactivity) which result from the oxidative stress that often accompanies AHFS. However, as evidenced by a series of preliminary trials (i.e., the COMPOSE [A Placebo Controlled, Randomized, Double-Blind, Fixed-dose, Multicenter, Phase IIb Study to Investigate the Efficacy and Tolerability of BAY 58-2667] studies), the vasodilator effects of cinaciguat are quite substantial and the risk of hypotension may be unacceptable for clinical use.

Tezosentan is an IV endothelin receptor antagonist that yields a rapid reduction in vascular resistance and PCWP while improving cardiac index. Tezosentan has proven effective for the management of pulmonary hypertension, and its hemodynamic effects have made it an attractive option for management of acute hypertensive HF. Despite this, tezosentan has not been found to be of benefit in AHFS in a number of randomized trials including the five RITZ (Randomized Intravenous TeZosentan) studies [51] and VERITAS (value of endothelin receptor inhibition with tezosentan in acute heart failure study) [52]. While this may relate to issues of patient selection, at present, there is no evidence to support the use of tezosentan in AHFS.

Excess Volume (Preload)

Volume overload is another common feature in patients presenting with AHFS, and relief of congestion through removal of excess fluid is an important goal of therapy [53]. Despite a lack of prospective, randomized trials, diuretics have remained the mainstay of therapy for decades and are used in the vast majority (~90%) of patients with acute HF symptoms. Several alternatives have been recently investigated, but none has been found to be superior in terms of safety or efficacy. Consequently, diuretics remain the de facto "standard" of care for AHFS in those with (and often without) hypervolemia.

Loop Diuretics

Intravenous loop diuretics (furosemide, bumetanide, torsemide, and ethacrynic acid) work by inhibiting the $Na^+–K^+–2Cl^-$ cotransport channel in epithelial cells which line the thick ascending limb of the loop of Henle [54] and are the most common class of medication used in the treatment of AHFS. They work to produce an osmotic diuresis and have an onset of action of approximately 30 min postadministration with a peak effect at 2–4 h. Furosemide is the agent used most frequently in the United States, and with typical dosing (40–80 mg IV every 8–12 h), in-hospital fluid losses can approach 4 L [55]. Furosemide has been noted to have hemodynamic effects as well, with nonsustained vasodilation occurring 5–15 min after administration [56]. Latent vasoconstriction has also been reported and appears to be related, at least in part, to activation of neurohormonal factors [57]. Despite this potential disadvantage, loop diuretics do effectively reduce filling pressures and induce symptomatic improvement [58], making them widely accepted for acute HF treatment.

Resistance to loop diuretics may be encountered while treating acute HF and is associated with a poor prognosis [59, 60]. Typically, patients experience diminished or absent response to high diuretic doses and refractory edema. Though such resistance is more common in those on long-term therapy, on occasion, it may be seen in diuretic naïve patients with profound volume depletion and decreased renal perfusion. Enhanced effect may be achieved through combining a loop diuretic with a thiazides diuretic (i.e., metolazone or chlorothiazide) [61, 62], but the specific applicability of this to the acute setting has been insufficiently explored.

The optimal approach to diuretic dosing and administration has been a source of ongoing controversy. Higher cumulative doses of furosemide have been associated with an increased risk of in-hospital death in one study [6], and in a Cochrane Collaborative review, continuous infusion was found to be more effective for than repeat bolusing, particularly for those patients with refractory edema or congestion [63]. The best evidence to date, however, has come from the recently completed diuretic optimization strategies evaluation (DOSE) study, which prospectively compared approaches to IV furosemide administration [64]. Using a 2×2 factorial design, patients ($n = 308$) were randomized to receive high (2.5 times daily oral) vs. low (daily oral) dosing and intermittent bolus (every 12 h) vs. continuous infusion for a period of at least 48 h. Results showed no statistical difference in global symptom relief or absolute change in renal function at 72 h for either level of comparison (i.e., low vs. high dose and intermittent bolus vs. continuous infusion), but there was a signal of greater improvement with use of a high-dose strategy in several secondary end points including dyspnea relief, weight loss and net volume loss, proportion free from signs of congestion, and reduction in biomarkers of myocardial stress (i.e., NT-proBNP). Of note, development of worsening renal function (defined as an increase in serum creatinine >3 mg/dL) was common, occurring in more than 15% by day 3 (with a greater incidence in those who received high [vs. low] dose, regardless of how it was administered—23% vs. 14%; $p = 0.041$) and close to 25% by day 7 (with no difference by dose or route). Moreover, such renal dysfunction appeared to persist postdischarge with an incidence of nearly 20% at day 60. Based on the DOSE data, there may be some clinical advantage to use of high-dose furosemide (albeit with an attendant risk of more profound renal dysfunction), but there is no benefit of continuous infusion over intermittent bolusing.

Vasopressin Antagonists (Vaptans)

Arginine vasopressin, also known as antidiuretic hormone, triggers manufacture and cell membrane insertion of aquaporin-2 molecules in renal collecting ducts and thus serves as a potent stimulus for free water reuptake by the kidneys. Vasopressin release is upregulated in HF, and its appearance contributes greatly to dysregulated fluid accumulation. While V1 receptors primarily regulate the effect of vasopressin in the vasculature (where it produces vasconstriction), V2 receptors function in the kidney. Antagonists of vasopressin (conivaptan [a dual V1/V2 receptor antagonist], tolvaptan [a V2 >> V1 receptor antagonist], and lixivaptan [a V2 >>> V1 receptor antagonist]) block this pathway, resulting in increased excretion of low-solute fluid, enabling reversal of hyponatremia (a known risk factor in acute HF) without adversely affecting glomerular filtration rate or renal blood flow [65]. This class of medications, therefore, has broad theoretical appeal for use in AHFS, offering a pharmacological approach to volume reduction that lacks the drawbacks of loop diuretics. Despite such potential, utility of the "vaptans" in EVEREST (Efficacy of Vasopressin Antagonism in hEart failuRE: Outcome Study With Tolvaptan), a two part investigation that enrolled over 4,000 patients with acute HF, was less than ideal offering a statistically significant (though clinically marginal) improvement in dyspnea, edema, serum sodium, and renal function without any long-term effect on mortality or HF-related morbidity [66, 67]. Consequently, there is no indication for use of vasopressin antagonism in AHFS at present, but pending results from THE BALANCE (Treatment of Hyponatremia Based on Lixivaptan in NYHA Class III/IV Cardiac Patient Evaluation) study, a limited role may exist in patients with acute HF complicated by hyponatremia [68].

A$_1$ Adenosine Receptor Antagonists

Acting through renal A$_1$ receptors, adenosine produces counter-regulatory effects in the kidney, working to decrease glomerular filtration rate through afferent arteriolar constriction and increase sodium reabsorption in the proximal tubule. Such actions are thought to contribute to chronic kidney disease and a progressive reduction in diuretic responsiveness, both of which are known to complicate treatment of acute HF. Preliminary study of adenosine A$_1$ receptor antagonism suggested promise as a potential therapy in AHFS, attenuating adverse effects on renal function by furosemide [69]. In the recently published PROTECT (Placebo-Controlled Randomized Study of the Selective A1 Adenosine Receptor Antagonist Rolofylline for Patients Hospitalized with Acute Decompensated Heart Failure and Volume Overload to Assess Treatment Effect on Congestion and Renal Function) trial, however, there was no demonstrable effect on primary (a composite of survival, heart failure status, and changes in renal function) or secondary (post-treatment development of persistent renal impairment and 60-day rate of death or readmission for cardiovascular or renal causes) end points with use of a selective adenosine A$_1$ receptor antagonist vs. placebo [70]. Despite sound theoretical principle, A$_1$ receptor antagonism appears to have no applicability in the management of AHFS.

Ultrafiltration

Mechanical fluid removal using ultrafiltration is an alternative to pharmacological diuresis and a viable option for the management of AHFS with volume overload, particularly in those with diuretic resistance or the cardiorenal syndrome. Ultrafiltration is an efficient yet costly (~$19,500 for device acquisition and $950 per filter, with 1–2 filters required per treatment) mechanism which uses venovenous hemoconcentration to extract up to 500 mL of isotonic fluid per hour. Although the UNLOAD (Ultrafiltration Versus Intravenous Diuretics for Patients Hospitalized for Acute Decompensated Heart Failure) study found an association with decreased readmissions [71], clear indications for the use of ultrafiltration in AHFS have not been defined. While clinical experience is limited, ultrafiltration is feasible in the ED and OU setting—in a recent case report, more than 7 L of fluid were removed from a patient over 19 h in an OU without adverse effect [72].

Diminished Cardiac Function

Cardiac output can be acutely reduced for a number of reasons, but ischemia, valvular dysfunction, and arrhythmia are among the most common. Each of these has inherent therapy which warrants a discussion that is beyond the scope of this chapter. It is important to remember, however, that when treating HF related to such causes, the primary intervention should be directed toward the inciting factor (i.e., reperfusion for ischemia, surgery for critical valve dysfunction, or rate control for atrial fibrillation) rather than the end manifestation.

On occasion (<5% of the time), reduced cardiac output with hypoperfusion will result from a simple, subacute progression of underlying, advanced HF, and intervention to improve pump function (i.e., inotropes) may be needed. In general, such patients are poor candidates for short-stay management of AHFS, but some, especially those with end-stage disease, may benefit from a brief "tune-up" with medications that augment cardiac function. For those without evidence of pulmonary congestion, a small bolus of isotonic normal saline (250–500 cc) may be attempted first, as these individuals frequently suffer from intravascular depletion as a result of chronic overdiuresis. It is important to remember that while inotropic agents can effectively transiently improve cardiac function, they should be used cautiously, especially in patients with coronary artery disease, as they increase myocardial oxygen demand and enhance the potential for arrhythmia development [31, 73–75].

The most commonly used inotropes are dobutamine and milrinone. Dobutamine acts through β_1 and β_2 adrenergic receptor stimulation to increase inotropy and chronotropy, and consequently, cardiac output [76]. Vascular effects include vasodilatation at low doses and vasoconstriction at higher doses. Patients with a history of beta-blocker usage at baseline may require increased dosing to achieve therapeutic effect [77]. Milrinone is a type III phosphodiesterase inhibitor (PDEI) which also improves hemodynamic function (i.e., stroke volume and cardiac output) but does so by preventing intracellular breakdown of cyclic adenosine monophosphate (cAMP) [78]. Though this activity is independent of adrenergic receptor stimulation, it produces similar net effects on the heart (i.e., inotropy, chronotropy, and lusitropy) [79]. In the peripheral circulation, however, vasodilatory effects predominate resulting in significant preload and afterload reduction. This latter response may cause a worsening of hypotension, particularly in patients with intravascular volume depletion [80]. Concurrent administration of dobutamine and milrinone (or an alternative PDEI such as amrinone or enoximone) yields an additive effect on cardiac function and may be a useful approach for those on chronic beta-blocker therapy [81, 82].

Positive inotropic effects can also be accomplished by targeting the myocardial contractile apparatus itself. Traditionally, this has been achieved through use of cardiac glycosides (i.e., digoxin) which produce their desired effect by inhibition of Na^+/K^+ ATPase. Mediated through an increase in intracellular sodium, this works to establish a gradient that promotes intracellular calcium ion accumulation, which subsequently enhances myocyte contractility, resulting in an incremental improvement in cardiac output. Digoxin was commonly used for management of AHFS two to three decades ago but has since fallen out of favor [83]. Digoxin, however, is one of the few medications which, when used in the ambulatory setting, has actually been shown to reduce rehospitalization for HF, and there is resurgent interest potential utility for patients with acute symptoms [84]. Other agents that enhance myocyte contractility include levosimendan (a calcium sensitizer that functions through K^+/ATP channels) [85], istaroxime (a concurrent inhibitor of Na^+/K^+ ATPase and stimulator of sarcoendoplasmic reticulum calcium ATPase) [86], and direct-acting cardiomyosin activators [87]. Of these, levosimendan has been most extensively studied, but in SURVIVE (Survival of Patients With Acute Heart Failure in Need of Intravenous Inotropic Support), the largest trial of the medication to date, no clinical benefit over dobutamine was found [88].

Is There a Role for Morphine Sulfate?

Perhaps the most common other medication used in the treatment of acute HF is morphine sulfate. Morphine is thought to produce mild vasodilatation (venous >> arterial) with a reduction in preload and, to a lesser extent, afterload. In addition, morphine may induce respiratory relaxation and exert a calming effect on those with agitated dyspnea. The evidence in support of morphine use for acute HF is limited with few if any trials demonstrating benefit and several actually showing potential harm with an increased risk of endotracheal intubation, need for intensive care unit admission, and prolonged hospital length of stay [89, 90]. Moreover, in ADHERE, morphine use was found to be an independent predictor of in-hospital mortality [adjusted odds ratio (95% CI) = 4.84 (4.52, 5.18)] [91]. Thus at best, morphine appears to be of marginal utility and, at worst, a possible contributor to suboptimal outcomes.

Oxygen Therapy and Ventilatory Support

Virtually, all AHFS patients will receive supplemental oxygen therapy. Nasal cannula delivery for mild dyspnea and a nonrebreather face mask for moderate dyspnea will generally be sufficient. For patients with profound dyspnea, early initiation of noninvasive positive airway pressure ventilation (NIPPV; either continuous [CPAP] of bi-level [BiPAP]) can dramatically reduce symptom severity and may decrease the need for endotracheal intubation. Though prior studies suggested a relative increase in the rate of myocardial infarction with use of BiPAP (vs. CPAP), several reviews [92, 93] and the recently completed prospective Three Interventions in Cardiogenic Pulmonary Oedema (3CPO) trial showed equivalence with regard to safety and efficacy (though neither appears to provide a mortality benefit when compared to face mask oxygen therapy) [94]. When using noninvasive ventilation, initial CPAP is typically set at 5–7 cm H_2O with BiPAP starting at 8–10 cm H_2O inspiratory and 4–5 cm H_2O expiratory with up (or down)-titration as needed (max = 15 cm H_2O for CPAP and 20/10 cm H_2O for BiPAP). In addition to reducing the work of breathing, NIPPV decreases preload helping to offset pulmonary congestion.

Approximately 5% of acute HF patients overall and up to 40% of those with cardiogenic pulmonary edema will require endotracheal intubation (ETI) [90, 95, 96]. For most of these individuals, signs of impending respiratory failure such as severe dyspnea, tachypnea, diaphoresis, muscle fatigue, and confusion will be readily apparent on arrival to the ED. In others, however, findings may be more subtle. Parameters which indicate potential need for ETI include persistent hypoxia ($SaO_2 < 80$) or hypoxemia ($PaO_2/FiO_2 < 200$) despite supplemental oxygen, hypercarbia ($PaCO_2 > 55$ mm Hg), and acidosis (pH < 7.25) [97]. The requirement for endotracheal intubation is associated with poor outcome [98] and decreases the risk of neurologically intact survival in patients with acute HF who suffer in-hospital cardiac arrest [99]. Such patients are clearly poor candidates for short-stay management of AHFS.

Other Considerations

Administration of chronic medications or refilling prescriptions may be required for some patients, particularly those who have been noncompliant. Though not specifically included in acute HF treatment, familiarity with oral dosing of common beta-blockers (i.e., atenolol, bisoprolol, metoprolol, nebivolol, and carvedilol), ACE inhibitors (i.e., benazepril, captopril, enalapril, lisinopril, and ramipril), angiotensin receptor blockers (i.e., candesartan, losartan, and valsartan), diuretics (loop, such as furosemide, bumetanide, and torsemide, and nonloop, such as hydrochlorothiazide and chlorthalidone), oral nitrates (isosorbide mononitrate, ISDN), and aldosterone antagonists (spironolactone and eplerenone), as well as single-agent classes such as hydralazine and digoxin, can be helpful and may facilitate disposition. Additionally, when prescribing medications to chronic HF patients, it is important to avoid non-steroidal anti-inflammatory drugs (NSAIDs) as they increase the risk of recurrent HF presentation [100].

Conclusions

The management of AHFS is rapidly evolving from an approach that is focused predominantly on diuresis for all to one that responds more directly to the complex interplay of underlying disease and acute precipitants. Recognition of divergent clinical profiles, despite homogeneity in presentation, will help ensure delivery of the most appropriate therapy for an individual patient and improve the likelihood of optimal outcome. Such therapy may involve a mixture of interventions, each ideally targeting a specific contributor to the acute decompensated state and administered during the appropriate phase of treatment. Despite the need for potentially differing specific therapy, the goals of intervention remain consistent: acute symptom relief without induction of cardiac or renal dysfunction.

References

1. Gheorghiade M, Pang PS. Acute heart failure syndromes. J Am Coll Cardiol. 2009;53(7): 557–73.
2. Lindenfeld J, Albert NM, Boehmer JP, et al. HFSA 2010 comprehensive heart failure practice guideline. J Card Fail. 2010;16(6):e1–194.
3. Mebazaa A, Gheorghiade M, Pina IL, et al. Practical recommendations for prehospital and early in-hospital management of patients presenting with acute heart failure syndromes. Crit Care Med. 2008;36(1 Suppl):S129–39.
4. Hunt SA, Abraham WT, Chin MH, et al. 2009 Focused update incorporated into the ACC/AHA 2005 guidelines for the diagnosis and management of heart failure in adults: a report of the American College of Cardiology Foundation/American Heart Association Task Force on Practice Guidelines: developed in collaboration with the International Society for Heart and Lung Transplantation. Circulation. 2009;119(14):e391–479.
5. Felker GM, Pang PS, Adams KF, et al. Clinical trials of pharmacological therapies in acute heart failure syndromes: lessons learned and directions forward. Circ Heart Fail. 2010;3(2):314–25.
6. Hasselblad V, Gattis Stough W, Shah MR. Relation between dose of loop diuretics and outcomes in a heart failure population: results of the ESCAPE trial. Eur J Heart Fail. 2007;9(10): 1064–9.
7. Weintraub NL, Collins SP, Pang PS, et al. Acute heart failure syndromes: emergency department presentation, treatment, and disposition: current approaches and future aims: a scientific statement from the American Heart Association. Circulation. 2010;122(19):1975–96.
8. Collins S, Storrow AB, Kirk JD, et al. Beyond pulmonary edema: diagnostic, risk stratification, and treatment challenges of acute heart failure management in the emergency department. Ann Emerg Med. 2008;51(1):45–57.

9. Nohria A, Tsang SW, Fang JC, et al. Clinical assessment identifies hemodynamic profiles that predict outcomes in patients admitted with heart failure. J Am Coll Cardiol. 2003;41(10): 1797–804.
10. De Luca L, Fonarow GC, Adams Jr KF, et al. Acute heart failure syndromes: clinical scenarios and pathophysiologic targets for therapy. Heart Fail Rev. 2007;12(2):97–104.
11. Gheorghiade M, Abraham WT, Albert NM, et al. Systolic blood pressure at admission, clinical characteristics, and outcomes in patients hospitalized with acute heart failure. JAMA. 2006;296(18):2217–26.
12. Peacock F, Emerman C, Costanzo M, et al. Early initiation of intravenous vasoactive therapy improves heart failure outcomes: an analysis from the ADHERE registry database. Ann Emerg Med. 2003;42:s29.
13. Kaluski E, Kobrin I, Zimlichman R, et al. RITZ-5: randomized intravenous TeZosentan (an endothelin-A/B antagonist) for the treatment of pulmonary edema: a prospective, multicenter, double-blind, placebo-controlled study. J Am Coll Cardiol. 2003;41(2):204–10.
14. Peacock F, Amin A, Granger CB, et al. Hypertensive heart failure: patient characteristics, treatment, and outcomes. Am J Emerg Med. 2010;29(8):855–62.
15. Ignarro LJ. After 130 years, the molecular mechanism of action of nitroglycerin is revealed. Proc Natl Acad Sci USA. 2002;99(12):7816–7.
16. Bussmann WD, Kaltenbach M. Sublingual nitroglycerin in the treatment of left ventricular failure and pulmonary edema. Eur J Cardiol. 1976;4(3):327–33.
17. Bussmann WD, Kaltenbach M. Sublingual nitroglycerin for left ventricular failure and pulmonary edema. Compr Ther. 1977;3(8):29–36.
18. Imhof PR, Ott B, Frankhauser P, et al. Difference in nitroglycerin dose–response in the venous and arterial beds. Eur J Clin Pharmacol. 1980;18(6):455–60.
19. Bayley S, Valentine H, Bennett ED. The haemodynamic responses to incremental doses of intravenous nitroglycerin in left ventricular failure. Intensive Care Med. 1984;10(3):139–45.
20. Herling IM. Intravenous nitroglycerin: clinical pharmacology and therapeutic considerations. Am Heart J. 1984;108(1):141–9.
21. Haber HL, Simek CL, Bergin JD, et al. Bolus intravenous nitroglycerin predominantly reduces afterload in patients with excessive arterial elastance. J Am Coll Cardiol. 1993;22(1):251–7.
22. Munir S, Guilcher A, Kamalesh T, et al. Peripheral augmentation index defines the relationship between central and peripheral pulse pressure. Hypertension. 2008;51(1):112–8.
23. Elkayam U, Akhter MW, Singh H, et al. Comparison of effects on left ventricular filling pressure of intravenous nesiritide and high-dose nitroglycerin in patients with decompensated heart failure. Am J Cardiol. 2004;93(2):237–40.
24. Gori T, Parker JD. Nitrate tolerance: a unifying hypothesis. Circulation. 2002;106(19): 2510–3.
25. Levy P, Compton S, Welch R, et al. Treatment of severe decompensated heart failure with high-dose intravenous nitroglycerin: a feasibility and outcome analysis. Ann Emerg Med. 2007;50(2):144–52.
26. Cotter G, Faibel H, Barash P, et al. High-dose nitrates in the immediate management of unstable angina: optimal dosage, route of administration, and therapeutic goals. Am J Emerg Med. 1998;16(3):219–24.
27. Sharon A, Shpirer I, Kaluski E, et al. High-dose intravenous isosorbide-dinitrate is safer and better than Bi-PAP ventilation combined with conventional treatment for severe pulmonary edema. J Am Coll Cardiol. 2000;36(3):832–7.
28. Breidthardt T, Noveanu M, Potocki M, et al. Impact of a high-dose nitrate strategy on cardiac stress in acute heart failure: a pilot study. J Intern Med. 2010;267(3):322–30.
29. Guiha NH, Cohn JN, Mikulic E, et al. Treatment of refractory heart failure with infusion of nitroprusside. N Engl J Med. 1974;291(12):587–92.
30. Eryonucu B, Guler N, Guntekin U, et al. Comparison of the effects of nitroglycerin and nitroprusside on transmitral Doppler flow parameters in patients with hypertensive urgency. Ann Pharmacother. 2005;39(6):997–1001.

31. Nieminen MS, Bohm M, Cowie MR, et al. Executive summary of the guidelines on the diagnosis and treatment of acute heart failure: the Task Force on Acute Heart Failure of the European Society of Cardiology. Eur Heart J. 2005;26(4):384–416.
32. Burger MR, Burger AJ. BNP in decompensated heart failure: diagnostic, prognostic and therapeutic potential. Curr Opin Investig Drugs. 2001;2(7):929–35.
33. Intravenous nesiritide vs nitroglycerin for treatment of decompensated congestive heart failure: a randomized controlled trial. JAMA. 2002;287(12):1531–40.
34. Peacock WFt, Holland R, Gyarmathy R, et al. Observation unit treatment of heart failure with nesiritide: results from the proaction trial. J Emerg Med. 2005;29(3):243–52.
35. Sackner-Bernstein JD, Kowalski M, Fox M, et al. Short-term risk of death after treatment with nesiritide for decompensated heart failure: a pooled analysis of randomized controlled trials. JAMA. 2005;293(15):1900–5.
36. Sackner-Bernstein JD, Skopicki HA, Aaronson KD. Risk of worsening renal function with nesiritide in patients with acutely decompensated heart failure. Circulation. 2005;111(12):1487–91.
37. Hauptman PJ, Schnitzler MA, Swindle J, et al. Use of nesiritide before and after publications suggesting drug-related risks in patients with acute decompensated heart failure. JAMA. 2006;296(15):1877–84.
38. O'Connor CM, Starloing RC, Hernandez AF, et al. Acute Study of clinical effectiveness of nesiritide in decompensated heart failure trial (ASCEND-HF). N Engl J Med. 2011;365:32–43.
39. Lisy O, Huntley BK, McCormick DJ, et al. Design, synthesis, and actions of a novel chimeric natriuretic peptide: CD-NP. J Am Coll Cardiol. 2008;52(1):60–8.
40. The CONSENSUS Trial Study Group. Effects of enalapril on mortality in severe congestive heart failure. Results of the Cooperative North Scandinavian Enalapril Survival Study (CONSENSUS). N Engl J Med. 1987;316(23):1429–35.
41. The SOLVD Investigators. Effect of enalapril on survival in patients with reduced left ventricular ejection fractions and congestive heart failure. N Engl J Med. 1991;325(5):293–302.
42. The SOLVD Investigattors. Effect of enalapril on mortality and the development of heart failure in asymptomatic patients with reduced left ventricular ejection fractions. N Engl J Med. 1992;327(10):685–91.
43. Hamilton RJ, Carter WA, Gallagher EJ. Rapid improvement of acute pulmonary edema with sublingual captopril. Acad Emerg Med. 1996;3(3):205–12.
44. Annane D, Bellissant E, Pussard E, et al. Placebo-controlled, randomized, double-blind study of intravenous enalaprilat efficacy and safety in acute cardiogenic pulmonary edema. Circulation. 1996;94(6):1316–24.
45. Epstein SE, Braunwald E. Beta-adrenergic receptor blocking drugs. Mechanisms of action and clinical applications. N Engl J Med. 1966;275(20):1106–12. contd.
46. Grossman E, Messerli FH, Grodzicki T, et al. Should a moratorium be placed on sublingual nifedipine capsules given for hypertensive emergencies and pseudoemergencies? JAMA. 1996;276(16):1328–31.
47. Peacock FWt, Varon J, Ebrahimi R, et al. Clevidipine for severe hypertension in acute heart failure: a VELOCITY trial analysis. Congest Heart Fail. 2010;16(2):55–9.
48. Teichman SL, Unemori E, Dschietzig T, et al. Relaxin, a pleiotropic vasodilator for the treatment of heart failure. Heart Fail Rev. 2009;14(4):321–9.
49. Teerlink JR, Metra M, Felker GM, et al. Relaxin for the treatment of patients with acute heart failure (Pre-RELAX-AHF): a multicentre, randomised, placebo-controlled, parallel-group, dose-finding phase IIb study. Lancet. 2009;373(9673):1429–39.
50. Mitrovic V, Hernandez AF, Meyer M, et al. Role of guanylate cyclase modulators in decompensated heart failure. Heart Fail Rev. 2009;14(4):309–19.
51. Rich S, McLaughlin VV. Endothelin receptor blockers in cardiovascular disease. Circulation. 2003;108(18):2184–90.

52. McMurray JJ, Teerlink JR, Cotter G, et al. Effects of tezosentan on symptoms and clinical outcomes in patients with acute heart failure: the VERITAS randomized controlled trials. JAMA. 2007;298(17):2009–19.
53. Pang PS, Levy P. Pathophysiology of volume overload in acute heart failure syndromes. Congest Heart Fail. 2010;16 Suppl 1:S1–6.
54. Brater DC. Diuretic therapy. N Engl J Med. 1998;339(6):387–95.
55. Steimle AE, Stevenson LW, Chelimsky-Fallick C, et al. Sustained hemodynamic efficacy of therapy tailored to reduce filling pressures in survivors with advanced heart failure. Circulation. 1997;96(4):1165–72.
56. Dikshit K, Vyden JK, Forrester JS, et al. Renal and extrarenal hemodynamic effects of furosemide in congestive heart failure after acute myocardial infarction. N Engl J Med. 1973;288(21):1087–90.
57. Francis GS, Siegel RM, Goldsmith SR, et al. Acute vasoconstrictor response to intravenous furosemide in patients with chronic congestive heart failure. Activation of the neurohumoral axis. Ann Intern Med. 1985;103(1):1–6.
58. Mebazaa A, Pang PS, Tavares M, et al. The impact of early standard therapy on dyspnoea in patients with acute heart failure: the URGENT-dyspnoea study. Eur Heart J. 2010;31(7): 832–41.
59. Kramer BK, Schweda F, Riegger GA. Diuretic treatment and diuretic resistance in heart failure. Am J Med. 1999;106(1):90–6.
60. Neuberg GW, Miller AB, O'Connor CM, et al. Diuretic resistance predicts mortality in patients with advanced heart failure. Am Heart J. 2002;144(1):31–8.
61. Channer KS, McLean KA, Lawson-Matthew P, et al. Combination diuretic treatment in severe heart failure: a randomised controlled trial. Br Heart J. 1994;71(2):146–50.
62. Dormans TP, Gerlag PG, Russel FG, et al. Combination diuretic therapy in severe congestive heart failure. Drugs. 1998;55(2):165–72.
63. Salvador DR, Rey NR, Ramos GC, et al. Continuous infusion versus bolus injection of loop diuretics in congestive heart failure. Cochrane Database Syst Rev. 2005;(3):CD003178.
64. Felker GM. On behalf of the heart failure research network: the diuretic optimization strategies evaluation (DOSE) study: a randomized, double blind, placebo-controlled trial of diuretic strategies in acute decompensated heart failure. Presented at the American College of Cardiology 59th Annual Scientific Session. Atlanta, GA; 14–16 March 2010.
65. De Luca L, Orlandi C, Udelson JE, et al. Overview of vasopressin receptor antagonists in heart failure resulting in hospitalization. Am J Cardiol. 2005;96(12A):24L–33.
66. Gheorghiade M, Konstam MA, Burnett Jr JC, et al. Short-term clinical effects of tolvaptan, an oral vasopressin antagonist, in patients hospitalized for heart failure: the EVEREST Clinical Status Trials. JAMA. 2007;297(12):1332–43.
67. Konstam MA, Gheorghiade M, Burnett Jr JC, et al. Effects of oral tolvaptan in patients hospitalized for worsening heart failure: the EVEREST outcome trial. JAMA. 2007;297(12): 1319–31.
68. Abraham WT, Aranda JM, Boehmer JP, et al. Rationale and design of the treatment of hyponatremia based on lixivaptan in NYHA Class III/IV cardiac patient evaluation (THE BALANCE) study. Clin Transl Sci. 2010;3(5):249–53.
69. Gottlieb SS, Brater DC, Thomas I, et al. BG9719 (CVT-124), an A1 adenosine receptor antagonist, protects against the decline in renal function observed with diuretic therapy. Circulation. 2002;105(11):1348–53.
70. Massie BM, O'Connor CM, Metra M, et al. Rolofylline, an adenosine A1-receptor antagonist, in acute heart failure. N Engl J Med. 2010;363(15):1419–28.
71. Costanzo MR, Guglin ME, Saltzberg MT, et al. Ultrafiltration versus intravenous diuretics for patients hospitalized for acute decompensated heart failure. J Am Coll Cardiol. 2007;49(6): 675–83.
72. Levy PD, Penugonda N, Guglin M. Treatment of massive fluid overload as a result of constrictive pericarditis with ultrafiltration in the emergency department. Ann Emerg Med. 2008;51(3): 247–50.

73. Burger AJ, Elkayam U, Neibaur MT, et al. Comparison of the occurrence of ventricular arrhythmias in patients with acutely decompensated congestive heart failure receiving dobutamine versus nesiritide therapy. Am J Cardiol. 2001;88(1):35–9.
74. Leier CV, Webel J, Bush CA. The cardiovascular effects of the continuous infusion of dobutamine in patients with severe cardiac failure. Circulation. 1977;56(3):468–72.
75. Hunt SA. ACC/AHA 2005 guideline update for the diagnosis and management of chronic heart failure in the adult: a report of the American College of Cardiology/American Heart Association Task Force on Practice Guidelines (Writing Committee to Update the 2001 Guidelines for the Evaluation and Management of Heart Failure). J Am Coll Cardiol. 2005; 46(6):e1–82.
76. Colucci WS, Wright RF, Braunwald E. New positive inotropic agents in the treatment of congestive heart failure. Mechanisms of action and recent clinical developments. 1. N Engl J Med. 1986;314(5):290–9.
77. Lowes BD, Tsvetkova T, Eichhorn EJ, et al. Milrinone versus dobutamine in heart failure subjects treated chronically with carvedilol. Int J Cardiol. 2001;81(2–3):141–9.
78. Colucci WS, Wright RF, Braunwald E. New positive inotropic agents in the treatment of congestive heart failure. Mechanisms of action and recent clinical developments. 2. N Engl J Med. 1986;314(6):349–58.
79. Colucci WS, Wright RF, Jaski BE, et al. Milrinone and dobutamine in severe heart failure: differing hemodynamic effects and individual patient responsiveness. Circulation. 1986;73(3 Pt 2):III175–83.
80. Cuffe MS, Califf RM, Adams Jr KF, et al. Short-term intravenous milrinone for acute exacerbation of chronic heart failure: a randomized controlled trial. JAMA. 2002;287(12):1541–7.
81. Gilbert EM, Hershberger RE, Wiechmann RJ, et al. Pharmacologic and hemodynamic effects of combined beta-agonist stimulation and phosphodiesterase inhibition in the failing human heart. Chest. 1995;108(6):1524–32.
82. Metra M, Nodari S, D'Aloia A, et al. Beta-blocker therapy influences the hemodynamic response to inotropic agents in patients with heart failure: a randomized comparison of dobutamine and enoximone before and after chronic treatment with metoprolol or carvedilol. J Am Coll Cardiol. 2002;40(7):1248–58.
83. Katz AM. The "modern" view of heart failure: how did we get here? Circ Heart Fail. 2008;1(1):63–71.
84. Gheorghiade M, Braunwald E. Reconsidering the role for digoxin in the management of acute heart failure syndromes. JAMA. 2009;302(19):2146–7.
85. Slawsky MT, Colucci WS, Gottlieb SS, et al. Acute hemodynamic and clinical effects of levosimendan in patients with severe heart failure. Study investigators. Circulation. 2000;102(18):2222–7.
86. Gheorghiade M, Blair JE, Filippatos GS, et al. Hemodynamic, echocardiographic, and neurohormonal effects of istaroxime, a novel intravenous inotropic and lusitropic agent: a randomized controlled trial in patients hospitalized with heart failure. J Am Coll Cardiol. 2008;51(23):2276–85.
87. Tavares M, Rezlan E, Vostroknoutova I, et al. New pharmacologic therapies for acute heart failure. Crit Care Med. 2008;36(1 Suppl):S112–20.
88. Mebazaa A, Nieminen MS, Packer M, et al. Levosimendan vs dobutamine for patients with acute decompensated heart failure: the SURVIVE Randomized Trial. JAMA. 2007;297(17): 1883–91.
89. Hoffman JR, Reynolds S. Comparison of nitroglycerin, morphine and furosemide in treatment of presumed pre-hospital pulmonary edema. Chest. 1987;92(4):586–93.
90. Sacchetti A, Ramoska E, Moakes ME, et al. Effect of ED management on ICU use in acute pulmonary edema. Am J Emerg Med. 1999;17(6):571–4.
91. Peacock WF, Hollander JE, Diercks DB, et al. Morphine and outcomes in acute decompensated heart failure: an ADHERE analysis. Emerg Med J. 2008;25(4):205–9.
92. Masip J, Roque M, Sanchez B, et al. Noninvasive ventilation in acute cardiogenic pulmonary edema: systematic review and meta-analysis. JAMA. 2005;294(24):3124–30.

93. Collins SP, Mielniczuk LM, Whittingham HA, et al. The use of noninvasive ventilation in emergency department patients with acute cardiogenic pulmonary edema: a systematic review. Ann Emerg Med. 2006;48(3):260–9. 269 e261-264.
94. Gray A, Goodacre S, Newby DE, et al. Noninvasive ventilation in acute cardiogenic pulmonary edema. N Engl J Med. 2008;359(2):142–51.
95. Pang D, Keenan SP, Cook DJ, et al. The effect of positive pressure airway support on mortality and the need for intubation in cardiogenic pulmonary edema: a systematic review. Chest. 1998;114(4):1185–92.
96. Yan AT, Bradley TD, Liu PP. The role of continuous positive airway pressure in the treatment of congestive heart failure. Chest. 2001;120(5):1675–85.
97. Masip J, Paez J, Merino M, et al. Risk factors for intubation as a guide for noninvasive ventilation in patients with severe acute cardiogenic pulmonary edema. Intensive Care Med. 2003;29(11):1921–8.
98. Adnet F, Le Toumelin P, Leberre A, et al. In-hospital and long-term prognosis of elderly patients requiring endotracheal intubation for life-threatening presentation of cardiogenic pulmonary edema. Crit Care Med. 2001;29(4):891–5.
99. Levy PD, Ye H, Compton S, et al. Factors associated with neurologically intact survival for patients with acute heart failure and in-hospital cardiac arrest. Circ Heart Fail. 2009;2(6):572–81.
100. Lage J, Henry D. Consumption of NSAIDs and the development of congestive heart failure in elderly patients: an underrecognized public health problem. Arch Intern Med. 2000;160(6):777–84.

Part IV
Observation Unit Entry Treatment and Disposition

Chapter 13
Observation Unit Admission Inclusion and Exclusion Criteria

Gregory J. Fermann and Sean P. Collins

Background

As more than 80% of AHFS patients present to the ED, significant pressures exist to manage patients efficiently in the acute care environment [1–7]. Selected patients may be eligible to receive care for AHFS in an observation unit (OU) which may provide a safe and effective means to lower costs by providing an alternative to an inpatient stay [1, 8]. There are two goals to risk-stratifying OU patients with AHFS (1) determining patient suitability for OU management and (2) determining endpoints of treatment. Other disease processes have predictive instruments which are helpful for determining subsequent risk at the time of ED decision-making. For example, patients with pneumonia can be risk-stratified using the PORT score, which can help determine the need for hospital admission [9]. Similarly, physicians can use the ACI-TIPI [10] or TIMI [11] risk score for triaging patients with possible acute coronary syndromes. However, no such prediction tool exists for ED patients with AHFS. The Society of Chest Pain Centers has published recommendations based on prior studies in AHFS risk stratification as well as previous publications about the OU management of AHFS. These recommendations are a good starting point for determining OU eligibility [11, 12] (Table 13.1). The goal for OU management of patients with AHFS is concurrent treatment and risk stratification in an effort to determine the need for hospital admission [13].

G.J. Fermann, MD (✉) • S.P. Collins, MSc, MD
Department of Emergency Medicine, University of Cincinnati,
231 Albert Sabin Way ML 0769, Cincinnati, OH 45267, USA
e-mail: Gregory.fermann@uc.edu; sean.collins@vanderbilt.edu

W. Frank Peacock (ed.), *Short Stay Management of Acute Heart Failure,*
Contemporary Cardiology, DOI 10.1007/978-1-61779-627-2_13,
© Springer Science+Business Media, LLC 2012

Table 13.1 Recommended inclusion and exclusion criteria for OU entry

	Recommended	Suggested
Inclusion criteria		
Blood pressure	SBP > 100 mmHg	SBP > 120 mmHg
Respiratory rate	< 32 Breaths/min	
Renal function	BUN < 40	
	Creatinine < 3.0	
ECG findings	No ischemic changes	
Natriuretic peptides		BNP < 1,000 pg/mL/
		NT-proBNP <5,000 pg/mL
Response to initial therapy		
Exclusion criteria		
ECG findings	Ischemic ECG changes	
Vasoactive medications	No active titration	
Social support		Adequate prior to OU admission

SBP systolic blood pressure, *BUN* blood urea nitrogen, *ECG* electrocardiogram, *BNP* B-type natriuretic peptide, *NT-proBNP* N-terminal pro B-type natriuretic peptide

Framingham Criteria

An ED diagnosis of AHFS is often based on history, physical examination, and ancillary tests such as biomarkers, plain radiography, echocardiography, or radionuclide scanning. The Framingham criteria, developed in 1971, are accepted criteria for establishing the etiology of undifferentiated dyspnea before ancillary studies have been performed [14]. For ED use, four of the criteria are eliminated, because they are not measured in the ED or rely on response to therapy. The remaining criteria are divided into major and minor. The clinical diagnosis of HF requires two major or one major and two minor criteria (Table 13.2). Entry criteria into a HF OU are established because an element of diagnostic certainty exists. Combining the modified Framingham criteria with immediately available diagnostic tests such as radiography and natriuretic peptides serves narrow the differential diagnosis. Some OUs require patients to have prior echocardiography to establish the HF diagnosis. Others place newly diagnosed HF patients in the OU and obtain an echocardiogram as part of the OU stay. The SCPC makes no formal recommendations about preexisting or new onset HF as part of the patient selection process. Thus, the recommendations made in this chapter serve as an adjunct to be used in those patients diagnosed with AHFS as the primary cause of their presenting symptoms.

Risk Stratification on Emergency Department Presentation

Clinical variables readily available to clinicians at the time of presentation are considered in the development of inclusion and exclusion criteria. Initial risk stratification has focused on the prediction of acute inpatient mortality as the primary endpoint. Early attempts at risk stratification focused on easily available parameters

Table 13.2 The modified Framingham criteria

Major	Minor
Paroxysmal nocturnal dyspnea	Extremity edema
Neck vein distention	Night cough
Pulmonary edema (on CXR)	Dyspnea on exertion
Rales	Hepatomegaly
Cardiomegaly	Pleural effusion
S₃ gallop	Tachycardia (≥130 beats/min)
Jugular venous distention	
Positive hepatojugular reflux	

CXR chest X-ray

such as demographics, hemodynamics, comorbidities, and 12-lead electrocardiography (ECG). More recently, biomarkers have been included in risk stratification, specifically cardiac troponin (cTn), high-sensitivity cardiac troponin (hsTn), the natriuretic peptides (NP) B-type natriuretic peptide (BNP) or N-terminal pro BNP (NT-proBNP), and markers of acute kidney injury (AKI). Clinical variables for risk stratification of ADHF are often categorized broadly into demographics, cognitive function/social services, comorbidities, hemodynamics, cardiac ischemia markers, electrolytes, and heart failure biomarkers.

Demographics. Although the current recommendations published by the Society of Chest Pain Centers (SCPC) do not specifically refer to age, sex, or race as inclusion/exclusion criteria, in two different analyses, neither Barsheshet nor Felker found that age greater than 65 was an independent predictor of inpatient mortality [15, 16].

Cognitive and Functional Status. Medical noncompliance, dietary indiscretion, and psychosocial factors play important causative roles in AHFS. Although such patients have a readily identifiable cause for their exacerbation, the complexity of their social needs may complicate the OU stay, although if there is readily reversible cause, such as an inability to secure their medications, these patients may be a logical choice for OU care. Others believe that the infrastructure, such as social workers, financial counselors, and patient educators, is beyond the scope of a 23-h OU stay. Institutional resources and policies should dictate whether a patient's social services needs should be an inclusion or exclusion criteria [17].

Hemodynamics. Selker [18] used patient's age, systolic blood pressure (SBP), and ECG findings to predict inpatient mortality. Although prospectively validated, the model was unable to include morbidity as an endpoint and could not discriminate a low-risk cohort. Chin and Goldman used similar criteria along with simple laboratory data and comorbidities to predict high-risk criteria. These early studies reflect the trend of attempting to describe a high-risk cohort using simple, rapidly available data points. Fonarow [19] studied 65,275 subjects enrolled in the ADHERE registry to identify 45 variables predicting inpatient mortality. They were able to risk stratify patients into high-, medium-, and low-risk groups, with the lowest-risk cohort having a 2.1% inpatient mortality. The limitations of this large-scale registry include a retrospective design and its use of several predictor variables that would be unknown at ED presentation. Other retrospective studies reveal similar findings regarding the high-risk AHFS patient. Patients with SBP of less than 120 mmHg had threefold higher inpatient mortality than those with SBP > 140 mmHg (7.2% vs. 2.5%, $p < 0.001$) [20].

The majority of patients who present with AHFS will require oxygen supplementation. The amount of oxygen that must be administered is often part of the inclusion/exclusion criteria to be admitted to an OU. After initial steps at symptom relief, patients can be titrated down to a nasal cannula that can easily be managed in an OU. Ventilatory support through endotracheal intubation or noninvasive ventilation (NIV) is a clinical decision made prior to OU enrollment and precludes OU admission. Noninvasive ventilatory support either through continuous positive airway pressure support (CPAP) or bi-level positive airway pressure (BiPAP) may reduce the need for intubation, improve physiologic parameters, shorten ICU stay, and reduce cost, but likely does not impact mortality [21, 22] (3CPO investigators). Patients on NIV are not candidates for OU protocols, as their care approaches ICU intensity. If they can be weaned off NIV in the ED, transitioning their care to an OU may be considered if other parameters are met [23].

Renal Function and Acute Kidney Injury. Elevated creatinine (SCr > 3.0 mg/dL) and blood urea nitrogen (BUN > 40 mg/dL) on hospital admission is strongly correlated to increased in-hospital and postdischarge mortality [24]. Patients admitted to the hospital with high blood pressure (>180/110 mmHg) or AKI, as defined by a >25% decrease in estimate glomerular filtration rate from baseline, have greater risk of heart failure, cardiac arrest ($p < 0.0001$), and higher 90-day mortality ($p > 0.003$) [25]. AKI, as measured by markers of tubular damage such as neutrophil gelatinase-associated lipocalin (NGAL), N-acetyl-beta-D-glucosaminidase (NAG), or kidney injury molecule 1 (KIM-1), is the subject of ongoing investigation in AHFS risk stratification [26].

Sodium and Potassium. Hyponatremia, as defined by a serum sodium <135 mmol/L, is associated with increased in-hospital mortality, postdischarge mortality, and readmission rates [27]. Hyperkalemia that may accompany renal insufficiency, resulting from excess repletion in the setting of diuretic use, or from potassium sparing diuretic use, can complicate OU management. Hypokalemia can be frequently encountered in this population, as most are taking loop diuretics. No specific studies exist that evaluate outcomes in AHFS patients with abnormal potassium levels, and the SCPC makes no recommendations regarding potassium levels and OU inclusion or exclusion criteria.

Cardiac Ischemia and Myocardial Necrosis Markers. Evidence of ischemia, as defined by ECG changes and troponin elevation, has been strongly associated with increased acute mortality, postdischarge mortality, and increased readmission rates. Peacock et al. found that AHFS patients with elevated cTn, all of whom had SCr < 2.0, had higher in-hospital mortality, lower blood pressure on admission, and a lower ejection fraction. The in-hospital mortality difference (8.7% vs. 2.0%,

$p < 0.001$) was independent of other predictive variables. The cut point for cTnI was 0.01 µg/L and for cTnT, 1.0 µg/L [28]. Diercks et al. studied an OU cohort of 160 patients and found that a SBP > 160 mmHg and a normal cTn identified a low-risk cohort that experienced no 30-day adverse events (death, readmission, myocardial infarction, or arrhythmias) [29]. Minimal troponin elevations using the high-sensitivity cTn assay have not been evaluated as extensively as the prior generation assays for their ability to predict poor outcome in this AHFS population.

Natriuretic Peptides

Natriuretic peptides are useful as a diagnostic tool in patients where there is still uncertainty after traditional testing [30, 31]. As such, patients with a BNP < 100 are unlikely to have AHFS. Elevated BNP levels have been associated with increased disease severity, but an absolute cutoff has not been established. The SCPC guidelines have suggested physicians should "consider" patients with a BNP level <1,000 pg/mL or a NT-proBNP level <5,000 pg/mL as good candidates for an OU stay. However, these levels are not an absolute cutoff, and patients with levels above these may still be good OU candidates, depending on the clinical scenario. BNP levels have been shown to decrease linearly as pulmonary capillary wedge pressure falls [32]. However, following BNP levels to indicate response to therapy and determining a "safe" discharge level has been met with mixed results [25, 33, 34]. For this reason, the SCPC OU AHFS guidelines suggest that BNP changes cannot be used as the sole marker on which to base OU discharge [12]. In summary, the NP's can be used to aid in identification of patients with AHFS and suggest who may be good OU candidates, but should not be used to identify those patients eligible for OU discharge.

Summary

Inclusion criteria for the observation unit thus require that patients have an initial systolic blood above 120 mmHg, no evidence of AKI as defined by a BUN < 40 mg/dL and a creatinine < 3.0 mg/dL, and a troponin below the 99th percentile as established by their hospitals' local lab evaluation. Patients excluded from observation unit heart failure management would consist of those with an unstable airway or vital signs, those with multiple morbidities, or ongoing evidence of myocardial ischemia. Despite the existence of a number of objective parameters, risk stratification of heart failure still requires a clinical impression by the physician of relative stability and a reasonable probability that the patient will be a discharge candidate in the next 24 h.

References

1. Ahmed A, et al. Incident heart failure hospitalization and subsequent mortality in chronic heart failure: a propensity-matched study. J Card Fail. 2008;14:211.
2. Rosamond W, et al. Heart disease and stroke statistics–2008 updated: a report from the American Heart Association Statistics Committee and Stroke Statistics Subcommittee. Circulation. 2008;117:e25.
3. Abraham WT, et al. Predictors of in-hospital mortality in patients hospitalized for heart failure: insights from the Organized Program to Initiate Lifesaving Treatment in Hospitalized Patients with Heart Failure (OPTIMIZE-HF). J Am Coll Cardiol. 2008;52:347.
4. Fonarow GC, et al. Association between performance measures and clinical outcomes for patients hospitalized with heart failure. JAMA. 2007;297:61.
5. O'Connor CM, et al. Predictors of mortality after discharge in patients hospitalized with heart failure: an analysis from the Organized Program to Initiate Lifesaving treatment in Hospitalized Patients with Heart Failure (OPTIMIZE-HF). Am Heart J. 2008;156:662.
6. Lee SL, et al. Early deaths in patients with heart failure discharged from the emergency department: a population-based analysis. Circ Heart Fail. 2010;3:228–35.
7. Schrock JW, Emerman CL. Observation unit management of acute decompensated heart failure. Heart Fail Clin. 2009;5(1):85. vii.
8. Collins SP, et al. Cost-effectiveness analysis of ED decision making in patients with non-high-risk heart failure. Am J Emerg Med. 2009;27(3):293.
9. Fine MJ, et al. A prediction rule to identify low-risk patients with community-acquired pneumonia. NEJM. 1997;336(4):243.
10. Selker HP, et al. Use of the Acute Cardiac Ischemia Time-Insensitive Predictive Instrument (ACI-TIPI) to assist with triage of patients with chest pain or other symptoms suggestive of acute cardiac ischemia. Ann Intern Med. 1998;129(11):845.
11. Pollack Jr CV, et al. Application of the TIMI risk score for unstable angina and non-ST elevation acute coronary syndrome to an unselected emergency department chest pain population. Acad Emerg Med. 2006;13(1):13–8.
12. Peacock WF, et al. Society of Chest Pain Centers recommendations for the evaluation and management of the observation stay acute heart failure patient—parts 1–6. Acute Card Care. 2009;11(1):3–42.
13. Collins SP, et al. Low-risk acute heart failure patients: external validation of the Society of Chest Pain Center's recommendations. Crit Pathw Cardiol. 2009;8(3):99–103.
14. McKee PA, et al. The natural history of congestive heart failure: the Framingham study. N Engl J Med. 1971;285(26):1441–6.
15. Felker GM, et al. Risk stratification after hospitalization for decompensated heart failure. J Card Fail. 2004;10(6):460–6.
16. Barsheshet A, et al. Admission blood glucose level and mortality among hospitalized nondiabetic patients with heart failure. Arch Intern Med. 2006;166(15):1613–9.
17. Fermann GJ, Collins SP. Observation units in the management of acute heart failure syndromes. Curr Heart Fail Rep. 2010;7(3):125–33.
18. Selker HP, Griffith JL, D'Agostino RB. A time-insensitive predictive instrument for acute hospital mortality due to congestive heart failure: development, testing, and use for comparing hospitals: a multicenter study. Med Care. 1994;32(10):1040–52.
19. Fonarow GC, et al. Risk stratification for in-hospital mortality in acutely decompensated heart failure: classification and regression tree analysis. JAMA. 2005;293(5):572–80.
20. Gheorghiade M, et al. Systolic blood pressure at admission, clinical characteristics, and outcomes in patients hospitalized with acute heart failure. JAMA. 2006;296(18):2217–26.
21. Vital FM, et al. Non-invasive positive pressure ventilation (CPAP or bilevel NPPV) for cardiogenic pulmonary edema. Cochrane Database Syst Rev. 2008;3:CD005351.
22. Masip J, et al. Non-invasive pressure support ventilation versus conventional oxygen therapy in acute cardiogenic pulmonary edema: a randomized trial. Lancet. 2000;356(9248):2126–32.

23. Mak S, et al. Effect of hyperoxia on left ventricular function and filling pressures in patients with and without congestive heart failure. Chest. 2001;120(2):467–73.
24. Formiga F, et al. Predictors of in-hospital mortality present at admission among patients hospitalised because of decompensated heart failure. Cardiology. 2007;108(2):73–8.
25. Szczech LA, et al. Acute kidney injury and cardiovascular outcomes in acute severe hypertension. Circulation. 2010;121(20):2183–91.
26. Damman K, et al. Tubular damage in chronic systolic heart failure is associated with reduced survival independent of glomerular filtration rate. Heart. 2010;96(16):1297–302.
27. Gheorghiade M, et al. Relationship between admission serum sodium concentration and clinical outcomes in patients hospitalized for heart failure: an analysis from the OPTIMIZE-HF registry. Eur Heart J. 2007;28(8):980–8.
28. Peacock IV WF, et al. Cardiac troponin and outcome in acute heart failure. N Engl J Med. 2008;358:2117.
29. Diercks DB, et al. ED patients with heart failure: identification of an observational unit-appropriate cohort. Am J Emerg Med. 2006;24(3):319–24.
30. Maisel AS, et al. Rapid measurement of B-type natriuretic peptide in the emergency diagnosis of heart failure. N Engl J Med. 2002;347(3):161–7.
31. McCullough PA, et al. B-type natriuretic peptide and clinical judgment in emergency diagnosis of heart failure: analysis from Breathing Not Properly (BNP) Multinational Study. Circulation. 2002;106(4):416–22.
32. Maisel AS, et al. Utility of B-natriuretic peptide as a rapid, point-of-care test for screening patients undergoing echocardiography to determine left ventricular dysfunction. Am Heart J. 2001;141(3):367–74.
33. Singer AJ, et al. Rapid Emergency Department Heart Failure Outpatients Trial (REDHOT II): a randomized controlled trial of the effect of serial B-type natriuretic peptide testing on patient management. Circ Heart Fail. 2009;2(4):287–93.
34. Lokuge A, et al. B-type natriuretic peptide testing and the accuracy of heart failure diagnosis in the emergency department. Circ Heart Fail. 2010;3(1):104–10.

Chapter 14
Acute Heart Failure in Observation Unit Treatment Protocols

J. Douglas Kirk and Michael Clarke

Introduction

Treatment of acute heart failure (AHF) patients who present with signs and symptoms of decompensation remains challenging. There is limited data from randomized controlled trials of these patients in the emergency department (ED), much less the observation unit (OU). As a result, there has been little consensus regarding their management, adding to the inconsistent care these patients receive. Only recently have guidelines emerged to provide clinicians a framework from which to work [1]. This chapter will focus on therapeutic management, with respect to general supportive measures, pharmacologic therapy, and, most importantly, specific treatment protocols or algorithms that can be implemented in your institution.

General Support

The majority of patients who present to the ED with AHF have a chief complaint of dyspnea, and supplemental oxygen should be reflexively administered in essentially all patients with a target of maintaining an oxygen saturation ≥95%. This may require high-flow oxygen by face mask in some patients, while others may only need oxygen by nasal cannula.

J.D. Kirk, MD, FACEP (✉)
Department of Emergency Medicine, University of California, Davis Medical Center,
4150 V Street, PSSB Suite 2100, Sacramento, CA 95817, USA
e-mail: jdkirk@ucdavis.edu

M. Clarke, MD
Department of Emergency Medicine, University of California, Davis Medical Center,
Sacramento, CA 95817, USA

W. Frank Peacock (ed.), *Short Stay Management of Acute Heart Failure*,
Contemporary Cardiology, DOI 10.1007/978-1-61779-627-2_14,
© Springer Science+Business Media, LLC 2012

In cases of flash pulmonary edema, often associated with severe hypertension and diastolic dysfunction, more aggressive airway maneuvers may be necessary.

In some cases, endotracheal intubation may be warranted or inevitable, but every attempt should be made to avoid this because of the transient nature of the requirement and the associated morbidity in these patients. Obviously, patients requiring invasive ventilation are not good candidates for OU care. However, the use of aggressive airway adjuncts such as noninvasive ventilation (NIV), consisting of either continuous positive airway pressure (CPAP) or bilevel positive airway pressure (BiPAP), may assist in avoiding the need for intubation while maintaining adequate oxygenation and ventilation. NIV should not be considered a substitute for intubation, but rather as a bridge to allow therapies directed at reducing filling pressures and pulmonary congestion to become efficacious. Further, brief periods of NIV should not exclude patients from the OU by definition, especially in patients with acute pulmonary edema related to severe hypertension, as these patients may rapidly improve with the combination of NIV and pharmacologic therapy.

While both methods of NIV appear to offer benefit, controversy exists regarding the relative superiority of either. Both interventions produce similar reductions in cardiac filling pressures and improve respiratory status, but a recent meta-analysis found a significant reduction in mortality for patients treated with CPAP, but not BiPAP, and no overall difference on intubation rates [2]. However, more recent data from a large, multicenter, randomized controlled trial demonstrated no significant outcome differences between the two methods, as well as no mortality benefit of NIV in general [3]. Based on the available evidence, it is difficult to distinguish either method as superior, and there is likely to be general equivalence in clinical practice. Hence, NIV should be considered as a useful adjunct in the management of patients with AHF.

Pharmacological Therapy

Although general supportive measures such as maintaining adequate oxygenation are critical, in the setting of hypertension, the mainstay of therapy for AHF is pharmacological, and the primary goal is to rapidly decrease filling pressures. Additional important goals include improving cardiac output through a reduction in afterload or improvement in contractility. Furthermore, given the large percentage of AHF patients with underlying diastolic dysfunction, improving the ventricle's ability to fill with blood through efforts to improve myocardial relaxation is crucial.

Initial Management of Acute Pulmonary Edema

Although many patients with acute pulmonary edema are too sick for subsequent OU management, a number will turn around quickly with aggressive ED treatment, particularly those with acute severe hypertension. Concurrent with the aforementioned airway maneuvers, all efforts should be directed at reducing pulmonary congestion. The most rapid improvement will be achieved with potent vasodilators such as nitroglycerin, nesiritide, or nitroprusside. Although each is quite effective, their immediate intravenous use often requires too much time to set up, a luxury these patients may not have on initial presentation. Initiation of sublingual nitroglycerin therapy, in doses larger than those typically used for chest pain (as many as twenty 0.4 mg tablets or sprays), can be quite effective [4]. One can achieve significant reductions in filling pressures and blood pressure (afterload) with a marked improvement in respiratory symptoms, often within minutes. Patients can then be transitioned to other formulations of a vasodilator (e.g., topical or intravenous) and typically become reasonable candidates for the OU.

The addition of an intravenous diuretic to this strategy is common and makes practical sense as it will result in significant diuresis and eventual drop in preload. However, a number of patients do not suffer from total fluid overload, but rather maldistribution of fluid into the pulmonary bed. Suffice it to say, the data is limited in the use of any of these agents in the setting of acute pulmonary edema and respiratory distress. However, there appears to be an immediate benefit from rapid administration of sublingual nitroglycerin with or without an intravenous loop diuretic. Further recommendations on the use of these agents cannot be made until further research elucidates the utility and safety of such an approach.

Diuretics

Diuretics are often the first-line therapy in the ED management of patients with AHF and have become a mainstay of many OU treatment protocols. The rationale that diuretics ameliorate total volume overload may be true; however, a reduction in elevated filling pressures may be more important. Nonetheless, diuretics are certainly effective at reducing preload and removing excess fluid. While they have demonstrated substantial clinical utility, the potential for harmful side effects is significant and must not be lost on the treating physician. In addition to electrolyte depletion (e.g., K^+, Mg^+), diuretics result in decreased renal perfusion and neurohormonal activation by increasing renin and norepinephrine [5, 6]. The short-term gains with diuretic therapy may be offset by these deleterious long-term effects.

The loop diuretic furosemide is most commonly used, although other loop diuretics are equally effective. Suggested starting doses are 20 mg of intravenous furosemide in diuretic-naive patients or an amount equivalent to the patient's total usual daily dose given intravenously. Peak diuresis should occur within 30–60 min, and urinary output should be monitored closely. Repeated doses, in some instances double the first dose, are often effective in patients who fail to respond initially. Doses greater than 160 mg of furosemide are likely to produce as many side effects as results and should be discouraged. The use of continuous dose loop diuretic (e.g., furosemide 5–10 mg/h) has also been advocated to temper the deleterious effects of intermittent boluses of higher doses. Although inconclusive, a Cochrane Review suggested greater diuresis and a better safety profile when loop diuretics were given as continuous infusion [7]. In patients with diuretic resistance, use of an additional diuretic that works on the proximal tubule, e.g., metolazone, may produce effective diuresis. Although large clinical trials evaluating timing and routes have not been performed, the use of diuretics remains a mainstay in the treatment of AHF.

Vasodilators

Oxygen therapy and loop diuretics may be sufficient therapy for mild AHF exacerbations, especially if their visit is due to brief periods of medical or dietary noncompliance. However, this frequently is not adequate, and the addition of vasodilators becomes necessary, particularly in patients with severe hypertension and/or diastolic dysfunction. Most hypertensive patients are well perfused and hence are best treated with vasodilators such as nitroglycerin, nesiritide, or nitroprusside. Some patients with mild AHF may respond to sublingual, oral, or topical nitrates, and several reports advocate this approach [4, 8]. Others have promoted the use of sublingual angiotensin-converting enzyme inhibitors (ACEI) in this setting, based largely on a small trial of 21 patients who showed symptomatic improvement after treatment with sublingual captopril [9]. Data from ADHERE, a multicenter heart failure registry, suggests that patients treated early (<6 h) with an intravenous vasodilator had lower 48-h in-hospital adjusted mortality [10]. This data generates enthusiasm that early goal-directed therapy initiated in the ED or OU may hold promise, and further study is warranted.

Despite their widespread acceptance as standard therapy, surprisingly, little clinical outcome data exist for nitroglycerin and nitroprusside to support their use in AHF. Physician familiarity with nitroglycerin use in patients with chest pain may contribute to its use (with diuretics) as frequent first-line therapy. The relatively predictable effect on filling pressures and blood pressure makes nitroglycerin an attractive choice. In this setting, dosing of intravenous nitroglycerin is typically higher than with chest pain, with usual starting doses of 50 mcg/min, depending upon initial blood pressure. It is not uncommon to need doses in excess of 200 mcg/min, with frequent (e.g., as often as every minute) titration. Nitroprusside can also be particularly useful in patients with acute pulmonary edema associated with severe hypertension, but its use has fallen out of favor and is usually reserved for those failing nitroglycerin.

There are several limitations to both of these therapies, including the deleterious effects of neurohormonal activation and the need for titration and hemodynamic monitoring. The latter two characteristics make these agents ill-suited for use in the OU. When employed in the OU, nitroglycerin's use is typically limited to a fixed, nontitratable dose. These drawbacks have led to a search for better therapeutic agents, ideally ones that improve acute symptoms and hemodynamics, as well as mortality.

Nesiritide

Nesiritide is identical to human endogenous B-type natriuretic peptide (BNP) and is the first commercially available natriuretic peptide used for the treatment of AHF. It serves as an antagonist to pathologic vasoconstrictive neurohormonal activation that occurs in AHF. A pivotal randomized, controlled trial demonstrated nesiritide decreased pulmonary capillary wedge pressure more than either nitroglycerin or placebo at 3 h and more than nitroglycerin at 24 h [11]. In addition, nesiritide's hemodynamic effects were longer lasting, without a need for uptitration, which was frequently necessary in the nitroglycerin group to maintain adequate reduction in wedge pressure [12]. Several characteristics emerged that suggested it was quite suitable for the ED or OU population, including a lack of proarrhythmic effect, no tachyphylaxis, and no need for titration [13]. Of all the vasodilators, only nesiritide has been specifically studied in the ED or OU. The PROACTION study was a blinded, randomized, standard therapy-controlled trial of standard therapy versus nesiritide for OU heart failure management. It reported that the addition to nesiritide to standard therapy resulted in a significant decrease in the rate of "days in-hospital" over the subsequent 30 days postdischarge [14].

However, the safety of nesiritide has been called into question as two meta-analyses suggested significant impairment of renal function and a trend toward increased risk of 30-day mortality which severely curtailed its use [15, 16]. More recent data from a large, randomized, placebo-controlled study reveals that nesiritide is not associated with an increase in serum creatinine or 30-day mortality; unfortunately, statistically significant improvements in dyspnea compared to standard therapy were also not found in this inpatient study [17]. Future research will be needed to further define the role of nesiritide in AHF.

Inotropes

The use of inotropes has essentially no role in the OU management of patients with AHF. While agents such as dobutamine and milrinone are effective at improving cardiac output and tissue perfusion, both cause neurohormonal activation, an increase in ventricular ectopy, and appear to be associated with an increase in long-term mortality [18, 19]. Patients exhibiting clear signs of decreased perfusion or overt cardiogenic shock should be managed in an intensive care unit with appropriate hemodynamic monitoring, and thus, further discussion here is not warranted.

Management Algorithms in the Observation Unit

A number of management algorithms for ED or OU care have recently appeared in the literature. Conclusive evidence identifying suitable patients who clearly benefit from a particular strategy is lacking, and only recently have specific recommendations to drive management been published [1]. It does appear, however, that patient risk stratification and initiation of aggressive treatment in the ED may limit potentially irreversible myocardial toxicity, especially in those with moderate to severe AHF [10, 20]. The algorithm depicted in Fig. 14.1 attempts to provide some guidance for the diagnostic and prognostic evaluation of the suspected AHF patient, in addition to recommendations for level of care and disposition decisions.

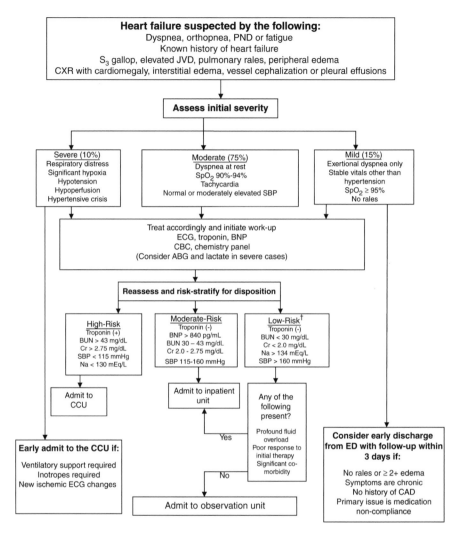

Fig. 14.1 Management algorithm developed by Phillip Levy, MD, MPH, and Jalal Ghali, MD for use at Detroit Receiving Hospital. *ABG* arterial blood gas, *BNP* B-type natriuretic peptide, *BUN* blood urea nitrogen, *CAD* coronary artery disease, *CCU* cardiac care unit, *CBC* complete blood count, *Cr* creatinine, *CXR* chest radiograph, *ECG* electrocardiogram, *JVD* jugular venous distention, *PND* paroxysmal nocturnal dyspnea, *SBP* systolic blood pressure, *SpO₂* saturation of peripheral oxygen. (*Dagger*) To meet this classification, all five criteria should be present

Using typical historical, physical examination, and key diagnostic test features, a clinical profile of AHF is defined. An assessment of initial severity is determined, based primarily upon level of respiratory distress and evidence of hypoperfusion. Further risk stratification is then derived after the initial workup from results of tests that have demonstrated important prognostic information such as serum sodium,

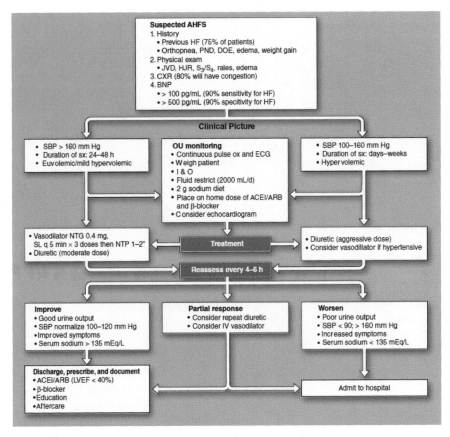

Fig. 14.2 Observation unit algorithm. *ACEI* angiotensin-converting enzyme inhibitor, *AHFS* acute heart failure syndrome, *ARB* angiotensin receptor blocker, *BNP* B-type natriuretic peptide, *CXR* chest radiograph, *DOE* dyspnea on exertion, *ECG* electrocardiogram, *HF* heart failure, *HJR* hepatojugular reflux, *I&O* intake and output, *IV* intravenous, *JVD* jugular venous distention, *LVEF* left ventricular ejection fraction, *NTG* nitroglycerin, *NTP* nitropaste, *OU* observation unit, *PND* paroxysmal nocturnal dyspnea, *SBP* systolic blood pressure, *SL* sublingual, *SX* symptoms (Adapted from Fermann GJ, Collins SP. Observation Units in the Management of Acute Heart Failure Syndromes. Curr Heart Fail Rep. 2010; 7:125–133)

renal function, troponin, BNP, and the initial systolic blood pressure [20–23]. For the purposes of this chapter's focus on OU care, sections pertaining to the potentially life-threatening complications of respiratory failure or cardiogenic shock will not be discussed in detail.

Figure 14.2 provides further detail of management strategies in patients with AHF who have a predominance of symptoms due to pulmonary congestion [24]. This algorithm divides patients into two clinical groups based upon the initial presenting blood pressure. Patients who are initially hypertensive may benefit more from aggressive vasodilator therapy and a modest dose of diuretics, while those who are initially normotensive are often substantially volume overloaded and require more aggressive diuretic therapy. Both groups may be candidates to undergo protocolized care and OU monitoring. In the OU, responses to treatment and achieving therapeutic targets determine disposition, whether to be discharged to home or admitted for inpatient care.

Another algorithm with more patient specific treatment recommendations for management of AHF in the OU is described in Fig. 14.3 [25]. In this strategy, treatment of AHF is generally based on the presence or absence of volume overload and an assessment of the patient's cardiac output. On the left side of Fig. 14.3 [A, C, D, E, F], treatment recommendations are given for patients with AHF experiencing signs and symptoms of volume overload, manifested by pulmonary congestion. One of the limitations of this algorithm is grouping all patients with pulmonary congestion together, regardless of the etiology. There is no consideration of the patient's blood pressure or whether systolic or diastolic dysfunction is present. Nonetheless, it is quite helpful with general management principles. The right side of the algorithm provides treatment recommendations for patients with low cardiac output, and since most OUs exclude these patients, little discussion of this component of the algorithm is warranted.

Volume overload is divided into mild and moderate–severe groups; patients with mild volume overload (Fig. 14.3 [C]) are treated with intravenous diuretic therapy, typically loop diuretics (Fig. 14.3 [D]). Dosages in patients previously taking diuretics are guided by the total home daily dose, given as an intravenous bolus. Therapy for patients not taking oral diuretics at home is based upon renal function, and clinicians should exercise caution with diuretic therapy in such patients to avoid further renal injury. Success of diuretic therapy is driven by urine output goals, and recommendations for repeat diuretic dosing are described in the algorithm. Again, caution should be exercised with extremely high doses of loop diuretics; prerenal azotemia and electrolyte abnormalities are common and should be recognized and treated quickly. A management strategy for electrolyte disturbances in this setting is included in the accompanying standing orders (Fig. 14.4).

The authors recognize that patients with more severe pulmonary congestion, which typically include those with severe hypertension and resultant acute pulmonary edema, are likely to have an inadequate response to intravenous diuretic therapy alone. In these patients, the initial pharmacologic regimen should be more aggressive and include both an intravenous diuretic and a parenteral vasodilator (Fig. 14.3 [F]) if the blood pressure allows. Intravenous nitroglycerin or nesiritide may be used to produce a more rapid response and more effectively relieve the signs and symptoms of congestion in these patients. No specific recommendations are provided as to which vasodilator should be used. Of note, the suggested starting dose of nitroglycerin (5–10 mcg/min) described in Fig. 14.3 [F] should be considerably higher.

Physician order sets for OU management of AHF are typically necessary to standardize the evaluation and treatment of these patients. Figures 14.4 and 14.5 represent two example order sets with slightly different components. While the former

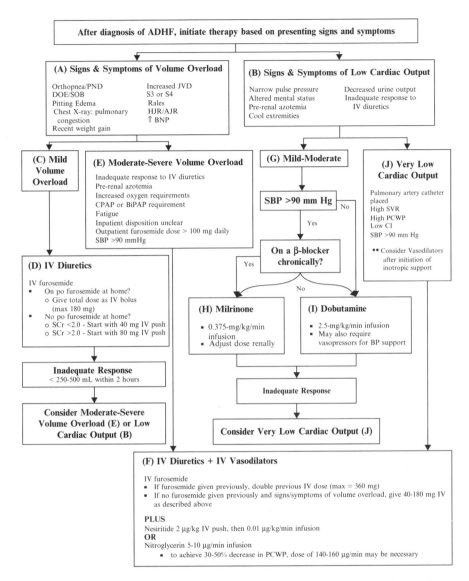

Fig. 14.3 Acute decompensated heart failure (ADHF) treatment algorithm. *AJR* abdominal jugular reflex, *BiPAP* bilevel positive airway pressure, *BNP* B-type natriuretic peptide, *BP* blood pressure, *CI* cardiac index, *CPAP* continuous positive airway pressure, *DOE* dyspnea on exertion, *HJR* hepatojugular reflex, *IV* intravenous, *JVD* jugular venous distention, *PCWP* pulmonary capillary wedge pressure, *PND* paroxysmal nocturnal dyspnea, *PO* by mouth, *SBP* systolic blood pressure, *SCr* serum creatinine, *SOB* shortness of breath, *SVR* systemic vascular resistance (Adapted from DiDomenico RJ, Park HY, Southworth MR, et al. Guidelines for acute decompensated heart failure treatment. Ann Pharmacother. 2004;38:649–660)

Congestive Heart Failure order Set
For Acute Decompensated Congestive Heart Failure Patients
Emergency Department Order Sheet

Date Time Primary Diagnosis: Acute Decompensated Congestive Heart Failure
             Secondary Diagnosis: _____
             Vital signs q4h and as directed by medications (see individual medications)

☐ Labs: Basic metabolic panel, calcium, magnesium, phosphorus, CBC, PT/INR, PTT,BNP,CK,CK-MB, Troponin, O_2 saturation
☐ Digoxin level (if outpatient medication)
☐ Patient Weight: _____
☐ Ins and Outs
☐ 12 Lead ECG
☐ AP and lateral
☐ Foley catheter prn heavy diuresis
☐ Diet: <2.4g Na, low fat
☐ Fluid restriction: 1800 mL/24h; if Na <131 mg/dL, restrict fluid to 1500 mL/24h

Intravenous Furosemide
☐ If furosemide naïve, furosemide 40 mg IVP × 1 dose
☐ If on furosemide as outpatient
      Total daily dose as IV_____mg: maximum 180 mg
      • Goal: >500 mL urine output within 2 hours for normal renal function
        >250 mL urine output within 2 hours if renal insufficiency
      • If goal urine output not met within 2 hours, double the furosemide dose to a maximum of 360 mg IV
      • Monitor symptom relief, vital signs, BUN, SCr, electrolytes

Nesiritide
☐ 2µg IV push followed by 0.01 µg/kg/min IV infusion
☐ If symptomatic hypotention during infusion, discontinue nesiritide
      • Monitor symptom relief, vital signs q15m × 1 hour, then q30min × 1 hour, then q4h, urine output, electrolytes, BUN, SCr, magnesium, calcium, phosphorus
☐ If poor symptom relief or diuretic response ≥ 3 hours after nesiritide therapy initiation AND SBP ≥90 mm Hg, may consider titration of nesiritide
      • Nesiritide 1 µg/kg IVP and increase infusion by 0.005 µg/kg/min
      • May increase infusion rate q1h after first dosage, increase to a maximum dose of 0.03 µg/kg/min

Nitroglycerin 50 mg/250 mL
☐ 5 µg/min IV infusion; titrate dose q5min by 10-20 µg/min to achieve symptom relief
      • Monitor Symptom relief, vital signs q15min until stable dose, then q30min × 1 hour, then q4h, ECG, urine output

Dobutamine 500 mg/250 mL
☐ 2.5 µg/kg/min IV infusion and titrate dose every 5 minutes to desired response to a maximum dose of 20 µg/kg/min
          • Monitor symptom relief, vital signs q15min until stable dose, then q30min × 1 hour, then q4h; ECG; urine output

Milrinone 20 mg/100mL
☐ 0.375 µg/kg/min
          • Monitor symptom relief, vital signs q15min until stable dose, then q30min × 1 hour, then q4h; ECG; urine output

Fig. 14.4 Physician order set for the initial management of acute decompensated heart failure in the emergency department/observation unit. *AP* anterior/posterior, *BNP* B-natriuretic peptide, *BUN* blood urea nitrogen, *CBC* complete blood count, *CK* creatine kinase, *CK-MB* creatine kinase MB isoenzyme, *ECG* electrocardiogram, *INR* international normalized ratio, *IV* intravenous, *IVP* intravenous push, *PO* by mouth, *PRN* as needed, *PT* prothrombin time, *PTT* partial thromboplastin time, *SBP* systolic blood pressure, *SCr* serum creatinine, *Clcr* creatinine clearance (Adapted from DiDomenico RJ, Park HY, Southworth MR, et al. Guidelines for acute decompensated heart failure treatment. Ann Pharmacother. 2004;38:649–660)

❑ Digoxin   _____
                        Dose   Route   Frequency

❑ Lisinopril PO _____
                        Dose   Frequency

❑ Losartan PO _____
                        Dose   Frequency

❑ Metoprolol PO _____
                        Dose   Frequency

❑ Spironolactone PO_____
                        Dose   Frequency

Electrolyte Replacement
❑   Potassium

level (mEq/L)	IV dose (over 1 h)	PO dose	When to recheck potassium
3.7–3.9	20 mEq	40 mEq	12 hours or next morning
3.4–3.6	20 mEq × 2 doses	40 mEq × 2 doses	6 hours or next morning
3.0–3.3	20 mEq × 4 doses	40 mEq × 3 doses	4 hours after last dose
<3.0	20 mEq × 6 doses	Give IV only	1 hour after last dose

• If Clcr <30 mL/min, reduce dose by 50%

❑   Magnesium

level (mEq/L)	IV dose	PO dose (Mg oxide)	When to recheck Megnesium
1.9	Give PO only	140 mg	Next morning
1.3–1.8	1 g MgSO$_4$ for every 0.1 below 1.9 (max 6 g)	Give IV only	Next morning
<1.3	8 g MgSO$_4$	Give IV only	6 hours after last dose or next morning

• MgSO$_4$ 1–2 g, infuse over 1 hour
• MgSO$_4$ 3–6 g, infuse ≤2 g/hour

_____   _____

Physician Signature   Date

Fig. 14.4 (continued)

represents a more exhaustive compilation, the latter illustrates a comparatively abbre-
viated order set, limited to one page, that was developed to maximize ease of use,
minimize errors, and meet key AHF clinical practice guidelines [26]. These orders
are for sample purposes only and should be modified accordingly to accommodate
institutional variations in practice. Again, the inclusion of orders for inotropic therapy
in Fig. 14.4 is not typically indicated in OU patients.

Conclusions

Evidence-based guidelines for the management of AHF patients in the ED and OU
are just now emerging [1]. While treatment protocols and management algorithms
appear vital to the success of any OU strategy, they are currently based largely on
anecdotal experience or at best, data from small trials. Cornerstones of these algorithms are appropriate patient risk stratification and recognition of those primarily
with pulmonary congestion versus those with cardiogenic shock. Further delinea-

Diuretics: **Give 1–2 x home daily dose.** ☐ **Contraindication to Furosemide:**   ☐ **Volume contracted** ☐ **Allergy**
☐ Patient already received furosemide by EMS
☐ Furosemide (Lasix).
     • IVP   ☐ 60 mg   ☐ 80 mg   ☐ _____ mg   ☐ Repeat this dose q 6 hours
     • IV continuous infusion   ☐ 10 mg/hr
☐ Measure urine output, implement below orders and notify physician of amount
     • **If urine output is less than 200 mL, 1 hour after initial administration, repeat the same dose.**
     • Total urine output goal generally 1,000 mL diuresis over 4 hours
     • Redraw K+ and Mg+ and notify physician after > 1,000 mL diuresis

Vasodilator: **Generally use one agent; or multiple agents with caution** ☐ **Contraindiction: Sildenafil (Viagra) in last 24 hours**
☐ IV Nitroglycerin (NTG) at 10 mcg/min. Titrate IV NTG q 5 minutes by 10 mcg/min to MAP drop of 20% from initial MAP or
                         to an SVR drop of around 1,000 and CI > 2 or
☐ Nitroglycerin paste: _____ inch(s) to chest wall (remove if MAP drops 20% from initial MAP) or   **Hold IV NTG for**
☐ Nesiritide (Natrecor)   ☐ no bolus   ☐ bolus: 2 mcg/kg over 1 minute, then:
                         ☐ Continuous infusion of   ☐ 0.01 mcg/kg/min   ☐ _____ mcg/kg/min   **SBP <90 – Notify MD**

ACE Inhibitor: **Early initiation improves outcome. Use patient's current dose or start other med**
☐ Contraindication to ACE: hypotension, dehydration, poor perfusion, allergy, angioedema, pregnancy,
                         renal insufficiency, renal artery stenosis, hyperkalemia
☐ Patient already took ACE within current dosing cycle
☐ Lisinopril (Prinivil/Zestril) _____ mg po   [start 10 mg daily] **or** | First dose okay without creatinine.
☐ Enalapril (Vasotec)   ☐ 1.25 mg IV infused over 1 hour   **or** |
☐ _____ mg po | Subsequent doses require creatinine.

ARB (Angiotensin Receptor Blocker) If ACE allergy.   **Early initiation improves outcome.**
                                       Use patient's current dose or start other med
☐ Contraindication to ARB: see ACE contraindications
☐ Patient already took ARB within current dosing cycle
☐ Losartan (Cozaar) _____ mg po   [start 25 mg daily] **or** | First dose okay without creatinine.
☐ _____ mg po | Subsequent doses require creatinine.

Respiratory:
☐ BiPAP: start at I 10/E 4. Adjust FiO2 to maintain O2 sat of ≥ 92%

☐ Respiratory med: ☐ Albuterol nebulizer 2.5 mg.   ☐ Atrovent nebulizer 0.5 mg

Treatments: **NOTIFY HEART FAILURE CENTER x3899**   **CONSIDER BIOIMPEDANCE**
☐ Scaled weight in ED in kilograms (kg) _____

☐ Saline lock IV access

☐ Foley to gravity if patient is unable to safely ambulate. Discontinue foley when able to safely ambulate.

☐ Strict I & O's

☐ Continuous pulse ox. Titrate to O2 sat of ≥ 92% by nasal cannula, ventimask or non-rebreather

☐ _____

☐ _____

MD Signature_____Date_____Time_____ Phone _____

RN Signature _____

✚ Advocate Christ Medical Center

EMERGENCY DEPARTMENT
CHF STANDING ORDERS

| Patient Name: _____
| MR Number: _____
| Patient Number: _____
| OR
| Affix Patient Label

010101

Green · Chart   Canary · Pharmacy

0101 · 5/05
Page 1 of 2
Divider # 8

Fig. 14.5 New congestive heart failure emergency department order set. *ACE* angiotensin-converting enzyme, *ARB* angiotensin receptor blocker, *EMS* emergency medical services, *IV* intravenous, *IVP* intravenous push, *MAP* mean arterial pressure, *NTG* nitroglycerin, *PO* by mouth, *SBP* systolic blood pressure, *SVR* systemic vascular resistance, *BiPAP* bilevel positive airway pressure, *I/E* inspiratory/expiratory, *I* intake, *O* output (Adapted from Reingold S, Kulstad E. Impact of Human Factor Design on the Use of Order Sets in the Treatment of Congestive Heart Failure. Acad Emerg Med. 2007; 14:1097–110)

tion based upon (1) severity of volume overload, (2) associated renal insufficiency, and (3) relationship to presenting blood pressure appears to aid with management decisions. Unfortunately, there is little consensus among authors regarding an overall approach. Suffice to say, systematic use of therapeutic agents (intravenous diuretics and vasodilators) with a priori clinical targets is a must. Further, in appropriate patients, data appear to support the early use of vasodilators [11]. Additional recommendations await publication of institutional experience with algorithms such as those presented here.

References

1. Peacock WF, Fonarow GC, Ander DS, et al. Society of Chest Pain Centers recommendations for the evaluation and management of the observation stay acute heart failure patient—parts 1–6. Acute Card Care. 2009;11:3–42.
2. Masip J, Roque M, Sánchez B, et al. Noninvasive ventilation in acute cardiogenic pulmonary edema: systematic review and meta-analysis. JAMA. 2005;294(24):3124–30.
3. Gray A, Goodacre S, Newby DE, et al. Noninvasive ventilation in acute cardiogenic pulmonary edema. N Engl J Med. 2008;359:142–51.
4. Bussmann W, Schupp D. Effect of sublingual nitroglycerin in emergency treatment of severe pulmonary edema. Am J Cardiol. 1978;41:931–6.
5. Gottlieb SS, Brater DC, Thomas I, et al. BG9719 (CVT-124), an A1 adenosine receptor antagonist, protects against the decline in renal function observed with diuretic therapy. Circulation. 2002;105(11):1348–53.
6. Brewster UC, Setaro JF, Perazella MA. The renin-angiotensin-aldosterone system: cardiorenal effects and implications for renal and cardiovascular disease states. Am J Med Sci. 2003;326(1):15–24.
7. Salvador DRK, Punzalan FE, Ramos GC. Continuous infusion versus bolus injection of loop diuretics in congestive heart failure. Cochrane Database Syst Rev. 2005;3:CD003178. doi:10.1002/14651858.
8. Cotter G, Metzkor E, Kaluski E, et al. Randomised trial of high-dose isosorbide dinitrate plus low-dose furosemide versus high-dose furosemide plus low-dose isosorbide dinitrate in severe pulmonary oedema. Lancet. 1998;351:389–93.
9. Hamilton RJ, Carter WA, Gallagher EJ. Rapid improvement of acute pulmonary edema with sublingual captopril. Acad Emerg Med. 1996;3:205–12.
10. Peacock WF, Emerman C, Costanzo MR, et al. Early vasoactive drugs improve heart failure outcomes. Congest Heart Fail. 2009;15:256–64.
11. Publication Committee for the VMAC Investigators. Intravenous nesiritide vs nitroglycerin for treatment of decompensated congestive heart failure: a randomized controlled trial. JAMA. 2002;287:1531–40.
12. Elkayam U, Akhter MW, Singh H, et al. Comparison of effects on left ventricular filling pressure of intravenous nesiritide and high-dose nitroglycerin in patients with decompensated heart failure. Am J Cardiol. 2004;93:237–40.
13. Fonarow GC, on behalf of the ADHERE Scientific Advisory Committee. The Acute Decompensated Heart Failure National Registry (ADHERE): opportunities to improve care of patients hospitalized with acute decompensated heart failure. Rev Cardiovasc Med. 2003;4 suppl 7:S21–30.
14. Peacock WF, Holland R, Gyamarthy R, Dunbar L, Klapholz M, Horton DP, deLissovoy G, Emerman CL. Observation unit treatment of heart failure with nesiritide: results from the PROACTION trial. J Emerg Med. 2005;29(3):243–52.

15. Sackner-Bernstein JD, Skopicki HA, Aaronson KD. Risk of worsening renal function with nesiritide in patients with acutely decompensated heart failure. Circulation. 2005;111: 1487–91.
16. Sackner-Bernstein JD, Kowalski M, Fox M, et al. Short-term risk of death after treatment with nesiritide for decompensated heart failure: a pooled analysis of randomized controlled trials. JAMA. 2005;293:1900–5.
17. Califf R. LBCT I, Abstract 21828. Presented at: American Heart Association Scientific Sessions 2010; Nov. 13-17; Chicago, IL.
18. Cuffe MS, Califf RM, Adams KF, et al. Short-term intravenous milrinone for acute exacerbation of chronic heart failure: a randomized controlled trial. JAMA. 2002;287:1541–7.
19. Abraham WT, Adams KF, Fonarow GC, et al. In-hospital mortality in patients with acute decompensated heart failure requiring intravenous vasoactive medications: an analysis from the ADHERE registry. J Am Coll Cardiol. 2005;46:57–64.
20. Fonarow GC, Adams KF, Abraham WT, et al., for the ADHERE Scientific Advisory Committee, Study Group, and Investigators. Risk stratification for in-hospital mortality in acutely decompensated heart failure: classification and regression tree analysis. JAMA. 2005;293:572–80.
21. Gheorghiade M, Abraham WT, Albert NM, for the OPTIMIZE-HF Organized Program to Initiate Lifesaving Treatment in Hospitalized Patients with Heart Failure Investigators and Coordinators, et al. Systolic blood pressure at admission, clinical characteristics, and outcomes in patients hospitalized with acute heart failure. JAMA. 2006;296:2217–26.
22. Peacock WF, De Marco T, Fonarow GC, et al. Cardiac troponin and outcome in acute heart failure. N Engl J Med. 2008;358:2117–26.
23. Fonarow GC, Peacock WF, Phillips CO, et al. Admission B-type natriuretic peptide levels and in-hospital mortality in acute decompensated heart failure. J Am Coll Cardiol. 2007;49: 1943–50.
24. Fermann GJ, Collins SP. Observation units in the management of acute heart failure syndromes. Curr Heart Fail Rep. 2010;7:125–33.
25. DiDomenico RJ, Park HY, Southworth MR, et al. Guidelines for acute decompensated heart failure treatment. Ann Pharmacother. 2004;38:649–60.
26. Reingold S, Kulstad E. Impact of human factor design on the use of order sets in the treatment of congestive heart failure. Acad Emerg Med. 2007;14:1097–110.

Chapter 15
Education Elements in the Observation Unit for Heart Failure Patients

Robin J. Trupp

Introduction

Heart failure (HF) is a complex chronic condition associated with great morbidity, mortality, and economic burden in the United States [1]. The vast majority of healthcare expenses related to HF occur as a result of hospitalizations for management of the decompensation [1]. Identification of the precipitant for the decompensation, such as tachyarrhythmias, sodium indiscretion, or ischemia, determines the treatment plan. Importantly, in most instances, the majority of hospitalizations could be avoided with adherence to medication and dietary regimens and careful symptom monitoring of changes in signs and symptoms of HF [2–4]. Although educational needs for the patient with HF are vast and include such topics as the pathophysiology and etiology of HF and necessary lifestyle modifications, in an observation unit, education must be directed and succinct, given the short-term nature of the interaction. However, during times of stress, as would be expected in patients presenting to an emergency department (ED) with acute dyspnea, retention of any information given is limited [5]. If the patient is ultimately hospitalized, the time urgency for providing information is lessened because the inpatient environment offers additional opportunity for, and reinforcement of, education. Therefore, patient and family education should take advantage of the "teachable moments" that occur across the spectrum of inpatient care, beginning in the ED and ending at discharge [6]. Since the majority of causes of decompensation are directly attributable to nonadherence to the medication and/or dietary regimens, this chapter concentrates on these topics as essential elements of patient education.

R.J. Trupp, PhD, ACNP-BC, CHFN (✉)
Society of Chest Pain Center, Columbus, OH, USA
e-mail: rtrupp@scpcp.org

W. Frank Peacock (ed.), *Short Stay Management of Acute Heart Failure*,
Contemporary Cardiology, DOI 10.1007/978-1-61779-627-2_15,
© Springer Science+Business Media, LLC 2012

Adherence to prescribed medical regimens, including both pharmacologic and nonpharmacologic interventions, significantly impacts both the short- and long-term management of HF. Despite strong evidence showing the efficacy of these interventions to halt or reverse disease progression, reduce hospitalizations, and improve quality of life and overall symptom control, numerous barriers to adherence exist. These barriers include, but are not limited to, the following: a lack of appreciation for the consequences of nonadherence and the importance of lifestyle modifications, an absence of social support, feelings of powerlessness or loss of control, and issues related to finances, resources, or time constraints. These barriers further complicate patients' ability and willingness to adhere to the complex treatment required for evidence-based HF care. In addition, in the haste to shorten length of stay and meet facility and national goals, clinicians may simply treat the symptoms, thus failing to identify the cause for the decompensation. By taking the time to do a thorough assessment to identify the precipitating event and any barriers, clinicians can better use the time spent with each patient, leading to a more individualized treatment plan and enhanced adherence [7].

Causes for Decompensation

Nonadherence to the medication schedule and volume overload, directly related to sodium indiscretion (willful or inadvertent) and excess fluid intake, are the major causes for decompensation, or worsening HF [3, 7]. To reduce postdischarge morbidity and mortality, a thorough evaluation and consideration of precipitating factors is encouraged [8]. Identification of reversible causes, such as coronary artery disease or valvular dysfunction during hospitalization, may shorten hospital lengths of stay and minimize postdischarge morbidity and mortality [9]. Patient education and close outpatient surveillance by the patient and family can reduce nonadherence and lead to the detection of early changes in clinical status so that interventions to prevent further clinical deterioration and ultimately ED care and hospitalization can be implemented [8].

Medication and Dietary Adherence

Dietary and medication adherence has profound implications for the management of HF. Lack of adherence as a contributor to decompensation and hospitalization has been well documented [3]. Poor adherence also has significant economic repercussions. For example, if insufficient medication is taken for the treatment to be fully effective, as when patients "ration" diuretics to extend the life of a prescription, hospital-based care may necessary. Not unexpectedly, better outcomes are seen with improved adherence to treatment plans. The role of education on medication and dietary adherence cannot be overemphasized and requires continual consistent reinforcement from all providers. Yet, strategies to increase adherence to diet and medication must be individualized. One size does not fit all here.

Dietary Instructions

The American Heart Association, the Institute of Medicine, and the US Department of Agriculture all advocate for Americans to restrict sodium intake to 2,300 mg per day [10–12]. For African Americans, those with heart disease, or those over the age of 40, this restriction drops to 1,500 mg per day. However, given American's consumption of processed products and fast food, this degree of sodium restriction is challenging for even the most dedicated individual. Since diuretics act by increasing sodium excretion in the urinary filtrate, which is followed by increased water excretion, a diet high in sodium makes diuretics essentially ineffective in controlling volume and symptoms. Patients must be taught and understand the relationship between fluid and sodium for managing volume and for controlling HF symptoms. Counseling should include repeated in-depth instruction on the components of a 2-g sodium diet, involving family members and caregivers as well. Having the patient complete a food diary over the course of several days will yield important insights into dietary habits, food preferences, and average fluid consumption. Reading food labels, low-sodium food choices when dining out, and cooking with herbs and spices to improve palatability are important aspects that should be included. Providing written materials or useful websites for low-sodium food choices and recipes is essential for home. As a note, salt substitutes should be used with caution, as many replace sodium chloride with potassium chloride, thus increasing the potential risk of hyperkalemia.

In advanced HF, further dietary sodium restriction may be necessary to attenuate expansion of extracellular fluid volume and the development of edema. Although sodium restriction may mitigate the development of edema, it cannot totally prevent it because the kidneys are capable of reducing urinary sodium excretion to less than 10 mmol per day. Hyponatremia should not be treated with sodium liberalization because this hyponatremia is typically dilutional in nature and occurs in the setting of free-water excess. Liberalized sodium intake or replacement should be reserved for overt cases of severe excessive diuresis and dehydration.

Within the emergency department, simple questions about recent dietary intake may yield the cause of decompensation. Accompanying family members are also good sources of information regarding food or fluid ingestion. Instructing patients to simply take an extra diuretic to relieve symptoms is no longer encouraged, as diuretics contribute to both increased neurohormonal stimulation and worsening renal function [7]. As discussed above, patients should understand that dietary indiscretion produces fluid retention and worsening symptoms. Thus, efforts should focus on helping patients make the association between behavior and symptoms. The challenge lies in doing this without preaching or condemning. Learning will not occur within that scenario. If a connection between a particular behavior and its negative consequences can be made, lifestyle changes are more likely to take place. However, behavioral changes do not happen overnight, and those who view the recommended changes as personal choices, rather than as edicts imposed by others, are more likely to make permanent lifestyle modifications [8].

Recognizing obvious sources of sodium, such as a salt shaker or potato chips, is evident for most patients, but in a typical diet, they constitute less than 25% of total sodium intake. Hidden sources of sodium play a greater role in dietary intake yet are often unrecognized. Good HF clinicians are also good detectives. Common high-sodium-content items include, but are not limited to, canned soups and vegetables, pickles, cheeses, softened water, tomato juice, antacids, and processed foods. As discussed above, a food diary provides important information on food choices and eating patterns. Having the patient start this diary after treatment in the emergency department affords the clinician next evaluating the patient much-needed information and the ability to discuss alternative lower sodium choices. The ED should be stocked with printed materials for patients and families to take home.

Medications

Pharmacologic interventions are vital to managing symptoms and halting disease progression in HF. Yet, medications for heart failure are both complex in their administration and costly. Polypharmacy, or the need for multiple medications, is a normal consequence of an evidence-based approach to managing heart failure because beta-blockers, angiotensin-converting enzyme (ACE) inhibitors and/or angiotensin receptor blockers, aldosterone inhibitors, electrolyte supplements, and diuretics must all be taken at different times throughout the day. No wonder patients become confused and fail to comply. Potential barriers to adherence should be identified and addressed. Besides financial barriers, other frequently missed obstacles include real or perceived side effects, depression, forgetfulness, and understanding the importance of and need for the medication [5, 6]. To improve patient adherence, ongoing discussions must occur between clinicians and patients to reach understanding and agreement on the necessity for medications and the appropriate regimen [6]. Rather than mandated or imposed views, this discussion may require some compromise from both parties, as a patient may agree to take more medications than initially desired or a clinician acknowledges the patient may be taking less than is ideal. What is most important is that health-care providers know about all medications being taken.

Medication reconciliation is the process of comparing medication orders to all of the medications the patient has been taking. This reconciliation is done to avoid medication errors such as omissions, duplications, dosing errors, or drug interactions. More than half of patients have at least one medication discrepancy on admission to a hospital [13]. In addition, there is an increased risk for discrepancy at every transition point: from home to ED, ED to admission, one unit to another, and inpatient to discharge. Recognizing that medication errors put patients at risk and are largely preventable, the Joint Commission named medication reconciliation as 2005

National Patient Safety Goal #8. The first step in medication reconciliation is to obtain the most accurate list of current medications prior to giving any medications in the ED (except in emergency or urgent scenarios). This includes prescription and over-the-counter medications, vitamins and supplements, noting the dose, route, frequency, indication, and time of last dose for each. Each facility likely has a specific form and process for documenting medication history and adherence. Besides the patient and family, the patient's pharmacy and previous medical records may be reliable sources of information. Patients should be instructed to bring all of their medications whenever seeking or receiving health care.

To assist with adherence, a variety of aids are available and may be helpful to some. These aids include pill boxes, medication trackers, timers, or interactive websites, to name few. For those with financial constraints, most major pharmaceutical companies offer assistance programs for individuals unable to afford medications. Many require documentation of medical necessity from the prescriber, and patients may need to submit documentation of financial need as well. Although this process is unlikely to be initiated in the emergency department, it is important to recognize resource options and to make the necessary referrals. Access to social worker or case management staff can be quite valuable in addressing these concerns.

Worsening Signs and Symptoms

Despite advanced warning signs and symptoms of decompensation, many patients either fail to recognize or fail to react to them. For example, Friedman reported that 90% of patients hospitalized due to worsening HF experienced dyspnea 3 days prior to hospitalization [14]. Additionally, 35% reported edema, and 33% had cough 1 week prior to admission [15]. This delay may be a failure to routinely monitor symptoms or an inability to recognize and interpret symptoms when they occur. Thus, when patients cannot recognize or acknowledge worsening signs and symptoms, clinicians lose the chance to intervene and potentially avert hospitalization. Therefore, educating patients and their families on both the signs and symptoms associated with worsening HF, and actions to take, provides an excellent opportunity to reduce hospitalizations and health-care expenditures.

Establishing self-care abilities is essential for patients with HF to participate in their own management, and that of their disease. Self-care involves patients' decisions about engaging in behaviors intended to maintain physiological stability and about changes in their HF status [16]. Self-care maintenance decisions include following the therapeutic regimen, i.e., taking medications, eating a low-sodium diet, exercise, engaging in preventive behaviors, and actively monitoring their condition. Self-care management refers to decisions that are made in response to changes in signs and symptoms, i.e., calling a health-care provider, taking an extra diuretic, or going to the ED. Table 15.1 lists self-care behaviors recommended for patients with HF.

Unfortunately, there is no one single sign or symptom indicative of worsening HF. Rather, patients experience a constellation of signs and symptoms, including increased

Table 15.1 Self-care behaviors recommended for all patients with HF

Maintain current immunizations, especially influenza and *Streptococcus pneumoniae*

Develop a system for taking all medications as prescribed

Monitor for changes in weight, increase or decrease

Monitor for changes in signs/symptoms of shortness of breath, swelling, fatigue, and other indicators of worsening HF

Restrict dietary sodium intake to 2,000 mg per day; learn to read labels

Restrict alcohol intake

Avoid other recreational toxins, especially cocaine

Cease all tobacco use and avoid exposure to second-hand smoke

Do not ignore emotional distress, especially depression and anxiety. Seek treatment early

Tell your provider about sleep disturbances, especially snoring, witnessed apnea, excessive daytime sleepiness

Achieve and maintain physical fitness

Visit your provider at regular intervals

Do not take over-the-counter medicines or herbal supplements without consulting with a provider

If diabetic, achieve diabetes mellitus treatment goals

Adapted from Riegel B, Moser DK, Anker SD, et al.; on behalf of the American Heart Association Council on Cardiovascular Nursing, Council on Clinical Cardiology, Council on Nutrition, Physical Activity, and Metabolism, and Interdisciplinary Council on Quality of Care and Outcomes Research. State of the science: promoting self-care in persons with heart failure: a scientific statement from the American Heart Association. *Circulation.* 2009;120:1141–1163

dyspnea and/or fatigue, weight gain, orthopnea, and paroxysmal nocturnal dyspnea. Efforts to improve patients' abilities to recognize, interpret, and act on the early signs and symptoms may be facilitated when patients receive simple consistent advice on what changes in symptoms are important and clear endpoints that should prompt them to seek help. Essential aspects of education are presented in Table 15.2.

Whenever special equipment is involved, instruction on proper use and when to seek help are required. For example, daily weights require that the patient owns a scale, that the scale has numbers that can be read by the patient, with a stable base large enough for them to stand on, and that the weights are obtained at approximately the same time each day. Education on when to call with weight changes is determined by the clinician and should be provided in written format and reinforced frequently. In all cases, patients and families should be diligent in monitoring physical signs and symptoms. Establishing plans for notifying health-care providers of any changes is the logical next step and should include the identification of emergency contact numbers for doing so.

Respiratory Symptoms

As mentioned above, the majority of patients with decompensated HF have evidence of excess extracellular volume or congestive signs and symptoms. However, typical respiratory complaints, such as dyspnea, have poor sensitivity and are nonspecific to HF [12]. In addition, many patients with HF also have significant comorbidities that

Table 15.2 Essentials of heart failure patient education

- Daily weights every day of your life
  - ☐ Use the same scale at the same time of the day wearing comparable clothing
  - ☐ Weigh first thing in the morning after going to the bathroom
  - ☐ Notify your health-care provider if you gain 3 or more pounds overnight or 5 pounds over 3 days OR if you lose weight and experience dizziness on standing up
- *Maintain a low-sodium diet to help avoid fluid retention*
  - ☐ A dietary intake of 2,000 mg of sodium per day is recommended
  - ☐ Ask for written materials that can help you make healthier choices
  - ☐ Salt is everywhere. Learn to read labels
- *Be conscious of fluid intake*
  - ☐ Do NOT drink 8 glasses of water per day if taking a diuretic (water pill). This defeats the purpose of the medication
  - ☐ Drink small sips when thirsty or when taking medications
  - ☐ Do NOT carry liquids with you
  - ☐ Fluid comes in a variety of formats: soup, Jell-O, ice, watermelon
- *Be as active as possible*
  - ☐ Engage in physical activity at least 3–4 times per week
  - ☐ Appropriate activities include walking or biking
- *Avoid any form of heavy lifting or isometric exercises*
  (Isometric exercises are those in which a force is applied to a resistant object, such as pushing against a brick wall)
  - ☐ Treatment of heart failure is directed at reducing the workload in your heart, not straining it. Do not lift anything heavier than 10 pounds
- *Notify your health-care provider of changes in your symptoms or weight*
  - ☐ This includes weight gain of 3 or more pounds overnight or 5 pounds over 3 days, increased fatigue or shortness of breath, dizziness, or fever, to name a few
  - ☐ Your physician or nurse will give you additional, specific instructions to follow
  - ☐ Keep their emergency number readily available in case of need
- *Bring all of your medications with you whenever you are seeking or receiving health care*
  - ☐ This includes both prescription medications and those purchased without a prescription, such as vitamins, pain medicines, or nutritional supplements

may further limit respiratory function, such as chronic pulmonary disease or obesity. When such comorbidities are present, the clinical importance of alterations from everyday respiratory limitations becomes the measure for pending decompensation. For example, using three pillows to sleep may be a normal sleep pattern for some and would not be considered as evidence of orthopnea, but for others, a change from one to two pillows may be indicative of congestion. Patients may report sleeping on one pillow but fail to mention that pillow is used in their recliner because they cannot tolerate lying flat in bed without severe respiratory distress. Additionally, emergency room clinicians may ask about sleep patterns, including hours of sleep, daytime sleepiness, the presence of snoring, witnessed apnea, and nocturia, to discover other possible sleep disturbances that impact HF [16].

Patients with chronic HF live with dyspnea, and breathlessness becomes "normal," or a part of everyday life [17]. Adjustments to constant dyspnea usually center on reducing physical activities to decrease breathlessness. In that scenario, seeking treatment occurs only when the usual strategies, such as rest or fresh air, fail to relieve symptoms and the patient becomes anxious or frightened. Initial treatment is aimed at rapidly alleviating air hunger and hypoxia. It is important to remember that substantial pulmonary congestion can occur without rales or jugular venous pressure being evident [18].

Changes in Weight

Just as diabetics monitor glucose levels to better manage their disease, so should patients with HF monitor their weight. While neither precise nor totally reflective of volume status, daily weights comprise the gold standard for the outpatient care and management of HF. However, less than half of HF patients report weighing themselves daily [19], even in the first week following a hospitalization for decompensation [20]. As previously discussed, daily weights will not occur or be accurate if the patient does not own a scale, devalues the necessity of performing the task, or fails to do so consistently and appropriately. Although the focus of weight monitoring is to detect weight gain, indicating fluid retention, patients should also pay attention to weight loss. Excessive weight loss can be the consequence of dehydration, result in electrolyte imbalances, or worsening renal function, and produce symptoms of dizziness, fatigue, and shortness of breath. In advanced HF, when the patient's appetite and caloric intake decline, excess volume may take place in the absence of any apparent weight gain, as true body mass is lost through muscle and fat catabolism.

Fatigue

Patients with HF experience chronic fatigue and reduce their physical activity accordingly to mitigate exhaustion. However, worsening or increasing fatigue, in the absence of increased physical activity, can be an early indicator of decompensation. Any increased fatigue that lasts longer than 2–3 days should be a source of concern for the patient and should prompt closer attention to sodium and medication adherence. Should additional symptoms develop, or the fatigue continues or worsens, patients should notify their clinician immediately so that treatment interventions can be initiated and hospitalization possibly avoided. However, as with dyspnea, fatigue is a vague, nonspecific symptom that is difficult to quantify and can be included in the differential diagnosis for many other conditions and diseases.

Nocturia

One of the earliest symptoms of excess extracellular fluid is nocturia. To maintain homeostasis, the heart attempts to eliminate excess volume through the secretion of natriuretic peptides from atrial and ventricular myocytes. These endogenous peptides act by dilating the renal afferent arteriole, preventing sodium reabsorption, and counteracting neurohormonal vasoconstriction effects. Atrial natriuretic peptide is secreted primarily at night, when right atrial pressures are highest as a result of supine positioning. Consequently, urinary volume is increased, and the patient is awakened to void. Patients should pay attention to new onset or increasing nocturia that occurs in the absence of changes in the medication, especially increased diuretics, or dietary regimen.

Reinforcement of Education

Information can be presented in different formats. Accordingly, a variety of educational materials must be accessible within the emergency department. Some examples of materials available include videotapes or CDs, pamphlets, or printed pages specifically distributed by the institution. Such materials should also be consistent with educational information given by other departments or community agencies. It is not unusual for patients to be given conflicting instructions on weight changes, such as call if you gain 2 pounds overnight, 3 pounds overnight, 5 pounds in 2–3 days, or 5 pounds in a week. When faced with conflicting advice, many simply opt to do nothing. Having these materials at hand provides patients and families the opportunity to read and have questions answered, resulting in an expedited education process.

Because high levels of relapse are likely to occur after short-term behavioral interventions, plans for reinforcement of the education must be established to improve long-term adherence and to prevent additional decompensation events [21]. Patients should be scheduled for a follow-up visit with the primary-care physician or other clinicians managing HF within days of discharge [9]. This quick appointment serves many purposes. The first is to ensure that treatment has been adequate in resolving the congestion and that no new issues have developed. The second is to closely compare the medications prescribed at discharge with the previous regimen to identify and correct any discrepancies. Finally, reinforcement of education can be provided, especially education specific to the precipitant of the exacerbation. If the cause was not identified, health-care providers more familiar with the patient may be able to discern it at this appointment and provide the requisite education.

Summary

For many, episodes of decompensated HF may be largely avoidable through self-monitoring of symptoms and enhanced adherence to treatment regimens. Unfortunately, during incidents of worsening HF, it can be difficult to provide education to patients on better managing their disease. A better plan in the emergency department is to begin by treating the excess volume and alleviating the symptoms. Once stabilized and in the observation unit, there are ample opportunity and teachable

Table 15.3 Example of wallet-sized patient reminder card

Medications				Medications		
MEDICATIONS	STRENGTH	DOSING		MEDICATION	STRENGTH	DOSING
___	___	___		___	___	___
___	___	___		___	___	___
___	___	___		___	___	___
___	___	___		___	___	___

CALL

Dr.——at (——)
if you have signs or symptoms of ——
worsening CHF

From The ADHERE®
Scientific Advisory
Committee

Appointments

DATE	TIME
___	___
___	___
___	___
___	___

- Increase in shortness of breath
- Swelling in the legs or ankles
- Weight gain ≥3 lbs within a few days
- Difficulty breathing when lying down
- Worsening tiredness
- Stomach bloating/fullness and loss of appetite
- Dry cough, especially when lying down

REMINDER
Always maintain a low-salt diet

Patient
Reminder
Card

Patient Name

Adhere
Acute Decompensated Heart Failure National Registry

BACK   FRONT

For best results, please print on heavyweight paper. Cut along black dotted lines and roll fold at blue dotted lines for a 4-paneled, threefold 2"×3.5" pocket card.

moments when educational content is likely to be better received and understood. Education and counseling that address specific concerns may provide knowledge, support, and impetus to adhere to treatment plans, recognize early signs of worsening HF, and ultimately reduce hospitalizations. Importantly, discharge instructions should include prompt follow-up with the established primary-care physician or cardiologist within days of ED treatment or hospital discharge [9]. Sending patients home with a wallet-sized card detailing these salient points further reinforces their importance (Table 15.3). Finally, in advanced or complex cases, referral to a HF specialist may be warranted [8].

References

1. O'Connell JB, Bristow M. Economic impact of heart failure in the United States: time for a different approach. J Heart Lung Transpl. 1994;13:107–12.
2. Evangelista LS, Dracup K. A closer look at compliance research in heart failure patients in the last decade. Progr Cardiovasc Nurs. 2000;15(3):97–103.
3. Dunbar SB, Clark PC, Deaton C, et al. Family education and support interventions in heart failure. Nurs Res. 2005;54(3):158–66.
4. Ni H, Nauman D, Donna Burgess D, et al. Factors influencing knowledge of and adherence to self-care among patients with heart failure. Arch Intern Med. 1999;159:1613–9.
5. Dominique JF, de Quervain DJF, Roozendaal B, et al. Acute cortisol administration impairs retrieval of long term declarative memory in humans. Nat Neurosci. 2000;3:313–4.
6. Williams S, Brown A, Patton R, Crawford MJ, Touquet R. The half-life of the 'teachable moment' for alcohol misusing patients in the emergency department. Drug Alcohol Depend. 2005;77:205–8.
7. Ryan RH, Deci EL. Self-determination theory and the facilitation of intrinsic motivation, social development, and well-being. Am Psychol. 2000;55:68–78.
8. Jessup M, Abraham WT, Casey DE, et al. 2009 Focused update: ACCF/AHA Guidelines for the diagnosis and management of heart failure in adults. Circulation. 2009;119(14):1977–2016.
9. Weintraub NL, Collins SP, Pang PS, on behalf of the American Heart Association Council on Clinical Cardiology and Council on Cardiopulmonary, Critical Care, Perioperative and Resuscitation, et al. Acute heart failure syndromes: emergency department presentation, treatment, and disposition: current approaches and future aims: a scientific statement from the American Heart Association. Circulation. 2010;122:1975–96.
10. Lichtenstein AH, Appel LJ, Brands M, et al. Diet and Lifestyle Recommendations Revision 2006A Scientific statement from the American Heart Association Nutrition Committee. Circulation. 2006;114:82–96.
11. Institute of Medicine. Dietary reference intakes for water, potassium, sodium chloride, and sulfate. 1st ed. Washington, DC: The National Academies Press; 2004. http://books.nap.edu/openbook.php?record_id=10925&page=r1.
12. US Department of Health and Human Services, US Department of Agriculture. Dietary guidelines for Americans 2005. 6th ed. Washington, DC: US Department of Health and Human Services, US Department of Agriculture; 2005. http://www.health.gov/dietaryguidelines/dga2005/document/pdf/dga2005.pdf.
13. Cornish PL, Knowles SR, Marchesano R, et al. Unintended medication discrepancies at the time of hospital admission. Arch Intern Med. 2005;165:424–9.
14. Friedman M, Griffin JA. Relationship of physical symptoms and physical functioning to depression in patients with heart failure. Heart Lung. 2001;30:98–104.

15. Parshall MB, Welsh JD, Brockopp DY, Heiser RM, Schooler MP, Cassidy KB. Dyspnea duration, distress, and intensity in emergency department visits for heart failure. Heart Lung. 2001;30:47–56.
16. Riegel B, Moser DK, Anker SD, et al; on behalf of the American Heart Association Council on Cardiovascular Nursing, Council on Clinical Cardiology, Council on Nutrition, Physical Activity, and Metabolism, and Interdisciplinary Council on Quality of Care and Outcomes Research. State of the science: promoting self-care in persons with heart failure: a scientific statement from the American Heart Association. *Circulation.* 2009;120:1141–1163.
17. Edmonds PE, Rogers A, Addington-Hall JM, et al. Patient descriptions of breathlessness in heart failure. Int J Cardiol. 2005;98:61–6.
18. Young JB, Mills RM. Clinical management of heart failure. West Islip, NY: Professional Communications; 2001.
19. Wright SP, Walsh H, Ingley KM, et al. Uptake of self-management strategies in a heart failure management programme. Eur J Heart Fail. 2003;5:371–80.
20. Moser DK, Doering LV, Chung ML. Vulnerabilities of patients recovering from an exacerbation of chronic heart failure. Am Heart J. 2005;150:984.
21. Rutledge DN, Donaldson NE, Pravikoff DS. Patient education in disease and symptom management in congestive heart failure. Online J Clin Innov. 2001;15(2):1–52.

Chapter 16
Emergency Department and Observation Unit Discharge Criteria

Rachel Rockford and Deborah B. Diercks

Heart failure (HF) causes substantial morbidity and mortality in the United States and is the most common principal discharge diagnosis in adults ≥65 years old [1, 2]. Over the last three decades, the number of admissions for heart failure has tripled [2]. A substantial number of these patients present to the emergency department for the initial treatment of their acute decompensation. It has been suggested that 80% of all patients who present with acute decompensated heart failure are admitted to the hospital [3]. A recent international study found this number to exceed 90% [4]. Identifying patients that are suitable for discharge home from the emergency department (ED) or be admitted to an observation unit (OU) may substantially reduce overall hospital costs. Discharge from the emergency department has been associated with a high rate of adverse events [5]. Accurate disposition is a challenge and perhaps more daunting than the management of these patients to emergency physicians.

Disposition decisions are often time-dependant and lack adequate time to assess response to treatment. This may result in inappropriate admissions and premature ED discharges with resultant increased cost and morbidity, respectively [6]. Although the ACC/AHA guidelines on the management of heart failure suggest that patients with mild to moderate symptoms generally do not require admission, risk assessment solely based on symptoms is often difficult [7]. In order to increase the number of patients discharged to home, effective treatment must be initiated in the ED as part of patient management or as an OU protocol. This early intervention and avoidance of hospital admission can result in significant cost savings. This saving benefit is particularly evident if patients with heart failure are at low risk for adverse events [8].

R. Rockford, MD • D.B. Diercks, MD, MSc, FACEP (✉)
Department of Emergency Medicine, University of California, Davis Medical Center,
Sacramento, CA, USA
e-mail: dbdiercks@ucdavis.eedu

W. Frank Peacock (ed.), *Short Stay Management of Acute Heart Failure*,
Contemporary Cardiology, DOI 10.1007/978-1-61779-627-2_16,
© Springer Science+Business Media, LLC 2012

Success of any protocol is dependent on accurate identification of patients suitable for an early discharge plan. Conversely, patients with a high probability of adverse outcomes, such as those with evidence of acute cardiac ischemia, should be admitted to the hospital as inpatients. Blood pressure and heart rate are two of the most significant independent predictors of acute mortality in patients with ADHF [9]. Thus, patients with unstable vital signs, including a heart rate >130 beats per minute, SBP <85 mm Hg or >175 mm Hg after initial ED treatment, and O_2 saturation <90%, are inappropriate for an early discharge strategy. In addition, those with airway instability, inadequate systemic perfusion, or cardiac arrhythmias requiring continuous IV intervention, as well as those requiring invasive hemodynamic monitoring or receiving medications that require frequent uptitration (e.g., nitroglycerin), are also not suitable for an heart failure OU admission [10].

As essential is the identification of appropriate patients for a rapid treatment protocol, so is the use of discharge criteria that results in a low rate of subsequent hospital readmissions soon after discharge. Unfortunately, there is a paucity of data addressing this issue in the ED, inpatient, or OU setting [11, 12]. The Society of Chest Pain Centers and Providers has established criteria for low-risk patients with heart failure [10]. These utilize parameters such as blood pressure and biomarkers to identify this cohort. The low risk of adverse events in patients meeting these criteria has been validated in a clinical trial [13]. While current methods of risk stratification have focused on identifying patients at risk for short- and long-term adverse events, in actuality, risk stratification is an ongoing process. It is dependent on clinical appearance, laboratory parameters, and response to acute therapies. Discharge to home should be considered from the perspective of an estimate of the acuity of the initial presentation of the patient, improvement after treatment, and risk of recidivism following discharge. Certain clinical features should then alter the initial estimate of acuity, and improvement in these parameters can identify patients suitable for discharge to home.

Consensus guidelines for discharge from the ED and OU have been developed [14]. These guidelines are based on the presence of factors associated with increased risk for adverse events. Although the lack of these parameters does not ensure a patient is ready for discharge, they are useful in identifying those with persistent decompensated heart failure who would benefit from additional treatment. Discharge criteria can be divided into three separate categories: patient-centered measures, hemodynamic and clinical measures, and laboratory measures (Table 16.1).

It has been well established that patient-centered outcome measures, such as a change in dyspnea, can be utilized to assess therapeutic success and improvement in symptoms. Although subjective, the measurement of dyspnea on a 7-point or 3-point scale is validated outcome measures [16]. In addition, the assessment of dyspnea has been shown to correlate with hemodynamic status and prognosis in clinical trials [17]. A recent clinical trial showed that dyspnea relief is often incomplete, and persistent symptoms are associated with worse prognosis and prolonged hospitalization [30].

Another patient-centered measure that should be present at the time of discharge is the lack of ongoing chest pain. It has been reported that ACS is a trigger for up to

Table 16.1 Discharge criteria: ideally, a candidate for discharge would make all of these criteria

Criteria
Presenting complaint
No chest pain that would raise concern for acute coronary syndrome (ACS) [15]
Quality-of-life indicators
Improvement in dyspnea [16, 17]
Ability to ambulate without dyspnea above baseline [18]
Free of symptoms of congestion [19]
Hemodynamic/clinical parameters
Systolic blood pressure <160 mm Hg, >90 mm Hg [20]
Improvement in thoracic electrical bioimpedance measurements [21]
Oxygen saturation >90% [10]
Urine output >1 L [22]
Decrease in weight/return to dry weight
Laboratory measurements
B type natriuretic peptide levels [23–25]
Stable creatinine [20, 26, 27]
Stable or declining troponin level [25, 28]
Return to normal or baseline of electrolytes and blood urea nitrogen (BUN) [11, 12, 29]

25% of patients with heart failure decompensation. Therefore, patients should be pain-free or have undergone an evaluation for ACS prior to discharge [15]. The last patient-centered measure is that the patient should be able to ambulate without an increase in dyspnea from baseline. Although there is no trial that has assessed this measure in an observation unit setting, it is effectively an inexpensive 6-minute exercise test. The distance that a patient can ambulate in a 6-minute period without excessive dyspnea and fatigue has been shown to correlate with long-term mortality [9, 31]. Unfortunately, many comorbid illnesses, such as obesity and lung disease, affect this outcome measure. It is important to assess a change from baseline.

While the prior studies did not specifically evaluate the ED, one recent investigation tested the feasibility of a 3-minute walk in the emergency department and found that 85% of all patients were able to complete the walk and the ability to walk 3 min was associated with outcomes [32]. In addition, freedom from symptoms of congestion has also been associated with improved long-term outcomes, although orthopnea can persist even after subjective improvement in dyspnea [19, 33].

Hemodynamic and clinical parameters can be a part of the data used to assess suitability for discharge. These comprise measures of perfusion, volume status, and oxygenation-based physical exam findings, as well as automated measures. Systolic blood pressure (SBP) is a useful predictor of adverse events at the time of presentation and discharge [20]. In the initial presentation of patients with decompensated HF, a hypertensive response is adaptive, although persistent elevation of SBP can correlate with increased risk of worsening renal function. In HF, any deterioration of renal function clearly correlates with morbidity and mortality; therefore, adjustment of medications to prevent hypertension is essential prior to discharge. While the ideal blood pressure at the time of hospital discharge is not clearly elucidated, patients should at least have a SBP <160 mm Hg [20]. Conversely, as medications are titrated, patients must be able to ambulate without symptoms of dizziness; therefore, the SBP should exceed 90 mm Hg [14].

Clinical findings can also be used to assess adequacy of acute interventions. These include a combination of changes in physical exam and easily obtained values such as pulse oximetry, weight, and urine output. Of all the clinical examination findings, the presence of an S_3 is most suggestive of acute decompensation [34]. Serial exams that document the resolution of an S_3 by auscultation can be used as a discharge criterion [34]. In the ED setting, this auscultatory finding has been shown to provide valuable diagnostic information in conjunction with B-type natriuretic peptide (BNP) [35]. However, the presence of a digitally recorded S_3 has not been shown to be associated with prognosis or improved diagnostic accuracy in one large clinical trial [36]. This physical exam finding, like an improvement in jugular venous distention, is dependent of physical attributes of the patient and careful physical exam assessment by the physician.

Another criterion, noted as part of the evaluation, is oxygen saturation. Patients should have an oxygen saturation greater than 90% [14]. No data exist to support this value; however, it is reasonable to only discharge patients who are able to maintain their oxygen saturation. Transient nighttime drops in oxygen saturations are common because HF is associated with an increased prevalence of obstructive sleep apnea. Therefore, pulse oximetry as a discharge criterion should be assessed when the patient is awake.

Urine output assessment is another parameter that can be used as a surrogate to assess treatment efficacy. Although there are no studies that compare the amount of urine output with outcomes, intuitively, this makes sense. Clinically, 1 L appears to be a significant amount. Closely linked to urine output is in the patient's weight [10, 14]. Dry weight is often one of the only baseline parameters that is known in the ED. Theoretically, a decline in the patient's weight can represent a resolution of the acute progression of the disease process; however, "overshooting" this parameter can lead to hypotension, hypoperfusion, and worsening renal function. Although not supported by clinical trials, it is reasonable to suggest that a patient's weight should be declining at the time of discharge; however, additional assessment may be warranted in patients who are below their dry weight at the time of discharge assessment.

Improvement in laboratory parameters may also be used to assess patients at the time of discharge. Studies have shown that a decline in B-type natriuretic peptide (BNP) levels is associated with improved morbidity and decreased hospital readmission rate [23, 24, 37]. It makes intuitive sense that a patient's BNP should be declining at the time of discharge assessment, although the exact amount of decline is not well established. Di Somma et al. studied BNP as predictor of adverse events in patients admitted for AHF. This multicenter observational study measured BNP at admission, at 24 h, at discharge, and 180 days after discharge. They found that a BNP absolute value of <300 pg/mL and a BNP reduction of >46% at discharge were powerful negative predictors for future cardiovascular outcomes [24].

Elevated troponin levels have been shown to be predictive of long-term prognosis in HF patients [25, 38, 39]. Patients with severe HF may have chronically elevated levels. However, a rise in troponin levels during an observation unit stay should provoke concern and may reflect inadequacy of treatment or the presence of ACS. In addition, patients with an elevated initial troponin have been shown to be more likely to stay in the hospital >24 h and have a high rate of 30-day hospital readmission [11, 40]. A recent study showed that increases in serial values of a high-sensitive troponin I were associated with an increased rate of 90-day mortality [28]. Therefore, patients with an elevated initial troponin level are probably not suitable for an early discharge strategy.

Traditional chemistry labs that are routinely assessed daily in patients with decompensated heart failure can also be used in the assessment at the time of discharge. A sodium level of <136 mEq/L or a serum BUN >43 mg/dL has been shown to correlate with 30-day and 1-year mortality [9, 41]. Therefore, improvement in the BUN and serum creatinine in patients with initially abnormal values is a potential marker of treatment success and may be useful in determining disposition [41]. However, at this point, there are no trials that have utilized these values in this capacity.

A significant amount of attention has been placed on the significance of worsening serum creatinine in the setting of treatment for decompensated heart failure [20, 26, 29]. An increase in creatinine level of >0.3 mg/dL from hospital admission correlates with in-hospital death, complications, and length of stay. The presence of worsening renal insufficiency, as defined by a creatinine change of >0.3 mg/dL from prior values, is concerning, and patients may warrant further treatment until the creatinine improves or stabilizes [20]. Extrapolation from these studies suggests that an increase in serum creatinine identifies a high-risk group of patients.

In addition, recent studies have shown an association between worsening renal function after discharge and poor prognosis [27]. Gotsman et al. studied the significance of serum urea and renal function in patients with heart failure. They found that serum urea may independently have prognostic importance for patients beyond renal function [29]. It may be a more comprehensive data point to measure the clinical status because it encompasses parameters such as renal function, fluid volume balance, hemodynamics, and neurohormonal axis. Since serum admission and discharge urea are predictors of 1-year survival, admission serum urea may be used as possible data point for admission given its probable prognosis for both short-term and long-term survival.

Another laboratory parameter associated with prognosis is the sodium level [42]. A sodium level of <136 mEq/L has been shown to correlate with 30-day and 1-year mortality [9, 41]. In patients with normal serum sodium and BUN at baseline, a decrease in sodium may be an indicator for the need of admission [9, 41]. In addition, an improvement in serum sodium during hospitalization is associated with reduce mortality [43].

Independent of the clinical presentation, the success of early discharge is related to the adequacy of outpatient follow-up and appropriate medication adjustment at the time of discharge. The initial improvements gained in the ED or observation unit

Table 16.2 Outpatient key components

Nursing case management
Physician follow-up (primary care coordinated with cardiology)
Optimization of medication regimen
Patient education
Social support (home health assessment)

can be quickly negated if the patient is discharged without suitable outpatient management plans. Key components include close follow-up to ensure adequate medication adjustment, dietary education, and a management plan (Table 16.2). Inclusion of a cohesive management plan as an outpatient has been show to result in a 25–75% reduction in hospitalization [44–46]. Optimizing the medical regimen is another complex portion of the disposition process, as it requires coordination between many providers, including the ED physician, OU physician, consultants, and the outpatient provider. Although beyond the scope of this chapter, medication considerations would include the titration of loop diuretic, spironolactone, angiotensin-converting enzyme inhibitor, B-blocker, and nitrates [7, 10, 47].

It should also be noted that every patient will not fit every criteria and that all recommendations must be interpreted in consideration of the patient's baseline status and follow-up care. The best recommendations contain a combination of these parameters adjusted for the individual patient. Utilizing a combination of patient-centered outcomes and more objective measures provides ample evidence that can help drive the disposition decision. Appropriate discharge from the emergency room or OU must be accompanied with adequate follow-up. Patient education is also extremely important on dietary recommendations, medication schedules, and tracking body weight to help prevent need for further emergency room visits or hospital admissions.

References

1. Ahmed A, Allman RM, Fonarow GC, et al. Incident heart failure hospitalization and subsequent mortality in chronic heart failure: a propensity-matched study. J Card Fail. 2008;14:211–8.
2. Rosamond W, Flegal K, Furie K, et al. Heart disease and stroke statistics–2008 update: a report from the American Heart Association Statistics Committee and Stroke Statistics Subcommittee. Circulation. 2008;117:e25–146.
3. Schrock JW, Emerman CL. Observation unit management of acute decompensated heart failure. Heart Fail Clin. 2009;5:85–100.
4. Collins SP, Pang PS, Lindsell CJ, et al. International variations in the clinical, diagnostic, and treatment characteristics of emergency department patients with acute heart failure syndromes. Eur J Heart Fail. 2010;12:1253–60.
5. Lee DS, Schull MJ, Alter DA, et al. Early deaths in patients with heart failure discharged from the emergency department: a population-based analysis. Circ Heart Fail. 2010;3:228–35.
6. Kosecoff J, Kahn KL, Rogers WH, et al. Prospective payment system and impairment at discharge. The 'quicker-and-sicker' story revisited. JAMA. 1990;264:1980–3.

7. Hunt SA, Abraham WT, Chin MH, et al. 2009 Focused update incorporated into the ACC/AHA 2005 Guidelines for the Diagnosis and Management of Heart Failure in Adults A Report of the American College of Cardiology Foundation/American Heart Association Task Force on Practice Guidelines Developed in Collaboration With the International Society for Heart and Lung Transplantation. J Am Coll Cardiol. 2009;53:e1–90.
8. Collins SP, Schauer DP, Gupta A, Brunner H, Storrow AB, Eckman MH. Cost-effectiveness analysis of ED decision making in patients with non-high-risk heart failure. Am J Emerg Med. 2009;27:293–302.
9. Fonarow GC, Adams Jr KF, Abraham WT, Yancy CW, Boscardin WJ. Risk stratification for in-hospital mortality in acutely decompensated heart failure: classification and regression tree analysis. JAMA. 2005;293:572–80.
10. Peacock WF, Fonarow GC, Ander DS, et al. Society of Chest Pain Centers recommendations for the evaluation and management of the observation stay acute heart failure patient—parts 1–6. Acute Card Care. 2009;11:3–42.
11. Diercks DB, Peacock WF, Kirk JD, Weber JE. ED patients with heart failure: identification of an observational unit-appropriate cohort. Am J Emerg Med. 2006;24:319–24.
12. Burkhardt J, Peacock WF, Emerman CL. Predictors of emergency department observation unit outcomes. Acad Emerg Med. 2005;12:869–74.
13. Collins SP, Lindsell CJ, Naftilan AJ, et al. Low-risk acute heart failure patients: external validation of the Society of Chest Pain Center's recommendations. Crit Pathw Cardiol. 2009;8:99–103.
14. Peacock WFT, Emerman CL. Emergency department management of patients with acute decompensated heart failure. Heart Fail Rev. 2004;9:187–93.
15. Khand AU, Gemmell I, Rankin AC, Cleland JG. Clinical events leading to the progression of heart failure: insights from a national database of hospital discharges. Eur Heart J. 2001;22:153–64.
16. Teerlink JR. Dyspnea as an end point in clinical trials of therapies for acute decompensated heart failure. Am Heart J. 2003;145:S26–33.
17. Metra M, Cleland JG, Weatherley BD, et al. Dyspnoea in patients with acute heart failure: an analysis of its clinical course, determinants, and relationship to 60-day outcomes in the PROTECT pilot study. Eur J Heart Fail. 2010;12:499–507.
18. Rostagno C, Gensini GF. Six minute walk test: a simple and useful test to evaluate functional capacity in patients with heart failure. Intern Emerg Med. 2008;3:205–12.
19. Lucas C, Johnson W, Hamilton MA, et al. Freedom from congestion predicts good survival despite previous class IV symptoms of heart failure. Am Heart J. 2000;140:840–7.
20. Forman DE, Butler J, Wang Y, et al. Incidence, predictors at admission, and impact of worsening renal function among patients hospitalized with heart failure. J Am Coll Cardiol. 2004;43:61–7.
21. Kazanegra R, Cheng V, Garcia A, et al. A rapid test for B-type natriuretic peptide correlates with falling wedge pressures in patients treated for decompensated heart failure: a pilot study. J Card Fail. 2001;7:21–9.
22. Peacock WF. Heart failure management in the emergency department observation unit. Prog Cardiovasc Dis. 2004;46:465–85.
23. Cheng V, Kazanegra R, Garcia A, et al. A rapid bedside test for B-type peptide predicts treatment outcomes in patients admitted for decompensated heart failure: a pilot study. J Am Coll Cardiol. 2001;37:386–91.
24. Disomma S, Magrini L, Pittoni V, Marino R, Peacock WF, Maisel A. Usefulness of serial assessment of natriuretic peptides in the emergency department for patients with acute decompensated heart failure. Congest Heart Fail. 2008;14:21–4.
25. Metra M, Nodari S, Parrinello G, et al. The role of plasma biomarkers in acute heart failure. Serial changes and independent prognostic value of NT-proBNP and cardiac troponin-T. Eur J Heart Fail. 2007;9:776–86.
26. Chittineni H, Miyawaki N, Gulipelli S, Fishbane S. Risk for acute renal failure in patients hospitalized for decompensated congestive heart failure. Am J Nephrol. 2007;27:55–62.

27. Damman K, Navis G, Voors AA, et al. Worsening renal function and prognosis in heart failure: systematic review and meta-analysis. J Card Fail. 2007;13:59–608.
28. Xue Y, Clopton P, Peacock WF, Maisel AS. Serial changes in high-sensitive troponin I predict outcome in patients with decompensated heart failure. Eur J Heart Fail. 2010;13:37–42.
29. Gotsman I, Zwas D, Planer D, Admon D, Lotan C, Keren A. The significance of serum urea and renal function in patients with heart failure. Medicine. 2010;89:197–203.
30. Metra M, Teerlink JR, Felker GM, et al. Dyspnoea and worsening heart failure in patients with acute heart failure: results from the Pre-RELAX-AHF study. Eur J Heart Fail. 2010;12:1130–9.
31. Rostagno C, Olivo G, Comeglio M, et al. Prognostic value of 6-minute walk corridor test in patients with mild to moderate heart failure: comparison with other methods of functional evaluation. Eur J Heart Fail. 2003;5:247–52.
32. Pan AM, Stiell IG, Clement CM, Acheson J, Aaron SD. Feasibility of a structured 3-minute walk test as a clinical decision tool for patients presenting to the emergency department with acute dyspnoea. Emerg Med J. 2009;26:278–82.
33. Mebazaa A, Pang PS, Tavares M, et al. The impact of early standard therapy on dyspnoea in patients with acute heart failure: the URGENT-dyspnoea study. Eur Heart J. 2010;31:832–41.
34. Marantz PR, Kaplan MC, Alderman MH. Clinical diagnosis of congestive heart failure in patients with acute dyspnea. Chest. 1990;97:776–81.
35. Collins SP, Lindsell CJ, Peacock WF, et al. The combined utility of an S3 heart sound and B-type natriuretic peptide levels in emergency department patients with dyspnea. J Card Fail. 2006;12:286–92.
36. Collins SP, Peacock WF, Lindsell CJ, et al. S3 detection as a diagnostic and prognostic aid in emergency department patients with acute dyspnea. Ann Emerg Med. 2009;53:748–57.
37. Knebel F, Schimke I, Diaz Ramirez I, et al. Hemodynamic improvement of acutely decompensated heart failure patients is associated with decreasing levels of NT-proBNP. Int J Cardiol. 2009;134:260–3.
38. Potluri S, Ventura HO, Mulumudi M, Mehra MR. Cardiac troponin levels in heart failure. Cardiol Rev. 2004;12:21–5.
39. Mueller C. Risk stratification in acute decompensated heart failure: the role of cardiac troponin. Nat Clin Pract Cardiovasc Med. 2008;5:680–1.
40. Parenti N, Bartolacci S, Carle F, Angelo F. Cardiac troponin I as prognostic marker in heart failure patients discharged from emergency department. Intern Emerg Med. 2008;3:43–7.
41. Lee DS, Austin PC, Rouleau JL, Liu PP, Naimark D, Tu JV. Predicting mortality among patients hospitalized for heart failure: derivation and validation of a clinical model. JAMA. 2003;290:2581–7.
42. Rusinaru D, Buiciuc O, Leborgne L, Slama M, Massy Z, Tribouilloy C. Relation of serum sodium level to long-term outcome after a first hospitalization for heart failure with preserved ejection fraction. Am J Cardiol. 2009;103:405–10.
43. Rossi J, Bayram M, Udelson JE, et al. Improvement in hyponatremia during hospitalization for worsening heart failure is associated with improved outcomes: insights from the Acute and Chronic Therapeutic Impact of a Vasopressin Antagonist in Chronic Heart Failure (ACTIV in CHF) trial. Acute Card Care. 2007;9:82–6.
44. Rich MW, Beckham V, Wittenberg C, Leven CL, Freedland KE, Carney RM. A multidisciplinary intervention to prevent the readmission of elderly patients with congestive heart failure. N Engl J Med. 1995;333:1190–5.
45. Hanumanthu S, Butler J, Chomsky D, Davis S, Wilson JR. Effect of a heart failure program on hospitalization frequency and exercise tolerance. Circulation. 1997;96:2842–8.
46. Kim YJ, Soeken KL. A meta-analysis of the effect of hospital-based case management on hospital length-of-stay and readmission. Nurs Res. 2005;54:255–64.
47. Dickstein K, Cohen-Solal A, Filippatos G, et al. ESC guidelines for the diagnosis and treatment of acute and chronic heart failure 2008: the Task Force for the diagnosis and treatment of acute and chronic heart failure 2008 of the European Society of Cardiology. Developed in collaboration with the Heart Failure Association of the ESC (HFA) and endorsed by the European Society of Intensive Care Medicine (ESICM). Eur J Heart Fail. 2008;10:933–89.

Chapter 17
Effective Discharge Planning

Ginger Conway

Discharge planning is the process of evaluation and planning for the patient's needs postdischarge. This begins at the time of admission and must be reevaluated throughout the treatment period [1]. The majority of research has been in the area of discharge planning from the inpatient setting; there is little data on discharge from the Emergency Department (ED) [2, 3]. However, there is obvious relevance to the ED [2, 3]. A comprehensive well-executed discharge plan can prevent unnecessary delays in discharge and ensure the availability of adequate support postdischarge [4, 5]. This is especially beneficial for the elderly [4, 5]. Inadequate discharge planning is linked to early readmissions [6].

Nearly all patients with heart failure will experience acute symptoms at least once necessitating evaluation in the ED [3]. The goal of therapy in the ED is to stabilize the patient, relieve congestion, and improve hemodynamics, as well as volume status, so that the patient can be transitioned to the next locus of care [3]. Many treated in the ED will be discharged home. This is a cost-saving approach but adds to the burden of the ED staff to provide comprehensive discharge planning [7]. Failure to meet this responsibility will result in repeated admissions.

Why Is Discharge Planning So Important for Heart Failure Patients?

Heart failure is the cause of nearly one million hospitalizations annually [8–12]. It is the most common discharge diagnosis among individuals 65 years of age and older and accounts for over one million ED visits per year [11–19]. All ages are at increased risk for readmission if they are inadequately prepared as a result of insufficient discharge planning. Those at increased risk for readmission need special attention.

G. Conway, MSN, RN, CNP (✉)
Division of Cardiovascular Disease, University of Cincinnati, Cincinnati, OH, USA
e-mail: conwaygg@ucmail.uc.edu

W. Frank Peacock (ed.), *Short Stay Management of Acute Heart Failure*,
Contemporary Cardiology, DOI 10.1007/978-1-61779-627-2_17,
© Springer Science+Business Media, LLC 2012

Readmission rates are extremely high among all individuals with heart failure. Approximately 20% are readmitted within 1 month of discharge and 50% within 6 months [10, 20–22]. However, as many as 50% of readmissions may be prevented with comprehensive discharge planning and after discharge follow-up [1, 23, 24]. Unplanned readmissions can be viewed as potential indicators of missed opportunities to improve and better coordinate care [25, 26].

Patients with heart failure often have a high prevalence of comorbid conditions which leads to polypharmacy and multiple health-care providers. This makes adherence to the medical plan more difficult [27–29]. The involvement of multiple care providers increases the need for the transfer of information after an ED visit. Different prescribers rarely have access to a comprehensive medication list, or the full medical record and communication failures contribute to poor outcomes [2, 30]. The average patient with heart failure and comorbid conditions takes 9–12 pills daily, and most do not understand why and how to take them [28]. Approximately one-third of patients with heart failure have dietary restrictions for at least two different conditions [28]. Discharge planning, home-based follow-up, and patient education have been proven to reduce readmission rates [25].

Effective Discharge Planning

The effective discharge plan starts with the first encounter in the ED, regardless of the final disposition of the patient [26, 31]. It begins with an assessment of the cause for this admission as well as an assessment of the patient's ability to recognize symptoms and to know what to do if symptoms worsen. The needs of the patient after discharge and their ability to meet those needs must also be evaluated [1, 3, 4, 19, 26, 32]. This assessment must involve the patient, all members of the health-care team, the family, and any other available caregivers during the ED stay [1, 4, 5, 26, 31, 33].

Addressing barriers to self-care (Table 17.1) by actively engaging the patient and all caregivers has been proven to improve outcomes [3]. Involvement of the caregiver will improve the patient's ability to achieve more sustainable skills [30]. If patients and caregivers believe that they can accomplish a given behavior, and that it will result in the desired effect, they are more likely to be compliant with the desired activity [33]. Individualized discharge plans improve adherence and outcomes by empowering patients to manage their health problems [27].

Table 17.1 Barriers to self-care [3, 18, 30, 34]

Conflicting medication instructions	Poverty
Inability to reach health-care provider	Complex medical regimen
Transportation limitations	Lack of access to adequate health care
Lack of support (living alone, nonsupportive family)	Minimal input from patient into plan of care
Low health-care literacy	Difficult home environment
Difficulty filling prescriptions	Lack of insurance
Comorbid conditions	

Contents of the Effective Discharge Plan (Table 17.2)

Assessment

Patients and their caregivers are often unprepared to care for themselves in the next care setting [30]. Causes for readmissions are multifactorial and include issues such as lack of adherence, inadequate discharge preparation, and education [31]. Additional causes include poor communication between the acute care team and the postacute care team, delayed discharge follow-up, and individual patient economics that may influence how patients use limited resources [31]. Many causes for readmission are items that patients and caregivers can be taught to recognize and avoid [35]. Their ability to learn must be assessed as they may or may not be able to absorb information early in their care due to anxiety, symptom severity, and fear [2, 3]. Heart failure education should employ a variety of methods including written, verbal, and visual aids to facilitate patient and caregiver understanding [26]. Inadequate patient education and nonadherence to the medical plan alone may account for as many as 40% of the readmissions [37].

The patient's and the caregiver's perceived needs must be assessed and met as this will facilitate their investment in the plan and the outcomes [4, 30]. Optimally, all members of the team are be involved in setting discharge goals, while encouraging caregivers and patients to assume a more active role in transitional care [30]. Patients have indicated they want to know why they should follow the medical regimen and what will happen if they do not. Individualizing the information and the method in which it is delivered is key [2]. The transition to home is fraught with confusion about medications, follow-up testing, and care. Many patients are discharged with an incomplete understanding of their care and instructions [2]. Patients especially need information on how to implement the discharge instructions [33]. Those who feel well prepared for discharge have lower rates of readmission [2].

As many as 90 million Americans have poor health literacy [28]. Health literacy is the ability to read and understand prescription labels and instructions, as well as appointment cards and health-related materials. As many as 62% of patients treated in

Table 17.2 Components of effective discharge instructions [3, 26–29, 35, 36]

Written at an appropriate reading level	Common heart failure symptoms
Customized educational materials	Medication reconciliation between admission medications and discharge medications
Activity guidelines	Follow-up appointment with contact information
Diet instructions	Follow-up plan for outstanding test results
Weight monitoring	Follow-up plan for scheduled/planned outpatient diagnostic test
Medication instructions including names, doses, and how and when to take	Who and when to call if symptoms worsen
Fluid restriction if appropriate	Smoking cessation
Avoidance of alcohol	Avoidance of nonsteroidal medications

the ED for heart failure are unable to read the label on a prescription bottle [28]. Low health literacy is a fundamental barrier to effective self-care. Formal education is not the same as health literacy [28]. Discharge instructions should be legibly written and in a patient friendly format [38]. It is recommended that they are written at the 6th grade reading level; however, most are written at a 9th–10th grade level [2]. Older individuals may need materials that are written in larger print.

Advanced age, complex medical plans, and multiple clinicians increase the risks of failure of the discharge plan [23, 29, 39]. Patients, like most individuals, do not realize what they do not know; therefore, they do not ask for help [2]. To improve comprehension, it is vital that the health-care provider identify what the patient does know and what they need to know. Individualized discharge plans improve adherence and outcomes by empowering patients to manage their health problems [27]. Nonadherence to lifestyle changes is reported to be as high as 50–80% [40]. The elderly are especially at risk for the inability to make necessary lifestyle changes [39].

Socioeconomic status is an independent risk factor for readmission with the highest risk for readmission being associated with the lowest income [34, 40]. Many individuals have no prescription coverage and must pay out of pocket for their medications [32]. The average number of medications taken by patients is 10.5 and increases as the severity of symptoms increase [32].

The home environment can also have an effect. It is important for the nurse to assess the level of involvement, ability, and willingness of the outpatient support team to assist the patient postdischarge. The lack of adequate support at home can increase the likelihood of readmissions [41]. The use of home health in Medicare-aged patients have been shown to reduce readmissions and costs significantly, regardless of the severity of heart failure [26].

Medications

It is important that the discharge plan includes medications that are evidence based [42]. The preadmission medication list must be reconciled with the discharge list, and clear written instructions should be given to the patient about what to stop and what to continue or add. An information sheet on each medication should be part of the discharge documents [35, 36]. Nonadherence with heart failure medications is reported to range between 30% and 60% and can lead to worsening symptoms and subsequent readmissions [27, 40, 42, 43]. The ED staff will need to ensure that the medications are available postdischarge [26].

Patients report reasons for nonadherence to be a lack of understanding of the discharge instructions, confusion about conflicting instructions given by different providers, costs, not being convinced of the utility of the medications, and side effects of the medications [28]. Patients take medications that were not prescribed because they were taking them previously, due to lack of confidence in the new medications or not realizing that two medications are the same [28]. Patients seldom tell the health-care provider about the over-the-counter medications and herbal therapies they are taking. Because there are many possible drug to drug interactions, it is best to encourage patients to discuss all medications and supplements that they are taking and to maintain a written record of all.

Diet

Nonadherence to dietary restrictions can lead to worsening symptoms and subsequent readmissions [27, 42, 43]. Few patients have the knowledge of how to follow a low sodium diet [44]. Slightly, over one-half of patients with heart failure report being told to decrease their sodium intake, and only 36% report following these recommendations [28]. Discharge instructions for the patient with heart failure should include a clear diet plan with examples of foods to avoid and how to read a food label. It has been reported that up to 42% of patients with heart failure are poor at reading food labels [28].

Some patients also need to restrict fluids. Alarmingly, 38% of patients with heart failure report thinking they are required to drink large quantities of fluids [45]. Those with persistent fluid retention or severe hyponatremia, despite a low sodium diet and diuretics, may benefit from a fluid restriction [28]. These individuals will need instructions on how to measure fluid intake and ways to address the sensation of thirst.

Activity

The activity plan should be tailored to the individual [28]. Patients need to be reassured that activity is beneficial and receive instructions on how to monitor their tolerance and symptoms. Exercise has been shown to improve oxygen delivery, decrease inflammation, increase peak oxygen uptake, and decrease depression [28].

Signs and Symptoms Monitoring

Patients delay seeking help for days, possibly due to failure to routinely monitor symptoms and/or failure to recognize and identify the symptom as related to heart failure [28]. Delays in seeking medical care may result in unnecessary readmissions [43].

Fewer than 50% of patients weigh themselves daily and those that do only do so intermittently [28]. Patients who weigh themselves are more likely to make appropriate adjustments in sodium intake and diuretic dosing [28]. Thus, the best discharge plans include written guidance on how, why, and when to weigh and when to notify a health-care provider of a change in weight.

Follow-up Care

Patients and their caregivers are at times the only common thread moving through the health-care system and often have to navigate their own way [19, 30]. It is essential that they are provided with adequate information to ensure that the team in the next setting will have a complete understanding of the care the patient received while in the ED and the discharge plan [26].

It is best that the written discharge summary includes the patient's functional status, medical history, baseline information, learning needs, care plans, and services provided while admitted [26]. The transfer of information from the hospital team to the outpatient team is important for continuity and transition of care. The patient should be given written instructions on their follow-up appointments with names, addresses, directions, and contact information [46]. They should also be given a list of pending diagnostic tests and procedures [46]. The discharge planning process and plan should be documented in the patient's medical record [4]. Many readmissions occur due to the lack of communication between the pre- and postdischarge health-care team [4, 17, 25, 41].

Ideally, a follow-up appointment is scheduled prior to the patient being discharged [3]. Early follow-up results in lower readmission rates [29]. Most patients need an outpatient follow-up visit within 1 week of discharge [3, 29]. The goal for high-risk patients, those with two admissions in the past year, is to be seen in 48 hours and those at moderate risk to be called within 48 hours and have an office visit with within 5 days [26]. If available, a multidisciplinary approach should be used as these have been shown to reduce mortality, cost, and admissions [26].

The time immediately following discharge is a particularly vulnerable period, especially with changes to the previous medical therapy [19, 29]. The utilization of both primary care provider (PCP) and cardiologist can be beneficial and may lead to improved adherence to evidence-based care [19]. The PCP may be able to see the patient earlier than the cardiologist and can provide care for noncardiac concerns [19].

Regional barriers to care including transportation, weather, economy, and the availability of affordable health care must be addressed [35]. Other barriers include overextended PCPs, lack of computerized records, and integrated systems [29, 46]. Each institution must assess the needs of their community and develop plans to ease the impact of these barriers for their patients.

How to Get It All Done

The ED is a unique high-acuity, fast-paced, rapid turnover environment which creates significant challenges for quality communication [2, 31]. There are time constraints, unpredictable interruptions, overcrowding, and frequent staff changes [2, 31]. Patients arrive in a state of increased stress with physical needs that may be life threatening. Anxiety levels are high which impairs cognition, motivation, and energy [2, 28]. This limits the patient's ability to learn and/or act on new information [28]. Repetition and reinforcement of the information improves the patient's understanding [2].

It is important for the ED staff to address the patient's concerns and maintain open, high-quality communication [2]. Discharge to the outpatient setting from the ED is especially challenging due to the limited time of the patient–clinician interaction. Many of the teachable moments are overlooked or missed. The ED staff must take advantage of these teachable moments. Opportunities for patients to ask questions and for staff to assess the patient's understanding of their condition must be utilized whenever possible [2].

Use of prepared discharge materials regarding medications, lifestyle modifications, and symptom assessment can facilitate comprehensive discharge instructions with less time [47]. Ancillary staff such as case managers (CM) can unburden the clinical staff [31]. These are often specially trained nurses who provide extra support for patients identified to be at increased risk and have been successful in improving outcomes [30]. Case managers can develop the individualized discharge plans, facilitate the transfer of information to the next care setting, schedule follow-up appointments, reinforce information to the patient and caregivers, and assist in meeting the needs of the home environment such as durable medical equipment or home care [31]. Patients treated in the ED may have a myriad of psychosocial issues such as homelessness, abuse or neglect, lack of insurance, and substance abuse. These often exceed the capabilities of the bedside nursing and medical staff [31]. Case managers can be extremely helpful in managing these complex situations.

Conclusions

Discharge planning is a process that begins with the first encounter in the ED and continues throughout the entire stay. Each institution needs to individually assess the requirements of the population they serve and the services provided by their institution and community. Unmet needs or gaps in the care should be identified and prioritized so as to address those with the greatest impact first [26]. The best discharge plans are individualized and involve all members of the health-care team. The plan is then communicated to the patient and their caregivers in a format that they can understand and use. It should include practical information as to how to implement the plan. It is important that the after discharge care team be included in the transfer of information. The discharge period has been identified as an opportunity to have a positive impact on patient outcomes [38]. More research is needed to ensure that interventions employed actually result in improved outcomes.

References

1. Grady KL, et al. Team management of patients with heart failure: a statement for healthcare professionals from the Cardiovascular Nursing Council of the American Heart Association. Circulation. 2000;102:2443–56.
2. Engel KG, et al. Communication amidst chaos: challenges to patient communication in the Emergency Department. J Clin Outcomes Manage. 2010;17(10):449–52.

3. Weintraub NL, et al. Acute heart failure syndromes: emergency department presentation, treatment, and disposition; current approaches and future aims: a scientific statement from the American Heart Association. Circulation. 2010;122:1966.
4. Naylor M, et al. Comprehensive discharge planning for the hospitalized elderly—A randomized clinical trial. Ann Intern Med. 1994;120:999–1006.
5. Kleinpell RM. Randomized trial of an intensive care unit-based early discharge planning intervention for critically ill elderly patient. Am J Crit Care. 2004;13:335–45.
6. Kossovsky MP, et al. Unplanned readmissions of patients with congestive heart failure: do they reflect in-hospital quality of care or patient characteristics? Am J Med. 2000;109:386–90.
7. Peacock WF. Emergency department observation unit management of heart failure. Crit Pathw Cardiol. 2003;2:207–20.
8. O'Connor CM, et al. Demographics, clinical characteristics, and outcomes of patients hospitalized for decompensated heart failure: observations from the IMPACT-HF registry. J Card Fail. 2005;11:200–5.
9. Capomolla S, et al. Heart failure case disease management program: a pilot study of home telemonitoring versus usual care. Eur Heart J. 2004;6(Suppl F):91–8.
10. Galbreath AD, et al. Long-term healthcare and cost outcomes of disease management in a large, randomized, community-based population with heart failure. Circulation. 2004;110: 3518–26.
11. Adams KF, et al. Characteristics and outcomes of patients hospitalized for heart failure in the United States: rational, design and preliminary observations from the first 100,000 cases in the acute decompensated heart failure national registry (ADHERE). Am Heart J. 2005;149:209–16.
12. Dunagan WC, et al. Randomized trial of a nurse-administered, telephone-based disease management program for patients with heart failure. J Card Fail. 2005;11:358–65.
13. Klienpell RM, Gawlinski A. Assessing outcomes in advance practice nursing. AACN Clin Issues. 2005;19:43–67.
14. Rich MW, et al. A multidisciplinary intervention to prevent the readmission of elderly patients with congestive heart failure. N Engl J Med. 1995;333:1190–5.
15. Stewart S, et al. Effects of a home based intervention among patients with congestive heart failure discharged from an acute care hospital. Arch Intern Med. 1998;158:1067–72.
16. DiSalvo TG, Stevenson LW. Interdisciplinary team based management of heart failure. Dis Manage Health Outcomes. 2003;11:87–94.
17. Phillips CO, et al. Comprehensive discharge planning with post-discharge support for older patients with congestive heart failure. JAMA. 2004;291:1358–67.
18. Ross JS, et al. Statistical models and patient predictors of readmission for heart failure. Arch Intern Med. 2008;168(13):1371–86.
19. Lee DS, et al. Improved outcomes with early collaborative care of ambulatory heart failure patients discharged from the Emergency Department. Circulation. 2010;122:1806–14.
20. Aghababian RV. Acutely decompensated heart failure: opportunities to improve care and outcomes in the emergency department. Rev Cardiovasc Med. 2002;3 suppl 4:S3–9.
21. Kleinpell R, Gawlinski A. Assessing outcomes in advanced practice nursing practice. AACN Clin Issues. 2005;16:43–57.
22. Butler J, et al. Outpatient utilization of angiotensin-converting enzyme inhibitors among heart failure patients after hospital discharge. J Am Coll Cardiol. 2004;43:2036–43.
23. Hardin S, Hussey L. AACN synergy model for patient care: case study of a CHF patient. Crit Care Nurse. 2003;23:73–6.
24. Barth V. A nurse managed discharge program for congestive heart failure patients: outcomes and costs. Home Health Care Manage Pract. 2001;13:436–43.
25. Ross JS, et al. Recent national trends in readmission rates after heart failure hospitalization. Circ Heart Fail. 2010;3:97–103.
26. Hines PA, et al. Preventing heart failure readmissions: is your organization prepared? Nurs Econ. 2010;28(2):74–85.
27. Atenza F, et al. Multicenter randomized trial of a comprehensive hospital discharge and outpatient heart failure management program. Eur J Heart Fail. 2004;6:643–52.

28. Reigel B, et al. State of the science promoting self-care in persons with heart failure: a scientific statement for the American Heart Association. Circulation. 2009;120:1141–63.
29. Hernandez AF, Greiner MA, et al. Relationship between early physician follow-up and 30 day readmission among medicare beneficiaries hospitalized for heart failure. JAMA. 2010;303(17):1716–22.
30. Coleman EA, et al. The care transitions intervention. Arch Intern Med. 2006;166:1822–8.
31. Sandy LP. Case management in the emergency room. Professional Case Manage. 2010;15(2): 111–3.
32. Hussey LC, et al. Outpatient costs of medications for patients with chronic heart failure. Am J Crit Care. 2002;11:474–8.
33. Cleland JG, Ekman I. Enlisting the help of the largest health care workforce: patients. JAMA. 2010;304(12):1383–4.
34. Bhala R, Kalkut G. Could medicare readmission policy exacerbate health care system inequity? Ann Intern Med. 2010;152:114–7.
35. McAlister et al. Multidisciplinary strategies for the management of heart failure patients at high risk for admission: a systematic review of randomized trials. JACC. 2004;44:810–9.
36. Koelling et al. Discharge education improves clinical outcomes in patients with chronic heart failure. Circulation. 2005;111:179–85.
37. Cline CMF et al. Cost effective management program for heart failure reduces hospitalization. Heart. 1998;80:442–6.
38. Fonarow G, et al. Association between performance measures and clinical outcomes for patients hospitalized with heart failure. JAMA. 2007;1:61–70.
39. Roe-Prior P. Variables predictive of poor post-discharge outcomes for hospitalized elders in heart failure. West J Nurs Res. 2004;26:533–46.
40. Powell LH, et al. Self-management counseling in patients with heart failure: the heart failure adherence and retention randomized behavioral trial. JAMA. 2010;304(12):1331–8.
41. Kee CC, Borchers L. Reducing readmission rates through discharge interventions. Clin Nurse Spec. 1998;12:206–9.
42. Jaarsma T. Inter-professional team approach to patients with heart failure. Heart. 2005;91: 832–8.
43. Krumholz HM, et al. Randomized trial of education and support intervention to prevent readmission of patient with heart failure. JACC. 2002;39:83–9.
44. Koelling TM, et al. Discharge education improves clinical outcomes in patients with chronic heart failure. Circulation. 2005;111:179–85.
45. Hanyu N, et al. Factors influencing knowledge of and adherence to self-care among patients with heart failure. Arch Intern Med. 1999;159:1613–9.
46. Jack BW, et al. A reengineered hospital discharge program to decrease rehospitalization. Ann Intern Med. 2009;150(3):178–87.
47. Anthony MK, Hudson-Barr D. A patient-centered model of care for hospital discharge. Clin Nurs Res. 2004;13:117–36.

Chapter 18
Outpatient Medication Titration in Acute Heart Failure

Khadijah Breathett and L. Kristin Newby

Background

Characterizing Heart Failure

Managing heart failure requires addressing both the American College of Cardiology/American Heart Association (ACC/AHA) stages and the New York Heart Association (NYHA) class at each visit. This assists in the prompt recognition of disease progression rather than stabilization or improvement. As a review, the ACC/AHA Task Force described heart failure as occurring in the following stages: Stage A, high risk for heart failure but without structural heart disease or symptoms of heart failure; Stage B, structural heart disease but without signs or symptoms of heart failure; Stage C, structural heart disease with prior or current symptoms of heart failure; and Stage D, refractory heart failure requiring specialized interventions [1]. The Stage A patient may have hypertension, atherosclerotic disease, diabetes, obesity, metabolic syndrome, be taking cardiotoxic medications, or have a strong family history of cardiovascular disease. Examples of Stage B patients include those with a previous myocardial infarction, left ventricular remodeling with left ventricular hypertrophy, a reduction in left ventricular ejection fraction (LVEF), or asymptomatic valvular disease. Stage C patients have known structural heart disease and shortness of breath, fatigue, or reduced exercise tolerance. Stage D patients

K. Breathett, MD
Department of Cardiology, The Ohio State University Medical Center, Columbus, OH, USA

L.K. Newby, MD, MHS (✉)
Department of Medicine, Division of Cardiovascular Medicine,
Duke Clinical Research Institute, Duke University Medical Center,
P.O. Box 17969, Durham, NC 27715-7969, USA
e-mail: newby001@mc.duke.edu

W. Frank Peacock (ed.), *Short Stay Management of Acute Heart Failure*,
Contemporary Cardiology, DOI 10.1007/978-1-61779-627-2_18,
© Springer Science+Business Media, LLC 2012

Intervention	Stage A High Risk	Stage B Asymptomatic	Stage C Symptomatic	Stage D Refractory
Ace Inhibitor or ARB	ACE: lisinopril 20 mg-40 mg daily(3 and expert opinion), enalapril 10-20 mg bid (4, 5), ramipril 1.25 mg-10 mg daily (6), captopril 25 mg bid- 50 mg tid (7, 8), quinapril 20 mg daily (7) (9 for all ACE) ARB:valsartan 160 mg bid (10), candesartan 32 mg daily (11)			
Beta-Blocker			carvedilol 25 mg bid (12), metoprolol extended release 200 mg daily (13), bisoprolol 5 mg- 10 mg daily (14, 15)	
Loop Diuretic				
Aldosterone Antagonist			spironolactone 25 mg-50 mg daily (16), eplerenone 25 mg-50 mg daily (17) (Limit:Cr>2.5 mg/dL or K>5 meq/L)	
Digitalis*			digoxin 0.125-0.5mg (18, 19)	
Hydralazine/Nitrate			hydralazine 75 mg tid and isosorbide dinitrate 40 mg tid (20)	
Sodium Restriction			2 g sodium (1, 21, 22)	
ICD			(24–26)	
CRT-ICD			(24, 27–29)	
Heart Txp, *Chronic Inotropes, Mechanical Support, Hospice*				
STOP THESE	Antiarrhythmics , (exception amiodarone, dofetilide)	Calcium Channel Blockers, (exception vasoselective ones)	NSAIDS (exception aspirin)	

Fig. 18.1 Outpatient management of heart failure. Interventions in *bold* reduce morbidity/mortality associated with heart failure. *Italic* interventions provide symptomatic care. The titrated target dosages for therapeutic benefit are listed based upon clinical trial. The *dashed gray* section represents the setting where the intervention risk may outweigh the benefit. The *asterisk* represents a setting where the medication may be considered for initiation for symptomatic care but provides morbidity/mortality benefit if initiated prior to onset of heart failure. ICD is implantable cardioversion defibrillation. *CRT* cardiac resynchronization therapy. Adapted from [1, 30]

usually have marked symptoms at rest despite maximal medical therapy and require recurrent hospitalizations. Rapid assessment of clinical history and review of prior echocardiograms, electrocardiograms, and possible heart catheterizations can properly place the patient in the appropriate stage.

The NYHA functional class is based solely on subjective information from patients who have known cardiac disease. Class I patients have no limitation of ordinary physical activity. Class II suffer slight limitation with ordinary physical activity. Class III has marked limitation with ordinary physical activity, and once in Class IV, patients are unable to do any physical activity without limitations. Unlike Classes I–III, Class IV patients may have symptoms of heart failure or anginal syndrome at rest and are worsened by physical activity [2]. Figure 18.1 depicts a model for treatment of patients with heart failure or at risk for heart failure according to ACC/AHA staging. Determining the patient's NYHA functional class assists the provider in initiating treatment or making medication titrations within these recommended interventions.

Managing Heart Failure in the Outpatient Setting

Outpatient management of heart failure has changed significantly over the past 20 years, with evolving concepts of what improves longevity, decreases hospitalizations, and optimizes functional capacity. Randomized controlled trials have confirmed the efficacy of most forms of angiotensin-converting enzyme (ACE) inhibitors or angiotensin receptor blockers (ARB), specific beta-blockers (carvedilol, metoprolol succinate, and bisoprolol), and aldosterone antagonists [3–17]. Careful dosing of digitalis has been demonstrated to reduce hospitalizations for heart failure [18]. On the contrary, while digitalis has no impact on mortality, patients who have been taking digoxin chronically may experience worsening symptoms after its discontinuation [19]. Secondary analyses have shown additional survival benefit in African Americans from the use of hydralazine and nitrates, potentially related to genetically reduced renin–angiotensin system activity; however, hydralazine and nitrates are not recommended to replace the use of a traditional regimen of ACE inhibitor or ARB, beta-blocker, and aldosterone antagonists [1, 20]. These medications are believed to exert their effects through mechanisms that result in changes in left ventricular remodeling, afterload reduction, and controlling the renin–angiotensin–aldosterone axis, yet not all patients have the same response to these therapies. There is great hope that as we enter the molecular era, genetic or other biomarkers will allow for more tailored treatment, but at present, treatment for heart failure is based on population data from randomized clinical trials. In this paradigm, an attempt should be made to initiate evidence-based therapies and to titrate them to the doses shown to be effective in clinical trials. Because these medications have many overlapping side effects, including the potential for hypokalemia and hypotension, it may be challenging to achieve evidence-based doses within a single hospitalization or outpatient visit. A stepwise approach to initiation of heart failure medication and titration to therapeutic doses is recommended and can be guided by considering both ACC/AHA Class and NYHA functional class of the patient (see Fig. 18.1).

Stage A Management: ACE Inhibitor or Angiotensin Receptor Blocker

The benefit of ACE inhibitors and ARBs in patients with heart failure is greater in Stage C and D patients. However, given the additional cardioprotection for patients with risk factors for heart disease, an ACE inhibitor or ARB is also recommended for Stage A or B patients with these cardiovascular risk factors [9]. Multiple clinical trials have shown morbidity and mortality reduction with various ACE inhibitors, leaving the physician with many options [9]. Finesse is required to reach therapeutic levels of ACE inhibitors or ARBs without causing undue side effects. Adjustment of medications at intervals of 1–4 weeks has been successful in clinical trials and can be done in the clinic or over the phone if appropriate follow-up is obtained to monitor for symptomatic hypotension, hyperkalemia, and worsening creatinine clearance (Table 18.1) [5]. Cough is a common side effect of treatment with ACE

Table 18.1 Titration of ACE inhibitors and ARBs

Medication	Initial dosage	Titration	Target dosage
Angiotensin Converting Enzyme inhibitor			
Lisinopril [3]	5 mg daily	Double every 4 weeks	20–40 mg daily
Enalapril [4, 5]	2.5–5 mg bid	Double every 1–2 weeks	10–20 mg bid
Ramipril [6]	1.25 mg daily	Double every 2 weeks	1.25–10 mg daily
Captopril [7, 8]	12.5 mg bid or tid	Double every 4 weeks	25 mg bid–50 mg tid
Quinapril [7]	10 mg daily	Double after 4 weeks	20 mg daily
Angiotensin Receptor Blocker			
Valsartan [10]	40 mg bid	Double every 2 weeks	160 mg bid
Candesartan [11]	4–8 mg daily	Double every 2 weeks	32 mg daily

inhibitors, occurring in up to 35% of patients, and more frequently in women, nonsmokers, and people of Chinese descent [31]. For patients who develop a cough on ACE inhibitor treatment, an ARB is a suitable replacement. Cough with an ARB occurs at similar frequency to placebo, 2–3% [32]. Angioedema is an absolute contraindication to use of both ACE inhibitors and ARBs. The direct renin inhibitors are still under evaluation for their effect on clinical endpoints, but they appear to promote reduction in left ventricular mass that is similar to ARBs [33].

In the case of persistent hypertension (systolic blood pressure ≥140 or diastolic blood pressure ≥90) after up-titrating ACE inhibitors or ARBs, additional antihypertensive medications should be considered to achieve reduction in blood pressure, with the exception of nonvasoselective calcium channel blockers which should be avoided [34]. In the setting of advancing heart failure class, care must be made to exchange medications that were used for blood pressure control with ones that reduce morbidity and mortality in this population (see Fig. 18.1).

Stage B Management: Angiotensin Converting Enzyme Inhibitor or Angiotensin Receptor Blocker, Beta-Blocker, Implantable Cardiac Defibrillator

Stage B patients should be first titrated to target doses of an ACE inhibitor or ARB before adding carvedilol, metoprolol succinate, or bisoprolol, which all have been demonstrated to benefit heart failure patients [12–15]. Titration of these medications should generally be made at 2-week intervals, holding dose titration in the setting of symptomatic hypotension or bradycardia (heart rate <60 beats/min, untreated second or third degree atrioventricular block) [12]. During titration of beta-blockade, systolic blood pressures in the 90–100 mmHg range may occur and should not cause alarm in the absence of presyncope or syncope (see Table 18.2).

Informing patients that beta-blockers can cause initial fatigue, but that it should improve with continued use, may help with compliance. In addition, consideration of switching between agents, or administration at bedtime, may reduce symptoms of fatigue. Patients should be taught how to monitor their blood pressure and heart rate at home on a regular basis, recognize abnormal blood pressure and heart rate, and have direct telecommunication of these data to their providers. Telecommunication

Table 18.2 Titration of beta-blockers

Medication	Initial dosage	Titration	Target dosage
Beta-blocker			
Carvedilol [12]	3.125 mg bid	Double every 2 weeks	25 mg bid
Metoprolol succinate [13]	12.5–25 mg daily	Double every 2 weeks	200 mg daily
Bisoprolol [14, 15]	1.25 mg daily	Increase by 1.25 mg weekly until dose of 5 mg reached. Then increase by 2.5 mg every 4 weeks	5–10 mg daily

systems with close provider follow-up have helped improve patient outcomes, quality of life, and compliance while reducing hospitalizations [35–37]. This becomes especially important as patients advance in heart failure stage.

Stage C Management: Angiotensin Converting Enzyme Inhibitor or Angiotensin Receptor Blocker, Beta-Blocker, Aldosterone Antagonist, Hydralazine and Nitrates, Loop Diuretic, Bi-ventricular Implantable Cardiac Defibrillator

The Stage C population is more precarious. Having close contact with the Stage C patient to detect changes in NYHA class will assist in improving patient satisfaction with care, quality of life, and reduce hospitalizations [35, 36]. Patients in this stage should be advised about the "Rule of 2s" (1) consume no more than 2 g of sodium daily, (2) weigh daily in the morning and double the dose of diuretic for that day if there is weight gain of >2 lbs in one day, and (3) call health provider to share new information. Finally, hyponatremic patients should also institute a daily 2-L fluid restriction [1, 21, 37, 38]. Robust trials are still lacking to provide evidence to support these recommendations for sodium and fluid restriction, but they are intuitively supported guidelines that may change over time with new data from pending trials [1, 22, 39]. A visit with a nutritionist or provider who can spend time educating heart failure patients about food labels and what products are high in sodium will also be helpful. These patients should contact their provider for complaints of new or recurrent heart failure symptoms (dyspnea, lower extremity swelling, inability to sleep lying flat) and new or recurrent angina symptoms. Structuring a clinic system to address patient complaints urgently can improve results [40].

Clinic visits should be tailored toward reaching target doses of medications, starting with ACE inhibitors and then beta-blockers. For the patients with NYHA functional class 3–4 heart failure, an aldosterone antagonist should also be initiated. Limitations to the use of aldosterone antagonists should be carefully considered, including rises in serum creatinine or potassium levels. In general, aldosterone antagonists may be initiated after the patient is on a stable dose of an ACE inhibitor, which can also affect creatinine level and cause retention of potassium. During initiation of an aldosterone antagonist, monitoring for an increase in creatinine to >2.5 mg/dL or potassium to >5 meq/L is important [1]. The ACE inhibitor dosage may be reduced by half or to every other day if tolerated without persistent rise in creatinine or potassium.

Table 18.3 Titration of aldosterone antagonists, digitalis, and hydralazine/nitrates

Medication	Initial dosage	Titration	Target dosage
Aldosterone antagonist			
Spironolactone [16]	25 mg daily	Double after 8 weeks	25–50 mg daily
Eplerenone [17]	25 mg daily	Double after 4 weeks	50 mg daily
Digitalis			
Digoxin [18, 19]		Based on CrCl, age, sex, and weight	0.125–0.5 mg daily (0.5–2.0 ng/ml serum)
Hydralazine/nitrates			
Hydralazine [20]	37.5 mg tid	Double after 2 weeks[a]	75 mg tid
Isosorbide dinitrate [20]	20 mg tid	Double after 2 weeks[a]	40 mg tid

[a]Titration time is not explicit in reported trials

African-American patients may also be treated with hydralazine and isosorbide dinitrate for its morbidity and mortality benefit [20]. In non-African-American patients with persistent heart failure symptoms who do not have symptomatic hypotension, hydralazine and isosorbide dinitrate can also be used to prevent hospitalizations [41]. Patients with contraindications to ACE inhibitor or ARB should also be considered to be hydralazine and isosorbide dinitrate candidates for additional symptom control [1]. Headache and gastrointestinal intolerance occasionally prevent titration and should be monitored for when assessing compliance [1].

As the number of medications and complexity of dosing intervals increase, medical adherence can decline. Medication reconciliation at each clinic visit is helpful to confirm what medications a patients is actually taking and to explore any side effects that may adversely affecting compliance. Having the patient describe how they take each medication, providing pillboxes, and addressing concerns with clinic pharmacy visits and social-service consultation can also improve care [1, 42, 43].

Digoxin can be considered for patients with persistent symptoms after appropriate titration of ACE inhibitor, beta-blocker, aldosterone inhibitor, hydralazine, and nitrates. There is no mortality benefit from the use of digoxin, but it has been demonstrated to reduce hospitalizations for heart failure [18]. For patients already taking digoxin, cessation of treatment has been associated with a worsening of heart failure symptoms and clinical parameters [19]. It may be preferential to use digoxin for rate control if effective rate control is not achieved with beta-blockade, rather than adding an alternate rate control medication, like verapamil or diltiazem, which could potentially worsen heart function [1, 44] (see Table 18.3). Similarly antiarrhythmics other than amiodarone or dofetilide should be avoided in this population, given their cardiodepressant and proarrhythmic effects [1, 44].

Diuresis

Diuresis provides symptomatic care that is usually needed to assist patients in maintaining a euvolemic state. Appropriate titration of the previously discussed medications

Table 18.4 Loop diuretic correlation table

Diuretic	Bioavailability (%)	IV-to-oral conversion	Relative potency (mg)
Bumetanide	75	1:1	1
Furosemide	50	1:2	40
Torsemide	80	1:1	20

Adapted from [48]

can sometimes reduce the need for diuretics. Generally, diuretics cannot be avoided in NYHA class 3–4 patients and those advancing to Stage D. Loop diuretics are most effective for diuresis but have not been demonstrated to have clinical outcome benefits in and of themselves [45, 46]. Initial dosing of the loop diuretic should be determined based upon creatinine clearance and response to a trial with the patient. For lack of efficacy at one dose, the dose can be doubled until urine output is satisfactory. Initiation of furosemide may be considered as first line unless the patient has significant bowel edema or ascites that might suggest better absorption with torsemide or bumetanide [46] (see Table 18.4). However, if a patient has substantial bowel edema, IV diuretic administration may become necessary.

A rise in serum creatinine can be expected while titrating diuretic therapy, but for a rise in serum creatinine of 40% or more, diuresis should be stopped or decreased, if possible [47]. The patient should keep a record of daily morning weights to assist in regulating diuretic dosing. When the patient has signs of hypervolemia, including pulmonary edema, elevated jugular venous pressure, S3 gallop, lower extremity edema, or ascites, the provider can target diuresis toward achieving dry weight. For example, a patient who usually takes furosemide 40 mg daily could, if still urinating well on furosemide 40 mg, change regimen to furosemide 40 mg bid or tid. If they were not responding to furosemide 40 mg daily, then an increase to furosemide 80 mg daily or higher would be appropriate. While adjusting diuresis, follow-up should be obtained within a few days after each dosing change to assess for appropriateness of diuresis and electrolyte alterations. Often potassium supplementation is required if the patient is not on an aldosterone antagonist. Hypo- and hyperkalemia are associated with higher morbidity in this population. Therefore, an objective is to keep the potassium close to 4 meq/L [1]. Occasionally, additional diuretic assistance is required and can be achieved by adding the thiazide diuretic, metolazone. This should generally be reserved for inpatient use given abrupt fluctuations in circulatory response, electrolytes, and creatinine clearance that can result from the use of metolazone. Progressively worsening creatinine clearance is associated with long-term morbidity in heart failure patients. Avoidance of nephrotoxic medications should be paramount, especially NSAIDS that effectively reduce renal blood flow.

Routine chest radiography and B-type natriuretic peptide levels are not indicated in the management of congestive heart failure. Repeat structural evaluation with echocardiogram is only needed when major clinical changes have occurred that result in a change in ACC/AHA stages or NYHA functional class [1].

Implantable Cardiac Defibrillator and Bi-ventricular Implantable Cardiac Defibrillator Therapy

There is mortality benefit from implantable cardioverter-defibrillator (ICD) devices in patients with ACC/AHA Stage C heart failure and persistent structural disease who are on appropriate medical therapy. It is important for the provider to monitor medication titration goals and advocate for ICD or resynchronization therapy when indicated. For primary prevention of sudden cardiac death, a mortality reduction has been demonstrated for ACC/AHA Stage C patients who have persistent LVEF ≤35% at least 40 days postmyocardial infarction, NYHA functional class II–III, and predicted survival >1 year [1, 23–25]. Secondary prevention ICD therapy should be provided in ACC/AHA Stage C patients with a history of cardiac arrest, ventricular fibrillation, or hemodynamically unstable ventricular tachycardia [1, 26].

Resynchronization is indicated for ACC/AHA Stage C patients with LVEF ≤35%, atrial fibrillation, dyssynchrony as evidenced by QRS ≥120 ms, NYHA functional class 3–4, and on optimal medical therapy. ACC/AHA Stage C patients with LVEF ≤35%, NYHA functional class 3–4, on optimal medical therapy who are dependent on frequent ventricular pacing may also benefit from biventricular synchronized pacing [1, 27–29].

Stage D Management: Angiotensin Converting Enzyme Inhibitor or Angiotensin Receptor Blocker, Beta-Blocker, Aldosterone Antagonist, Hydralazine and Nitrates, Loop Diuretic, Bi-ventricular Pacemaker, Heart Transplant, Hospice

Evaluation of ACC/AHA Stage D patients is geared toward palliation, unless heart transplant is an option. Life expectancy at this stage is greatly reduced. ICD therapy no longer provides benefit, as death is usually impending [1]. Beta-blockers can cause more harm than benefit and may need to be discontinued in the presence of symptomatic bradycardia, symptomatic hypotension, worsening fatigue, worsening dyspnea, or other signs of decompensated heart failure. ACE inhibitors, aldosterone antagonists, hydralazine and nitrates, and digoxin may still be useful if hypotension and renal function are not limiting, and effective diuresis becomes a mainstay of providing comfort. Given the high mortality among Stage D patients, readdressing patient goals of care becomes very important. Options may include hospice, palliation with or without ICD deactivation, chronic inotropes, mechanical support with "bridge" or "destination therapy," and heart transplant. Referrals to end-stage heart failure specialists can assist the provider in communicating best care options to the patient.

Failure of Outpatient Management

Many reasons for heart failure readmission can be addressed and prevented in the outpatient setting with a good care plan (see Fig. 18.1). Common reasons for readmission include noncompliance with medical regimen and/or sodium and fluid restrictions, acute myocardial infarction, uncorrected high blood pressure, atrial fibrillation and other arrhythmias, addition of negative inotropic medications, pulmonary embolus, NSAIDS use, excessive alcohol or illicit drug use, endocrine abnormalities (diabetes mellitus, hyperthyroidism, hypothyroidism), and concurrent infections [1]. As above, a good telecommunication system and contact with providers (nurses, nurse practitioners or physicians assistants, or physicians) can help to identify issues before outpatient management fails [35–37].

Summary

Outpatient management is the crux of heart failure care and has a large influence on short- and long-term morbidity, mortality, and quality of life in heart failure patients. Understanding the results of major clinical trials of heart failure therapies and applying proven therapies at tested doses are of prime importance in successful outpatient management of heart failure. Key goals include:

- Determine ACC/AHA heart failure stage and NYHA functional class at each visit.
- Titrate medications to goal doses that were tested in clinical outcome trials with close monitoring for adverse effects.
- Address patient concerns early and provide means for easy communication in order to improve medical adherence.
- Teach patients the "Rule of 2s."
- Stage A patients should take an ACE inhibitor or ARB.
- Stage B patients should take an ACE inhibitor or ARB and a beta-blocker that has been shown to be efficacious in clinical outcomes trials.
- Stage C patents should take an ACE inhibitor or ARB, beta-blocker, and aldosterone antagonist. Hydralazine and nitrates should be added for African Americans and used in patients who cannot tolerate ACE inhibitor or ARB. Consider adding digoxin. Determine diuretic dose needed. Consider indications for ICD and/or CRT-ICD therapy.
- Stage D patients should take an ACE inhibitor or ARB, aldosterone antagonist, hydralazine and nitrates, and possibly digoxin. Consider discontinuation of beta-blocker if decompensated heart failure occurs. Refer to an appropriate specialist for assistance with end-stage heart failure goals of care.

References

1. Jessup M, et al. 2009 Focused update: ACCF/AHA guidelines for the diagnosis and management of heart failure in adults. Circulation. 2009;119:1977–2016.
2. The Criteria Committee of the New York Heart Association. Nomenclature and criteria for diagnosis of diseases of the heart and great vessels. London: Little Brown; 1994. p. 253–256.

3. Lewis GR. Lisinopril versus placebo in older congestive heart failure patients. Am J Med. 1988;85:48–54.
4. SOLVD Investigators. Effect of enalapril on survival in patients with reduced left ventricular ejection fractions and congestive heart failure. N Engl J Med. 1991;325:293–302.
5. Ljungman S, et al. Renal function in severe congestive heart failure during treatment with enalapril (the Cooperative North Scandinavian Enalapril Survival Study CONSENSUS Trial). Am J Cardiol. 1992;70:479–87.
6. Heintz B, et al. Efficacy and safety of ramipril in long-term treatment of congestive heart failure. Curr Ther Res. 1994;95:489–99.
7. Acanfora D, et al. Quinapril in patients with congestive heart failure: controlled trial versus captopril. Am J Ther. 1997;4:181–8.
8. Giles TD, et al. Short- and long-acting angiotensin-converting enzyme inhibitors: a randomized trial of lisinopril versus captopril in the treatment of congestive heart failure. The Multicenter Lisinopril-Captopril Congestive Heart Failure Study Group. J Am Coll Cardiol. 1989;13:1240–7.
9. Garg R, et al. Overview of randomized trials of angiotensin-converting enzyme inhibitors on mortality and morbidity in patients with heart failure. JAMA. 1995;273:1450–6.
10. Maggioni AP, et al. Effects of valsartan on morbidity and mortality in patients with heart failure not receiving angiotensin-converting enzyme inhibitors. J Am Coll Cardiol. 2002;40: 1414–21.
11. Granger CB, et al. Effects of candesartan in patients with chronic heart failure and reduced left-ventricular systolic function intolerant to angiotensin-converting enzyme inhibitors: the CHARM-alternative trial. Lancet. 2003;362:772–6.
12. Poole-Wilson PA, et al. Comparison of carvedilol and metoprolol on clinical outcomes in patients with chronic heart failure in the carvedilol or metoprolol European trial: randomized controlled trial. Lancet. 2003;362:7–13.
13. Wikstrand J. Metoprolol CR/XL randomized intervention trial in heart failure, MERIT-HF: Description of the trial. Basic Res Cardiol. 2000;190–197.
14. Leizorovicz A, et al. Bisoprolol for the treatment of chronic heart failure: a meta-analysis on individual data of two placebo-controlled studies—CIBIS and CIBIS II. Am Heart J. 2002;143:301–7.
15. CIBIS II Investigators and Committees. The cardiac insufficiency bisoprolol study II: a randomized trial. Lancet. 1999;353:9–13.
16. Pitt B, et al. The effect of spironolactone of morbidity and mortality in patients with severe heart failure. N Engl J Med. 1999;341:709–17.
17. Pitt B, et al. The EPHESUS trial: eplerenone in patients with heart failure due to systolic dysfunction complicating acute myocardial infarction. Card Drugs Ther. 2001;15(1):79–87.
18. The Digitalis Investigation Group. The effect of digoxin on mortality and morbidity in patients with heart failure. N Engl J Med. 1997;336:525–33.
19. Packer M, et al. Withdrawal of digoxin from patients with chronic heart failure treated with angiotensin-converting-enzyme inhibitors. N Engl J Med. 1993;329:1–7.
20. Taylor AL, et al. Combination of isosorbide dinitrate and hydralazine in blacks with heart failure. N Engl J Med. 2004;351:2049–57.
21. Arcand J, et al. A high-sodium diet is associated with acute decompensated heart failure in ambulatory heart failure patients: a prospective follow-up study. Am J Clin Nutr. 2011;93: 2332–337.
22. Kollipara UK, et al. Relation of lack of knowledge about dietary sodium to hospital readmission in patients with heart failure. Am J Cardiol. 2008;102:1212–5.
23. Moss AJ, et al. Prophylactic implantation of a defibrillator in patients with myocardial infarction and reduced ejection fraction. N Engl J Med. 2002;346:877–83.
24. Epstein AE, et al. ACC/AHA/HRS 2008 guidelines for device-based therapy of cardiac rhythm abnormalities: a report of the American College of Cardiology/American Heart Association of Task Force on Practice Guidelines. J Am Coll Cardiol. 2008;51:1–62.
25. Cleland JGF, et al. Clinical trials update and cumulative meta-analyses from the American College of Cardiology: WATCH, SCD-HeFT, DINAMIT, CASINO, INSPIRE, STRATUS-US,

RIO-Lipids and Cardiac Resynchronisation Therapy in Heart Failure. Eur J Heart Fail. 2004;6:501–8.

26. Bokhari F, et al. Long-term comparison of the implantable cardioverter defibrillator versus amiodarone: eleven-year follow-up of a subset of patients in the Canadian Implantable Defibrillator Study. Circulation. 2004;110:112–6.

27. Cleland JG, et al. Longer-term effects of cardiac resynchronization therapy on mortality in heart failure. The Cardiac Resynchronization – Heart Failure trial Extension. Eur Heart J. 2006;27:1928–32.

28. Young JB, et al. Combined cardiac resynchronization and implantable cardioversion defibrillation in advanced chronic heart failure. The MIRACLE ICD Trial. JAMA. 2003;289:2685–94.

29. Bristow MR, et al. Cardiac-resynchronization therapy with or without an implantable defibrillator in advanced chronic heart failure. COMPANION. New Engl J Med. 2004;350:2140–50.

30. Nohria A, et al. Medical management of advanced heart failure. JAMA. 2002;287:628–40.

31. Dicpinigaitis PV. Angiotensin-converting enzyme inhibitor-induced cough. ACCP Evidence-Based Clinical Practice Guidelines. Chest. 2006;129:169S–73S.

32. Pylypchuk G. ACE inhibitor- versus angiotensin II blocker-induced cough and angioedema. Ann Pharmacother. 1998;32:1060–6.

33. Soloman SD, et al. Effect of the direct renin inhibitor aliskiren, the angiotensin receptor blocker losartan, or both on left ventricular mass in patients with hypertension and left ventricular hypertrophy. Circulation. 2009;119:530–7.

34. Chobanian AV, et al. The Seventh Report of the Joint National Committee on Prevention, Detection, Evaluation, and Treatment of High Blood Pressure. The JNC7 Report. JAMA. 2003;289:2560–72.

35. Louis AA, et al. A systematic review of telemonitoring for the management of heart failure. Eur J Heart Fail. 2003;5:583–90.

36. Chaudhry SI, et al. Telemonitoring for patients with chronic heart failure: a systematic review. J Card Fail. 2007;13:56–62.

37. Shah NB, et al. Prevention of hospitalizations for heart failure with an interactive home monitoring program. Am Heart J. 1998;135:373–8.

38. Chatterjee K. Hyponatremia in heart failure concluding remarks. Heart Fail Rev. 2009;14:87–8.

39. Song EK et al. Less than 2 g of dietary sodium intake is associated with shorter event-free survival in patients with compensated heart failure (Abstract). Circulation. 2010; 122.

40. O'Connor CM, et al. Predictors of mortality after discharge in patients hospitalized with heart failure: an analysis from the organized program to initiate lifesaving treatment in hospitalized patients with heart failure (OPTIMIZE-HF). Am Heart J. 2008;156:662–73.

41. Loeb HS, et al. Effect of enalapril, hydralazine plus isosorbide dinitrate, and prazosin on hospitalization in patients with chronic congestive heart failure. The V-HeFT VA Cooperative Studies Group. Circulation. 1993;87:V178–187.

42. Rich MW, et al. A multidisciplinary intervention to prevent the readmission of elderly patients with congestive heart failure. N Engl J Med. 1995;333:1190–5.

43. Phibin EF. Comprehensive multidisciplinary programs for the management of patients with congestive heart failure. J Gen Intern Med. 1999;14:130–5.

44. Packer M, et al. Hemodynamic consequences of antiarrhythmic drug therapy in patients with chronic heart failure. J Cardiovasc Electrophysiol. 1991;2:S240–7.

45. Felker GM, et al. Loop diuretics in acute decompensated heart failure. Necessary? Evil? A Necessary Evil? Circ Heart Fail. 2009;2:56–62.

46. Chiong JR, Cheung RJ. Loop diuretic therapy in heart failure: the need for solid evidence on a fluid issue. Clin Cardiol. 2010;33:345–52.

47. Vasavada N, et al. A double-blind randomized crossover trial of two loop diuretics in chronic kidney disease. Kidney Int. 2003;64:632–40.

48. Young JB, Mills RM. Clinical management of heart failure. 2nd ed. New York: Professional Communications; 2004.

Part V
Complications and Future Research

Chapter 19
Drugs to Avoid in Acute Heart Failure: Contraindicated Medications and Interactions

James McCord

Vasodilators

The long-term use of angiotensin-converting enzyme (ACE) inhibitors is associated with improved symptoms and lower mortality in patients with systolic heart failure. However, the benefits of early IV ACE inhibitors in acute heart failure (AHF) have not been established and may actually be harmful. In the CONSENSUS 2 trial, early IV enalaprilat was studied in patients with acute myocardial infarction (AMI). In patients with AMI and acute decompensated heart failure (ADHF), IV enalaprilat was associated with worse outcomes [1]. The American College of Emergency Physicians supports the early use of IV ACE inhibitors [2] while the European Society of Cardiology does not [3]. Until studied further, IV ACE inhibitors should be avoided in the setting of ADHF. Nitroprusside has not been well studied in ADHF but also has been associated with worse outcomes in patients with AMI and ADHF [4] and likely should be avoided unless the clinical picture is one of hypertensive crisis and prompt blood pressure control is clinically indicated.

Nesiritide was approved by the FDA in 2001, but retrospective data raised the issue of worsening renal function and increased mortality which led to a dramatic decrease in the use of this medication [5, 6]. The ASCEND-HF trial was a randomized multicenter, placebo-controlled trial that studied the use of nesiritide in 7,141 patients with ADHF [7]. ASCEND-HF demonstrated that nesiritide had a non-significant impact on dyspnea, and no impact on mortality, worsening of renal function, or rehospitalization. Based on ASCEND-HF there is no clear benefit from nesiritide in the setting of ADHF.

J. McCord, MD (✉)
Henry Ford Hospital, Detroit, MI, USA
e-mail: jmccord1@hfhs.org

W. Frank Peacock (ed.), *Short Stay Management of Acute Heart Failure*,
Contemporary Cardiology, DOI 10.1007/978-1-61779-627-2_19,
© Springer Science+Business Media, LLC 2012

Calcium Channel Blockers

Calcium channel blockers have negative inotropic properties and, as a general rule, should be avoided in ADHF. In one study, post-AMI patients with an ejection fraction <40% that received diltiazem were more likely to develop clinical heart failure as compared to placebo [8]. Verapamil use also has been associated with hemodynamic and clinical deterioration in patients with ejection fractions <35%. Finally, the dihydropyridines, such as nifedipine, have also been associated with clinical deterioration in patients with systolic heart failure [9].

Conversely, patients with diastolic heart in the setting of hypertension may benefit from diltiazem or verapamil by controlling blood pressure and slowing heart rate, which can improve diastolic filling in this group of patients. Diltiazem can also be considered in patients with ADHF and atrial fibrillation with rapid ventricular response when there is not an adequate clinical response to digoxin, amiodarone, or procainamide.

Beta-Blockers

Beta-blockers, in general, have been avoided in patients with ADHF. In clinical trials of beta-blockers for AMI, patients with significant heart failure have been excluded. Many patients with ADHF are taking beta-blockers, and most of these can have the beta-blocker continued. In patients presenting with hypotension or end-organ hypoperfusion where inotropic therapy is being considered, beta-blocker may need to be discontinued. However, there is overwhelming data to support the long-term benefits of beta-blockers in patients with systolic heart failure. After patients have been compensated, an attempt should be made to reinstitute the beta-blocker. Short acting beta-blocker therapy can be considered, but used with caution, in ADHF when uncontrolled cardiac ischemia is present or for control of tachyarrhythmias as necessary.

Antiarrhythmics

Class I antiarrhythmic drugs in the Vaughn Williams classification system produce a greater negative inotropic and more frequent proarrhythmic effects in patients with systolic heart failure and, in general, should not be used in such patients [10]. The cardiac arrhythmia suppression trial (CAST) demonstrated that the Class Ic agents (flecainide and moricizine) were associated with proarrhythmia and increased mortality in patients that suffered an AMI and had decreased systolic function [11, 12]. Another Class Ic agent, propafenone, should also be avoided. Class Ia drugs (procainamide, quinidine, disopyramide) have also been associated with increased mortality in patients with decreased LV systolic function. Amiodarone has proven to be safe in patients with systolic HF and is recommended to be used in patients with heart failure accompanied by atrial fibrillation when clinically indicated [13].

Glycosides

Digitalis can be used as a rate control drug in atrial fibrillation and leads to improved symptoms in patients with chronic systolic HF. However, caution is warranted in the setting of AHF as it has been associated with adverse effects in AMI accompanied by HF [14]. In a study in patients with AMI and AHF, the use of digoxin was a predictor of life-threatening proarrhythmic events [15]. The use of digoxin may be considered in AHF associated with atrial fibrillation with rapid ventricular response [16].

Inotropes

Inotropes should be avoided in ADHF and only considered in the minority of cases when there is significant systemic hypotension or end-organ hypoperfusion. In clinical trials, inotropes have been associated with worse outcomes. Inotropes increase oxygen demand and may worsen arrhythmias or myocardial ischemia [17, 18]. In one randomized trial, short-term use of milrinone (a phosphodiesterase inhibitor) did not improve signs or symptoms of ADHF and was associated with severe hypotension and arrhythmias [19]. Other trials have demonstrated that the beta-agonist dobutamine is associated with adverse cardiac events when used in ADHF [20, 21].

When either atrial or ventricular arrhythmias are of clinical concern, milrinone is preferred over dobutamine which more commonly worsens tachyarrhythmias [22, 23]. Since the site of action of milrinone is distal to the beta-adrenergic receptors, milrinone is preferred over dobutamine during concomitant beta-blocker therapy [24–26]. However, there is particular concern over safety of milrinone in the setting of ischemic heart failure, and it should be avoided in this situation [19, 27, 28].

Miscellaneous

There are numerous medications that can exacerbate heart failure and should be avoided or discontinued if clinically possible. NSAIDS act by inhibiting prostaglandin synthesis by blocking cyclooxygenase. Lower renal prostaglandin levels may reduce glomerular filtration rate leading to sodium and water retention [29]. The cyclooxygenase II inhibitors, which block cyclooxygenase II, also can lead to fluid retention and do not appear to offer any advantage over standard NSAIDS. Similarly, corticosteroids lead to fluid retention and elevated blood pressure [30].

Other drugs that should be avoided in patients with a history of heart failure include the thiazolidinediones (rosiglitazone and pioglitazone), which are used to treat type II diabetes. These agents may increase intravascular volume by 7% [31] and may lead to ADHF [32]. Finally, cilostazol inhibits type III phosphodiesterase and is used for the treatment of intermittent claudication. The use of cilostazol is contraindicated in patients with ADHF as the drug may lead to increased heart rate and ventricular tachycardia [33].

References

1. Swedberg K, et al. Effects of the early administration of enalapril on mortality in patients with acute myocardial infarction. Results of the Cooperative New Scandinavian Enalapril Survival Study II (CONSENSUS II). N Engl J Med. 1992;327(10):678–84.
2. Silvers SM, et al. Clinical policy: critical issues in the evaluation and management of adult patients presenting to the emergency department with acute heart failure syndromes. Ann Emerg Med. 2007;49(5):627–69.
3. Dickstein K, et al. ESC Guidelines for the diagnosis and treatment of acute and chronic heart failure 2008: the Task Force for the Diagnosis and Treatment of Acute and Chronic Heart Failure 2008 of the European Society of Cardiology. Developed in collaboration with the Heart Failure Association of the ESC (HFA) and endorsed by the European Society of Intensive Care Medicine (ESICM). Eur Heart J. 2008;29(19):2388–442.
4. Cohn JN, et al. Effect of short-term infusion of sodium nitroprusside on mortality rate in acute myocardial infarction complicated by left ventricular failure: results of a Veterans Administration cooperative study. N Engl J Med. 1982;306(19):1129–35.
5. Sackner-Bernstein JD, et al. Short-term risk of death after treatment with nesiritide for decompensated heart failure: a pooled analysis of randomized controlled trials. JAMA. 2005;293(15):1900–5.
6. Sackner-Bernstein JD, Skopicki HA, Aaronson KD. Risk of worsening renal function with nesiritide in patients with acutely decompensated heart failure. Circulation. 2005;111(12):1487–91.
7. O'Connor CM, et al. Effect of Nesiritide in patients with acute decompensated heart failure. N Engl J Med. 2011;365;32–43.
8. Goldstein RE, et al. Diltiazem increases late-onset congestive heart failure in postinfarction patients with early reduction in ejection fraction. The Adverse Experience Committee; and the Multicenter Diltiazem Postinfarction Research Group. Circulation. 1991;83(1):52–60.
9. Elkayam U, et al. A prospective, randomized, double-blind, crossover study to compare the efficacy and safety of chronic nifedipine therapy with that of isosorbide dinitrate and their combination in the treatment of chronic congestive heart failure. Circulation. 1990;82(6):1954–61.
10. Kottkamp H, et al. Clinical significance and management of ventricular arrhythmias in heart failure. Eur Heart J. 1994;15(Suppl D):155–63.
11. Echt DS, et al. Mortality and morbidity in patients receiving encainide, flecainide, or placebo. The Cardiac Arrhythmia Suppression Trial. N Engl J Med. 1991;324(12):781–8.
12. Hallstrom AP, et al. Time to arrhythmic, ischemic, and heart failure events: exploratory analyses to elucidate mechanisms of adverse drug effects in the Cardiac Arrhythmia Suppression Trial. Am Heart J. 1995;130(1):71–9.
13. Hunt SA, et al. ACC/AHA guidelines for the evaluation and management of chronic heart failure in the adult: executive summary A report of the American College of Cardiology/ American Heart Association Task Force on Practice Guidelines (Committee to revise the 1995 Guidelines for the Evaluation and Management of Heart Failure). J Am Coll Cardiol. 2001;38(7):2101–13.
14. Spargias KS, Hall AS, Ball SG. Safety concerns about digoxin after acute myocardial infarction. Lancet. 1999;354(9176):391–2.
15. McClements BM, Adgey AA. Value of signal-averaged electrocardiography, radionuclide ventriculography, Holter monitoring and clinical variables for prediction of arrhythmic events in survivors of acute myocardial infarction in the thrombolytic era. J Am Coll Cardiol. 1993;21(6):1419–27.

16. Khand AU, et al. Systematic review of the management of atrial fibrillation in patients with heart failure. Eur Heart J. 2000;21(8):614–32.
17. Katz AM. Potential deleterious effects of inotropic agents in the therapy of chronic heart failure. Circulation. 1986;73(3 Pt 2):III184–90.
18. Packer M, et al. Double-blind, placebo-controlled study of the efficacy of flosequinan in patients with chronic heart failure. Principal Investigators of the REFLECT Study. J Am Coll Cardiol. 1993;22(1):65–72.
19. Cuffe MS, et al. Short-term intravenous milrinone for acute exacerbation of chronic heart failure: a randomized controlled trial. JAMA. 2002;287(12):1541–7.
20. Follath F, et al. Efficacy and safety of intravenous levosimendan compared with dobutamine in severe low-output heart failure (the LIDO study): a randomised double-blind trial. Lancet. 2002;360(9328):196–202.
21. O'Connor CM, et al. Continuous intravenous dobutamine is associated with an increased risk of death in patients with advanced heart failure: insights from the Flolan International Randomized Survival Trial (FIRST). Am Heart J. 1999;138(1 Pt 1):78–86.
22. Caldicott LD, et al. Intravenous enoximone or dobutamine for severe heart failure after acute myocardial infarction: a randomized double-blind trial. Eur Heart J. 1993;14(5):696–700.
23. Burger AJ, et al. Effect of nesiritide (B-type natriuretic peptide) and dobutamine on ventricular arrhythmias in the treatment of patients with acutely decompensated congestive heart failure: the PRECEDENT study. Am Heart J. 2002;144(6):1102–8.
24. Lowes BD, et al. Milrinone versus dobutamine in heart failure subjects treated chronically with carvedilol. Int J Cardiol. 2001;81(2–3):141–9.
25. Metra M, et al. Beta-blocker therapy influences the hemodynamic response to inotropic agents in patients with heart failure: a randomized comparison of dobutamine and enoximone before and after chronic treatment with metoprolol or carvedilol. J Am Coll Cardiol. 2002;40(7):1248–58.
26. Bohm M, et al. Improvement of postreceptor events by metoprolol treatment in patients with chronic heart failure. J Am Coll Cardiol. 1997;30(4):992–6.
27. Thackray S, et al. The effectiveness and relative effectiveness of intravenous inotropic drugs acting through the adrenergic pathway in patients with heart failure-a meta-regression analysis. Eur J Heart Fail. 2002;4(4):515–29.
28. Loh E, et al. A randomized multicenter study comparing the efficacy and safety of intravenous milrinone and intravenous nitroglycerin in patients with advanced heart failure. J Card Fail. 2001;7(2):114–21.
29. Feenstra J, et al. Association of nonsteroidal anti-inflammatory drugs with first occurrence of heart failure and with relapsing heart failure: the Rotterdam Study. Arch Intern Med. 2002;162(3):265–70.
30. Whitworth JA, et al. The nitric oxide system in glucocorticoid-induced hypertension. J Hypertens. 2002;20(6):1035–43.
31. Kennedy FP. Do thiazolidinediones cause congestive heart failure? Mayo Clin Proc. 2003;78(9):1076–7.
32. Misbin RI. The phantom of lactic acidosis due to metformin in patients with diabetes. Diabet Care. 2004;27(7):1791–3.
33. Gamssari F, et al. Rapid ventricular tachycardias associated with cilostazol use. Tex Heart Inst J. 2002;29(2):140–2.

Chapter 20
Implications of Atrial Fibrillation in Heart Failure Management

Chad E. Darling and Richard V. Aghababian

Background

Atrial fibrillation (AF) and congestive heart failure (HF) are comorbidities that coexist in many patients with underlying cardiovascular disease and in patients with certain acute medical conditions such as hyperthyroidism. The number of individuals who present to the Emergency Department (ED) with clinical symptoms based on AF and HF is likely to remain high as demographics of the population of the United States (USA) trend to an older age [1]. Both AF and HF can play a causative role in the development of each other. The fast, irregular heart rates often seen with AF may lead to the development of acute HF, or in patients with a history of HF, may result in clinical instability. In this chapter, we will focus on patients that present with both HF and AF with regard to epidemiology, ED evaluation, treatment, and implications for potential short-stay management.

Epidemiology

There are over 5.5 million people with HF [2] in the USA. Moreover, acute HF episodes are the leading cause of hospital admissions in the elderly [3], and over three quarters of all these admissions are initially cared for in the ED [4]. AF is also

C.E. Darling, MD ✉)
Department of Emergency Medicine, University of Massachusetts Medical School,
Worcester, MA, USA
e-mail: chad.darling@umassmed.edu

R.V. Aghababian, MD
University of Massachusetts Medical School, Worcester, MA, USA

W. Frank Peacock (ed.), *Short Stay Management of Acute Heart Failure*,
Contemporary Cardiology, DOI 10.1007/978-1-61779-627-2_20,
© Springer Science+Business Media, LLC 2012

Table 20.1 Potential complications of AF and HF

Acute
  Sudden death
  Ischemic stroke
  Thromboembolic events
  Ventricular ectopy
  Acute respiratory failure
  Cardiogenic shock
Subacute
  Cognitive dysfunction
  Diminished quality of life
  Chronic renal failure
  Peripheral edema
Chronic
  Stasis ulcers
  Shortened life span
  Syncopal episodes

highly prevalent with over 2.2 million cases in the USA [5]. The incidence of AF has steadily increased in the past decade as the average age of the population has increased [6], and it often coexists with HF [7, 8]. Data from the Framingham Heart Study have found the cumulative incidence of AF in patients with HF approximates 25 % [8]. Unpublished data from the ongoing Worcester Heart Failure Study [7] have demonstrated that roughly a third of 4,536 patients hospitalized with acute HF had a medical history of AF, and 25 % had electrocardiograms documenting AF on admission. It is generally felt that the combination of AF and HF portends a worse prognosis than having either disease alone although there is conflicting evidence in the literature. For instance, many studies have suggested that the survival of HF patients is decreased in patients with concomitant AF [8–11] while other studies have found that no difference in survival in HF patients with or without AF [12, 13]. There is significant heterogeneity in these studies which may, in part, explain these results. What is clear is that over time, a range of clinical complications can develop in these patients (Table 20.1).

Etiologies

There are several conditions associated with both AF [14] and HF [15] such as essential hypertension, diabetes mellitus, coronary heart disease, valvular heart disease, dilated and hypertrophic cardiomyopathies, and bronchopulmonary disease. Most importantly, both AF and HF are risk factors for the development of each other (Table 20.2).

Table 20.2 Common and overlapping conditions associated with AF and HF

Toxins (alcohol, cocaine)
Coronary heart disease
Valvular heart disease
Cardiomyopathies (dilated, hypertrophic)
Diabetes mellitus
Essential hypertension
Bronchopulmonary disease
Thyroid abnormalities
Obesity
Stress/elevated catecholamines
Metabolic disturbances
Cardiac surgery

Patient Evaluation

History and Presentation

The presenting symptoms for AF and HF are relatively similar and nonspecific. Typical symptoms of AF include chest pain, light-headedness, fatigue, palpitations, nausea, and dyspnea [16]. The most common symptoms and signs of HF include dyspnea, peripheral edema, cough, orthopnea, chest pain, weakness, nausea/vomiting, and fatigue [17]. The characteristic ECG findings of AF, along with an irregular pulse, are likely to be recognized early on in patients presenting with AF and HF. Once AF is recognized, and assuming the patient is not unstable, there are several useful pieces of historical information to obtain. First, it is helpful to ascertain the history of the patient's current symptoms with a focus on whether or not the AF is a long-standing condition, new in onset (e.g., <48 h), and whether or not the onset can be accurately identified. In patients with prior episodes of AF, a quick investigation of past ED treatment approaches may also be useful. If HF is suspected clinically, then it is important to gather information regarding prior episodes, potential precipitating factors such as diet, medication omissions/errors, and echocardiogram results (e.g., does the patient have primarily systolic or diastolic dysfunction). Lastly, other comorbidities, and current medications the patient is taking, including anticoagulant, antiplatelet, and other cardiovascular (e.g., beta-blockers, digoxin, calcium channel blockers) medications will help inform subsequent decision making.

With or without concomitant HF, AF presentations have been categorized in numerous ways such as *asymptomatic, paroxysmal, persistent, permanent, perioperative, lone, and recurrent* (Table 20.3). All of these categories refer to the timing of onset and/or duration of AF. For patients not requiring urgent cardioversion due to instability, the duration of AF is the most important factor in determining whether chemical or electrical cardioversion can be safely attempted in the ED.

Table 20.3 Types of AF

AF type	Definition
Asymptomatic	AF without symptoms or patient awareness
Paroxysmal	A self-limited AF episode lasting <7 days
Persistent	AF continuing >7 days
Permanent	AF lasting >1 year or with cardioversion that has failed or not been tried
Perioperative	AF developing within 48 h after cardiac surgery
Lone	AF not caused by underlying heart disease
Recurrent	Having a history of two or more independent episodes of AF

Exam

For any patient with AF and HF, acquiring vital signs on presentation, setting up critical care monitoring, obtaining IV access, and performing a rapid exam are central to the initial assessment. The focus for patients with AF and HF needs to first be directed at determining if there are signs of instability such as hypotension, respiratory failure, ischemic chest pain, severe HF, or altered mental status. If these, or other signs of instability, are present and the patient is experiencing a rapid heart rate due to AF, then urgent synchronized cardioversion based on Advanced Cardiac Life Support [18] (see below) is indicated. At the same time, if HF is felt to be playing a significant role in the patient's presentation, then respiratory and pharmacologic therapies directed at the HF should be started. If the patient is stable, a thorough exam focusing on mental acuity, neurologic status, heart and lung auscultation, abdomen, peripheral perfusion, and edema should be undertaken. Paying particular attention to the heart exam may uncover significant valvular disease which may be contributing to the present symptoms and, depending on the severity of the presentation, require an echocardiogram in the ED for diagnostic purposes.

Diagnostic Testing

For many patients who meet the clinical criteria for AF and HF, more than one underlying disorder may be contributing to the patients presenting symptoms. Thorough appreciation of all the underlying causes for the patient's signs and symptoms requires a careful diagnostic workup to achieve the best possible outcomes. In general, the diagnostic testing in patients with AF and HF does not differ significantly from that of patients with HF alone. All patients should receive an electrocardiogram (ECG), cardiopulmonary monitoring, and a chest X-ray on arrival. On the ECG, you would look for the abnormalities such as the characteristic findings of AF, evidence of ischemia, and signs of preexcitation. Laboratory tests may vary with suspicion of certain etiologies for AF and HF but often will include basic hematology tests, serum markers of myocardial injury, a natriuretic peptide, electrolytes, and kidney function. Thyroid function tests, which may often be considered, have been found to be abnormal in many patients with AF but are only rarely (<1% in a large registry [16]) felt to be the cause of the AF itself. In patients where there are concerns based on history, exam, or ECG for ongoing myocardial ischemia, valvular disease, or pericardial effusion, it may be useful to obtain an urgent echocardiogram in the ED.

Treatment of Symptomatic Patients with Atrial Fibrillation and Heart Failure

Hemodynamically Unstable Patient

The hemodynamically unstable patient with AF and HF needs urgent cardioversion if the instability is deemed to be related to AF-mediated tachycardia. Significant acute HF may be a sign of instability in the AF patient regardless of whether the AF caused the HF or vice versa. In either case, converting the AF to sinus rhythm, even transiently, may normalize vital signs and facilitate treatment of the HF.

The preparation for emergent cardioversion includes administering analgesics and sedatives when possible. However, if the patient is suffering a severe decompensation, this step may have to be omitted. In addition for patients whose AF has lasted ≥48 h, intravenous heparin should be administered at the time of cardioversion and continued after the procedure as a bridge to 4 weeks of total anticoagulation [14]. The placement of the defibrillator pads is somewhat controversial but the anterior–posterior position is likely to be the most efficacious in the majority of AF patients [19]. The amount of energy required to convert the patient to sinus rhythm from AF is generally higher than that for atrial flutter [14] and also varies depending on whether the defibrillator is monophasic or biphasic. For monophasic, 200 J is a reasonable starting point, whereas for biphasic, 100 J is likely to be more effective [14, 20, 21]. For patients with implanted pacemakers, cardioversion can proceed as usual, but care should be taken to avoid placing the defibrillator pad over the generator [14]. Although therapy with antiarrhythmic agents prior to cardioversion has been shown to increase efficacy of elective cardioversion [22], in the unstable patient, this is generally not an option.

In the setting of concomitant decompensated HF, the rate of recurrence of AF after successful cardioversion is likely to be high [23], so therapies aimed at improving HF should be started immediately once the patient is more stable. The use of antiarrhythmic agents, such as amiodarone, after cardioversion may help to prevent early recurrence, but in the acute setting, the decision to use these agents should be made on a patient by patient basis [14] in conjunction with a consultant.

After cardioversion, in addition to treating underlying HF, it is important to obtain another ECG to evaluate for the presence of an acute coronary syndrome (ACS). Furthermore, this reevaluation should maintain a broad differential diagnosis so as not to miss other contributing conditions such as adverse medication reactions, alcohol or drug toxicity (e.g., digoxin), electrolyte disturbances, valvular heart disease, pulmonary emboli, and sepsis/septic shock.

Hemodynamically Stable Patient with Atrial Fibrillation and Heart Failure

Although HF in the setting of AF can be considered a sign of instability, many cases will be of milder severity and not require urgent cardioversion. These patients may fall into various categories such as rapid AF with mild HF, HF with only a history of AF, or HF with AF without tachycardia. In cases where urgent cardioversion is not needed, strategies to control rate, initiate anticoagulation if indicated, potentially convert the rhythm (electrical or chemical), and treat the underlying HF, will all need to be considered and instituted where appropriate.

Rate Control

Due to the risk of venous thromboembolism, initial heart rate (HR) control, rather than acute rhythm conversion, is likely to be the preferred treatment in the majority of cases. There are several rate-control agents that may be considered and include digoxin, calcium channel blockers, beta-blockers, and amiodarone. In cases where the onset of the AF episode is not clearly within 48 h, then anticoagulation should be initiated early on unless there is a specific contraindication. A reasonable target for rate control is ≤120 beats/min over the first few hours of treatment [24].

Digoxin

When considering rate control for patients with rapid AF and HF, digoxin may be particularly useful agent as it already has an established role in treating HF [25]. In the AF and HF patient, it may be considered a first-line agent [14, 24] and may be most efficacious when used in conjunction with typical AF rate-control agents, such as beta-blockers and diltiazem [14, 26]. The mechanism by which digoxin slows the HR in AF appears to be due to its effect on increasing vagal activity on the AV node [27–29]. In patients who are not on digoxin, it is administered acutely in a series of loading doses over several hours to approximately 1–1.5 g total dose, depending on clinical response [14, 30].

Several trials have examined digoxin use acutely for rapid AF. In the Digitalis in Acute Atrial Fibrillation (DAAF) trial, 239 patients with rapid AF were randomized to receive either digoxin or placebo and then followed over 16 h to determine effect on HR and conversion to sinus rhythm [31]. In this trial, digoxin was not found to facilitate conversion to sinus rhythm but had a significant rate effect rate at 2 h compared to placebo (mean HR 105 vs. 117 bpm). A smaller randomized trial of digoxin versus placebo for rate control found that digoxin's ability to slow HR was not evident until over 5 h after the first dose was given [29]. Hou et al. compared the ability of digoxin versus amiodarone to slow HR in patients with AF (approximately half of which had NYHA class IV HF) and found that after 1 h, digoxin slowed HRs approximately 10–15 beats/min compared to 30 for amiodarone. There are a number of conditions that either warrant caution or represent contraindications to the use of digoxin. First, AV nodal blocking agents such as digoxin care contraindicated in situations where a preexcitation syndrome such as Wolff–Parkinson–White is known or suspected. Other situations where digoxin should be used cautiously are with renal impairment, electrolyte disturbances, and with the risk of toxicity when loading patients already on digoxin [30]. Lastly, digoxin may not work as well in the setting of high sympathetic tone [24, 28].

Calcium Channel Blockers

The calcium channel blockers diltiazem and verapamil have both been studied as agents for rate control in rapid AF. Both agents act within 5–10 min to decrease heart rate [28, 32]. In patients with AF and HF (particularly with a low EF), diltiazem is a better choice of agent to use than verapamil as it has less of a negative inotropic effect and is less likely to lead to worsening HF and hypotension [27, 28, 33]. Goldenberg et al. examined the effectiveness of diltiazem versus placebo to reduce heart rate in patient with NYHA grade III or IV HF. In this study, 36/37 patients responded to the diltiazem with reduced rates within a median of 15 min compared to 0/15 placebo patients. Furthermore, there were only three adverse events (hypotension) suggesting that in many patients diltiazem may be safe [34]. Theoretically, the negative inotropic effects of calcium channel antagonists may be offset when these agents are used in combination with digoxin [27], but in patients with acute AF and HF, this has not been established. As mentioned, when compared to digoxin, diltiazem is significantly more efficacious in controlling heart rate over the first few hours of acute treatment [35, 36].

Beta-Blockers

Beta-blockers have a well-established role in the treatment of chronic HF [37]. However, in the presence of acute HF and AF, beta-blockers should be used carefully, if at all, with small incremental dosing [24] and close monitoring of the patient's vital signs. Demerican et al. compared intravenous metoprolol and diltiazem with regard to slowing HR in patients with rapid AF and found that at 20 min, 80% of the metoprolol patients had significant HR control versus 90% in the diltiazem group (defined as either HR < 100 or a 20% decrease from baseline). Furthermore, at all time points, diltiazem resulted in more HR slowing than metoprolol. However, in this trial, patients with class IV HF were excluded, and it is unclear how much HF was present overall. Where there is concern regarding the negative inotropic effects of beta-blockers in patients with HF, the ultra short-acting beta-blocker esmolol may be a good choice [38]. Esmolol has a 9-min half-life, and therefore, if it needs to be stopped due to worsening HF or hypotension, its effects will rapidly diminish. It has been used in the setting of rapid AF after coronary artery bypass, where some degree of myocardial dysfunction is likely to be present, and appears to be more effective than diltiazem and as safe [39, 40]. Esmolol has also been shown to be safe and effective when used in conjunction with digoxin for rapid AF [26].

Amiodarone

Amiodarone may also be considered for rate control in the AF and HF patient unless they are on other antiarrhythmics that should not be combined with amiodarone [24, 41, 42]. The 2006 AHA/ACC guidelines recommend that amiodarone or digoxin be used to acutely control rate in patients with AF and HF (Class I recommendation) [14]. However, as it may facilitate conversion to sinus rhythm, it would ideally be used in cases where the patient either meets anticoagulation guidelines for cardioversion or will be given anticoagulants [24]. Amiodarone is also a common choice of agent to be used to maintain sinus rhythm in the AF and HF patient after cardioversion [14]. Dronedarone is a newer antiarrhythmic drug similar in structure to amiodarone. It has been studied in a number of trials looking at its ability to affect rhythm control for AF over the long term [43–45]. It currently has no role for acute rate or rhythm control. In addition, one clinical trial found excess cardiovascular mortality in a dronedarone-treated group of AF patients with poor left ventricular function (EF $\leq 35\%$) [44].

Summary

In summary, HR control for patients with AF and HF can be approached with the usual medications used in patients without HF provided vital signs are monitored closely [14]. The use of digoxin with other rate-control agents may be beneficial, and amiodarone also has a heightened role in these patients [14]. Diltiazem rather than verapamil would be the best choice if calcium channel blockers are used and incremental beta-blocker dosing or use of esmolol may help avoid complications with these agents.

Rhythm Control/Conversion

A recent editorial examining rate versus rhythm-control strategies for AF in the ED [46] concluded that there was not enough evidence to support a rhythm-control strategy as opposed to the standard HR control for new onset AF in the ED. However, Stiell and others have published on the safety and efficacy of acute cardioversion in the ED for rapid AF patients, but these studies have excluded patients with more significant HF [47, 48]. Their results suggest that cardioversion of AF alone appears to be safe, and it is likely that at least a small percentage of the patients that have undergone cardioversion have had some degree HF. It is worth noting, however, that in these studies, an antiarrhythmic agent such as procainamide is often given as a first attempt at cardioversion, which may not be feasible in patients with concomitant acute HF or low blood pressure [49]. This "preloading" with an antiarrhythmic may also be influencing their high success rates of electrical cardioversion. Vernakalant is an investigational, relatively atrial selective, antiarrhythmic agent (approved in Europe but not by the FDA) that appears to be successful in converting

AF to sinus rhythm. However, one published ED-based study had only a small minority (≤5%) of patients with HF [50]. It is worth noting that if pharmacologic agents are given, the risk of thromboembolism and stroke appears to be the same as in patients who receive electric cardioversion [14].

The main concern with acute rhythm conversion is the risk of venous thromboembolism, which appears to be the same in patients who receive electrical or chemical cardioversion [14]. However, in carefully selected AF patients (e.g., acute onset <48 h of AF), the risk is very low. One study of 357 admitted patients with AF ≤48 h who underwent electrical, chemical, or spontaneous cardioversion were found to have a risk of thromboembolism of less than 1% [51]. This study did not include any patients with reduced EF where the risk of complications may be higher. As one potential treatment option, it seems reasonable to consider acute rhythm conversion in HF and AF patients who have either a history of HF and/or milder acute HF. This decision will need to be made on a case-by-case basis taking into account each patients presentation, history, anticoagulation status, and personal preferences.

Disposition Decisions

Disposition of the AF and HF patient may include any of the following: hospital admission, short-stay unit (SSU) admission, or discharge to home, rehabilitation hospital, or other extended care facility including hospice. Despite the fact that acute coronary syndromes rarely present as AF alone [52], most patients with AF and HF are likely to require an admission to the hospital as the presence of both entities complicates their evaluation and treatment (see Fig. 20.1). However, the SSU may have a role in these patients as opportunities to reduce cost and improve the quality of care among Medicare recipients are sought as part of current health reform efforts. Among many others, there is likely to be a focus on strategies that can identify patients who can be managed in a SSU and also prevent repeat ED visits and subsequent readmissions.

Transfer of Symptomatic Atrial Fibrillation and Heart Failure Patients to Short-Stay Unit

The most likely candidates for admission to the SSU are those that have rate-controlled AF with either historical or mild HF amenable to a short course (≤24 h) of observation care and treatment. Due to the presence of AF and HF and other associated comorbidities, the treatment plan will need to be individualized for each patient. Key data for risk stratification of these patients include their response to treatment in the ED, prior medical history (e.g., AF, HF, and ejection fraction), results of ED tests [e.g., troponin (associated with increased mortality in patients with HF [53])], electrolytes, renal function, overall patient appearance, and mental status. In the future, there is also likely to be an increasing number of patients with advanced HF, AF, and

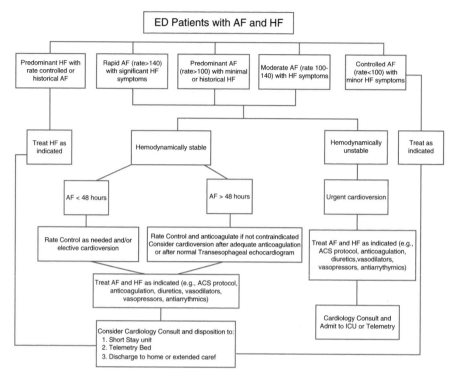

Fig. 20.1 Clinical management of patients with AF and HF

Table 20.4 General management for patients with AF and HF in the SSU

Continue critical care monitoring and establish treatment objectives for Atrial Fibrillation and Heart Failure

Evaluate response to Emergency Department treatment and adjust therapy as needed

Rule out and identify precipitating etiologies (e.g., renal failure, electrolyte disturbances, anemia, ischemia)

Consult with primary care and cardiology as appropriate

Consider provocative cardiac testing

Consider echocardiography

Arrange for patient and family education (e.g., disease-specific education, medications, diet, self-care)

Arrange follow-up care (e.g., specialists, primary care)

left ventricular assist devices [54–56]. Although the information on the care of patients with these devices is lacking, their presence is likely to rule out observation admissions for the foreseeable future. While in the SSU, many issues will need to be addressed, and (Table 20.4) consultations with appropriate specialists should be arranged as indicated to help with pharmacotherapy options for AF and HF and to evaluate for potential invasive treatment (e.g., pacemaker insertion, radiofrequency ablation, cardiac surgery evaluation). Primary care providers should also be contacted and kept abreast of the treatment and follow-up plans. As with admitted patients, the SSU should also provide patients with disease-specific education, review medication lists and address errors and issues of compliance, discuss dietary habits, and provide advice on self-management strategies. In addition, referral to HF management programs may cut costs and reduce readmissions [57–59].

Long-Term Management Considerations for Patients with Atrial Fibrillation and Heart Failure

There are a multitude of options for the long-term management of the patient with AF and HF. One of the first questions that may be addressed is whether a rate-control or rhythm-control strategy should be used for those with persistent or recurrent AF. For rhythm control, there are several long-term antiarrhythmic options to choose from based on the results of clinical trials and FDA approval such as β-blockers, flecainide, sotalol, amiodarone, and dronedarone, with amiodarone being the agent of choice in patients with advanced HF [14]. Long-term rhythm control may improve myocardial function, avoid anticoagulation, and prevent complications related to thromboembolism [60]. The advantages of a rate-control strategy are that antiarrhythmic drugs can be avoided and cardioversion procedures can be avoided [60]. Several studies have compared these two strategies and found no significant differences in outcomes over time [61–63]. Specifically, in AF patients, the AFFIRM and RACE trials found a trend toward a decrease in mortality and/or in combined adverse outcomes associated with rate control rather than a rhythm-control strategy [62, 63]. In an analogous fashion, Roy et al. studied rate versus rhythm control in 1,376 patients with EF < 35%, HF symptoms, and a history of AF. Follow-up found no difference in the rates of death or other secondary outcomes between either strategy [61]. Current guidelines suggest that, in patients with AF and HF, decisions regarding rate versus rhythm control will need to be individualized and it is reasonable to use either approach [25].

   Another potential long-term treatment is catheter ablation of AF foci. Hsu et al. studied the efficacy and safety of catheter ablation in patients with both AF and HF (reduced EF <45%) as compared to patients with AF alone. They found that maintenance of sinus rhythm was achieved in over 3/4 of both groups, and this was associated with improved left ventricular function [64]. Biventricular pacing (often with AV-node ablation) has also been shown to be beneficial for patients with AF and HF [65, 66] and may be offered to carefully selected patients. Lastly, some patients may be referred for surgical treatment (Maze procedure) for their AF [67]. Due to the number of treatment options, consultations with specialists are a key component of treatment.

Use of Anticoagulant and Antiplatelet Therapies

Another key long-term therapy question to address in the SSU is the need for oral anticoagulation therapy. Concomitant HF increases the risk of stroke, and therefore, the need for consideration of pharmacologic prophylaxis is even more important in the patient with AF and HF. The decision to use long-term anticoagulants such as warfarin is based on an evaluation of various risk factors (e.g., age, hypertension, presence of HF, and valvular heart disease) for stroke along with other factors (e.g., fall risk), and patient preferences. Several studies have described the features associated with stroke in patients with AF [68–71], and there are scoring systems such as $CHADS_2$ [69, 72] which can help with stroke risk stratification. Some patients will be deemed low risk, and only aspirin may be recommended, whereas higher risk individuals may be prescribed long-term anticoagulation.

A newer anticoagulant option to consider is dabigatran which is an oral direct thrombin inhibitor. A recent study randomized anticoagulation treatment of dabigatran at two different fixed doses (110 mg and 150 mg) and compared it to adjusted dose warfarin with respect to rates of subsequent stroke, systemic embolism, or bleeding complications. Dabigatran use was found to result in similar or decreased rates of stroke and systemic embolism and similar rates of major bleeding events. The incidence of HF in this group was approximately 1/3 in each treatment arm [73]. Lastly, in patients who are not candidates for anticoagulation, antiplatelet medications may provide some protection against stroke. Aspirin plus clopidogrel has been found to result in lower rates of stroke/year in AF patients compared with aspirin alone but at the trade-off of an increased risk of bleeding (2.0% vs. 1.3% per year). These decisions must be made in consultation with a cardiologist or responsible primary care physician who will be following the patient after discharge from the SSU.

Summary/Conclusions

As the US population ages, the number of patients presenting with AF and HF will increase. Because of the number of etiologies and frequency of comorbidity, patients with concurrent AF and HF comprise a heterogeneous group that requires customized treatment strategies. Despite their complexity, management of a small percentage of patients presenting with AF and HF in an observation/SSU setting may be feasible provided that there is access to necessary consultants and that patients are provided with detail education and discharge planning. Determining selection criteria for entry into the SSU treatment pathway and evaluating outcomes of treatment will be key to determining the safety of this form of outpatient management for this growing population of patients.

References

1. United States Census Bureau. International database. Table 094. Midyear population by age and sex. http://www.census.gov/population/www/projections/natdet-D1A.html. Accessed 1 Dec 2011.
2. Roger VL, Go AS, Lloyd-Jones DM, et al. Heart disease and stroke statistics—2011 update: a report from the American Heart Association. Circulation. 2011;123(4):e18–209.
3. Cardozo L, Aherns S. Assessing the efficacy of a clinical pathway in the management of older patients hospitalized with congestive heart failure. J Healthc Qual. 1999;21:12–6. quiz 16–7.
4. Emerman CL, Peacock WF, for the ADHERE™ Scientific Advisory Committee and Investigators. Evolving patterns of care for decompensated heart failure: Implications from the ADHERE™ Registry Database [abstract 200]. Acad Emerg Med. 2004;11:503.
5. Go AS, Hylek EM, Phillips KA, et al. Prevalence of diagnosed atrial fibrillation in adults: national implications for rhythm management and stroke prevention: the AnTicoagulation and Risk Factors in Atrial Fibrillation (ATRIA) Study. JAMA. 2001;285:2370–5.
6. Lloyd-Jones D, Adams R, Carnethon M, et al. Heart disease and stroke statistics—2009 update. A report from the American Heart Association Statistics Committee and Stroke Statistics Subcommittee. Circulation. 2008;108:191–261.
7. Goldberg RJ, Ciampa J, Lessard D, Meyer TE, Spencer FA. Long-term survival after heart failure: a contemporary population-based perspective. Arch Intern Med. 2007;167:490–6.
8. Wang TJ, Larson MG, Levy D, et al. Temporal relations of atrial fibrillation and congestive heart failure and their joint influence on mortality: the Framingham Heart Study. Circulation. 2003;107:2920–5.
9. Aronow WS, Ahn C, Kronzon I. Prognosis of congestive heart failure after prior myocardial infarction in older persons with atrial fibrillation versus sinus rhythm. Am J Cardiol. 2001;87(224–5):A8–9.
10. Dries DL, Exner DV, Gersh BJ, Domanski MJ, Waclawiw MA, Stevenson LW. Atrial fibrillation is associated with an increased risk for mortality and heart failure progression in patients with asymptomatic and symptomatic left ventricular systolic dysfunction: a retrospective analysis of the SOLVD trials. Studies of Left Ventricular Dysfunction. J Am Coll Cardiol. 1998;32:695–703.
11. Middlekauff HR, Stevenson WG, Stevenson LW. Prognostic significance of atrial fibrillation in advanced heart failure. A study of 390 patients. Circulation. 1991;84:40–8.
12. Carson PE, Johnson GR, Dunkman WB, Fletcher RD, Farrell L, Cohn JN. The influence of atrial fibrillation on prognosis in mild to moderate heart failure. The V-HeFT Studies. The V-HeFT VA Cooperative Studies Group. Circulation. 1993;87:VI102–110.
13. Mahoney P, Kimmel S, DeNofrio D, Wahl P, Loh E. Prognostic significance of atrial fibrillation in patients at a tertiary medical center referred for heart transplantation because of severe heart failure. Am J Cardiol. 1999;83:1544–7.
14. Fuster V, Ryden LE, Cannom DS, et al. ACC/AHA/ESC 2006 Guidelines for the Management of Patients with Atrial Fibrillation: a report of the American College of Cardiology/American Heart Association Task Force on Practice Guidelines and the European Society of Cardiology Committee for Practice Guidelines (Writing Committee to Revise the 2001 Guidelines for the Management of Patients With Atrial Fibrillation): developed in collaboration with the European Heart Rhythm Association and the Heart Rhythm Society. Circulation. 2006;114:e257–354.
15. Dickstein K, Cohen-Solal A, Filippatos G, et al. ESC Guidelines for the diagnosis and treatment of acute and chronic heart failure 2008: the Task Force for the Diagnosis and Treatment of Acute and Chronic Heart Failure 2008 of the European Society of Cardiology. Developed in collaboration with the Heart Failure Association of the ESC (HFA) and endorsed by the European Society of Intensive Care Medicine (ESICM). Eur Heart J. 2008;29:2388–442.
16. Kerr C, Boone J, Connolly S, et al. Follow-up of atrial fibrillation: the initial experience of the Canadian Registry of Atrial Fibrillation. Eur Heart J. 1996;17(Suppl C):48–51.

17. Goldberg RJ, Spencer FA, Szklo-Coxe M, et al. Symptom presentation in patients hospitalized with acute heart failure. Clin Cardiol. 2010;33:E73–80.
18. Neumar RW, Otto CW, Link MS, et al. Part 8: adult advanced cardiovascular life support, American Heart Association Guidelines for Cardiopulmonary Resuscitation and Emergency Cardiovascular Care. Circulation. 2010;122:S729–67.
19. Botto GL, Politi A, Bonini W, Broffoni T, Bonatti R. External cardioversion of atrial fibrillation: role of paddle position on technical efficacy and energy requirements. Heart. 1999;82: 726–30.
20. Niebauer MJ, Brewer JE, Chung MK, Tchou PJ. Comparison of the rectilinear biphasic waveform with the monophasic damped sine waveform for external cardioversion of atrial fibrillation and flutter. Am J Cardiol. 2004;93:1495–9.
21. Page RL, Kerber RE, Russell JK, et al. Biphasic versus monophasic shock waveform for conversion of atrial fibrillation: the results of an international randomized, double-blind multicenter trial. J Am Coll Cardiol. 2002;39:1956–63.
22. Opolski G, Stanislawska J, Gorecki A, Swiecicka G, Torbicki A, Kraska T. Amiodarone in restoration and maintenance of sinus rhythm in patients with chronic atrial fibrillation after unsuccessful direct-current cardioversion. Clin Cardiol. 1997;20:337–40.
23. Kanji S, Stewart R, Fergusson DA, McIntyre L, Turgeon AF, Hebert PC. Treatment of new-onset atrial fibrillation in noncardiac intensive care unit patients: a systematic review of randomized controlled trials. Crit Care Med. 2008;36:1620–4.
24. DiMarco JP. Atrial fibrillation and acute decompensated heart failure. Circ Heart Fail. 2009;2:72–3.
25. Hunt SA, Abraham WT, Chin MH, et al. 2009 focused update incorporated into the ACC/AHA 2005 Guidelines for the Diagnosis and Management of Heart Failure in Adults: a report of the American College of Cardiology Foundation/American Heart Association Task Force on Practice Guidelines: developed in collaboration with the International Society for Heart and Lung Transplantation. Circulation. 2009;119:e391–479.
26. Shettigar UR, Toole JG, Appunn DO. Combined use of esmolol and digoxin in the acute treatment of atrial fibrillation or flutter. Am Heart J. 1993;126:368–74.
27. Tamariz LJ, Bass EB. Pharmacological rate control of atrial fibrillation. Cardiol Clin. 2004;22: 35–45.
28. Micromedex 2.0. Thomson Reuters. Ann Arbor, MI. 2011. Accessed 25 Jan 2011.
29. Falk RH, Knowlton AA, Bernard SA, Gotlieb NE, Battinelli NJ. Digoxin for converting recent-onset atrial fibrillation to sinus rhythm. A randomized, double-blinded trial. Ann Intern Med. 1987;106:503–6.
30. Information P. Lanoxin(R) oral tablets, digoxin oral tablets. Research Triangle Park, NC: GlaxoSmithKline; 2009.
31. Intravenous digoxin in acute atrial fibrillation. Results of a randomized, placebo-controlled multicentre trial in 239 patients. The Digitalis in Acute Atrial Fibrillation (DAAF) Trial Group. Eur Heart J. 1997;18:649–54.
32. Milne JR. Verapamil in cardiac arrhythmias. Br Med J. 1972;2:348–9.
33. Salerno DM, Dias VC, Kleiger RE, et al. Efficacy and safety of intravenous diltiazem for treatment of atrial fibrillation and atrial flutter. The Diltiazem-Atrial Fibrillation/Flutter Study Group. Am J Cardiol. 1989;63:1046–51.
34. Goldenberg IF, Lewis WR, Dias VC, Heywood JT, Pedersen WR. Intravenous diltiazem for the treatment of patients with atrial fibrillation or flutter and moderate to severe congestive heart failure. Am J Cardiol. 1994;74:884–9.
35. Siu CW, Lau CP, Lee WL, Lam KF, Tse HF. Intravenous diltiazem is superior to intravenous amiodarone or digoxin for achieving ventricular rate control in patients with acute uncomplicated atrial fibrillation. Crit Care Med. 2009;37:2174–9. quiz 80.
36. Schreck DM, Rivera AR, Tricarico VJ. Emergency management of atrial fibrillation and flutter: intravenous diltiazem versus intravenous digoxin. Ann Emerg Med. 1997;29:135–40.
37. Aronow WS. Effect of beta blockers on mortality and morbidity in persons treated for congestive heart failure. J Am Geriatr Soc. 2001;49:331–3.

38. Barbier GH, Shettigar UR, Appunn DO. Clinical rationale for the use of an ultra-short acting beta-blocker: esmolol. Int J Clin Pharmacol Ther. 1995;33:212–8.
39. Hilleman DE, Reyes AP, Mooss AN, Packard KA. Esmolol versus diltiazem in atrial fibrillation following coronary artery bypass graft surgery. Curr Med Res Opin. 2003;19:376–82.
40. Mooss AN, Wurdeman RL, Mohiuddin SM, et al. Esmolol versus diltiazem in the treatment of postoperative atrial fibrillation/atrial flutter after open heart surgery. Am Heart J. 2000;140: 176–80.
41. Clemo HF, Wood MA, Gilligan DM, Ellenbogen KA. Intravenous amiodarone for acute heart rate control in the critically ill patient with atrial tachyarrhythmias. Am J Cardiol. 1998;81: 594–8.
42. Hou ZY, Chang MS, Chen CY, et al. Acute treatment of recent-onset atrial fibrillation and flutter with a tailored dosing regimen of intravenous amiodarone. A randomized, digoxin-controlled study. Eur Heart J. 1995;16:521–8.
43. Hohnloser SH, Crijns HJ, van Eickels M, et al. Effect of dronedarone on cardiovascular events in atrial fibrillation. N Engl J Med. 2009;360:668–78.
44. Kober L, Torp-Pedersen C, McMurray JJ, et al. Increased mortality after dronedarone therapy for severe heart failure. N Engl J Med. 2008;358:2678–87.
45. Zimetbaum PJ. Dronedarone for atrial fibrillation–an odyssey. N Engl J Med. 2009;360: 1811–3.
46. Decker WW, Stead LG. Selecting rate control for recent-onset atrial fibrillation. Ann Emerg Med. 2011;57:32–3.
47. Michael JA, Stiell IG, Agarwal S, Mandavia DP. Cardioversion of paroxysmal atrial fibrillation in the emergency department. Ann Emerg Med. 1999;33:379–87.
48. Stiell IG, Clement CM, Perry JJ, et al. Association of the Ottawa Aggressive Protocol with rapid discharge of emergency department patients with recent-onset atrial fibrillation or flutter. CJEM. 2010;12:181–91.
49. Stiell IG, Birnie D. Managing recent-onset atrial fibrillation in the emergency department. Ann Emerg Med. 2011;57:31–2.
50. Stiell IG, Dickinson G, Butterfield NN, et al. Vernakalant hydrochloride: a novel atrial-selective agent for the cardioversion of recent-onset atrial fibrillation in the emergency department. Acad Emerg Med. 2010;17:1175–82.
51. Weigner MJ, Caulfield TA, Danias PG, Silverman DI, Manning WJ. Risk for clinical thromboembolism associated with conversion to sinus rhythm in patients with atrial fibrillation lasting less than 48 hours. Ann Intern Med. 1997;126:615–20.
52. Friedman HZ, Weber-Bornstein N, Deboe SF, Mancini GB. Cardiac care unit admission criteria for suspected acute myocardial infarction in new-onset atrial fibrillation. Am J Cardiol. 1987;59:866–9.
53. Peacock WFt, De Marco T, Fonarow GC, et al. Cardiac troponin and outcome in acute heart failure. N Engl J Med. 2008;358:2117–26.
54. Fang JC. Rise of the machines–left ventricular assist devices as permanent therapy for advanced heart failure. N Engl J Med. 2009;361:2282–5.
55. Landzaat LH, Sinclair CT, Rosielle DA. Continuous-flow left ventricular assist device. N Engl J Med. 2010;362:1149.
56. Slaughter MS, Rogers JG, Milano CA, et al. Advanced heart failure treated with continuous-flow left ventricular assist device. N Engl J Med. 2009;361:2241–51.
57. Fonarow GC, Stevenson LW, Walden JA, et al. Impact of a comprehensive heart failure management program on hospital readmission and functional status of patients with advanced heart failure. J Am Coll Cardiol. 1997;30:725–32.
58. Gonseth J, Guallar-Castillon P, Banegas JR, Rodriguez-Artalejo F. The effectiveness of disease management programmes in reducing hospital re-admission in older patients with heart failure: a systematic review and meta-analysis of published reports. Eur Heart J. 2004;25:1570–95.
59. Rich MW, Beckham V, Wittenberg C, Leven CL, Freedland KE, Carney RM. A multidisciplinary intervention to prevent the readmission of elderly patients with congestive heart failure. N Engl J Med. 1995;333:1190–5.

60. Nattel S, Opie LH. Controversies in atrial fibrillation. Lancet. 2006;367:262–72.
61. Roy D, Talajic M, Nattel S, et al. Rhythm control versus rate control for atrial fibrillation and heart failure. N Engl J Med. 2008;358:2667–77.
62. Van Gelder IC, Groenveld HF, Crijns HJ, et al. Lenient versus strict rate control in patients with atrial fibrillation. N Engl J Med. 2010;362:1363–73.
63. Wyse DG, Waldo AL, DiMarco JP, et al. A comparison of rate control and rhythm control in patients with atrial fibrillation. N Engl J Med. 2002;347:1825–33.
64. Hsu LF, Jais P, Sanders P, et al. Catheter ablation for atrial fibrillation in congestive heart failure. N Engl J Med. 2004;351:2373–83.
65. Leclercq C, Walker S, Linde C, et al. Comparative effects of permanent biventricular and right-univentricular pacing in heart failure patients with chronic atrial fibrillation. Eur Heart J. 2002;23:1780–7.
66. Gasparini M, Bocchiardo M, Lunati M, et al. Comparison of 1-year effects of left ventricular and biventricular pacing in patients with heart failure who have ventricular arrhythmias and left bundle-branch block: the Bi vs. Left Ventricular Pacing: an International Pilot Evaluation on Heart Failure Patients with Ventricular Arrhythmias (BELIEVE) multicenter prospective randomized pilot study. Am Heart J. 2006;152:155.e1.
67. Kong MH, Lopes RD, Piccini JP, Hasselblad V, Bahnson TD, Al-Khatib SM. Surgical Maze procedure as a treatment for atrial fibrillation: a meta-analysis of randomized controlled trials. Cardiovasc Ther. 2010;28:311–26.
68. Risk factors for stroke and efficacy of antithrombotic therapy in atrial fibrillation. Analysis of pooled data from five randomized controlled trials. Arch Intern Med. 1994;154:1449-57.
69. Gage BF, Waterman AD, Shannon W, Boechler M, Rich MW, Radford MJ. Validation of clinical classification schemes for predicting stroke: results from the National Registry of Atrial Fibrillation. JAMA. 2001;285:2864–70.
70. van Walraven C, Hart RG, Wells GA, et al. A clinical prediction rule to identify patients with atrial fibrillation and a low risk for stroke while taking aspirin. Arch Intern Med. 2003;163:936–43.
71. Wang TJ, Massaro JM, Levy D, et al. A risk score for predicting stroke or death in individuals with new-onset atrial fibrillation in the community: the Framingham Heart Study. JAMA. 2003;290:1049–56.
72. Rietbrock S, Heeley E, Plumb J, van Staa T. Chronic atrial fibrillation: Incidence, prevalence, and prediction of stroke using the Congestive heart failure, hypertension, age >75, Diabetes mellitus, and prior Stroke or transient ischemic attack (CHADS2) risk stratification scheme. Am Heart J. 2008;156:57–64.
73. Connolly SJ, Ezekowitz MD, Yusuf S, et al. Dabigatran versus warfarin in patients with atrial fibrillation. N Engl J Med. 2009;361:1139–51.

Chapter 21
Implantable Cardiac Devices

Brian Hiestand and William Abraham

In regard to implantable devices, there are three types of heart failure patients managed in the short-stay setting: those who have implantable cardiac devices, those who meet criteria for having an implantable device but do not know it, and those who may qualify for an implantable cardiac device at some point in the future. We will briefly discuss the indications for the various implantable cardiac devices, as referral for consideration of such devices can be done on a nonemergent outpatient basis. It should be noted, however, that this encounter in the emergency department or the short-stay setting may be the one opportunity for uniting the appropriate patient with the appropriate device treatment modality. We will also discuss in more detail the data that can be extracted from implantable devices and describe how this information can assist with the diagnosis and treatment of acutely decompensated heart failure.

Therapeutic Functions

The active functions of implantable devices can be broadly divided into two categories—arrhythmia termination and primary pacing. Defibrillation is the primary mode for termination of malignant ventricular tachydysrhythmias, although overdrive pacing may be attempted based on the functionality and programming capabilities of the device. Patients with heart failure are at substantial risk for both atrial and ventricular tachydysrhythmias, with subsequent clinical deterioration.

B. Hiestand, MD, MPH, FACEP (✉)
Department of Emergency Medicine, Wake Forest University Health Sciences,
Winston Salem, NC, USA
e-mail: bhiestan@wfubmc.edu

W. Abraham, MD, FACC
The Ohio State University, Columbus, OH, USA

W. Frank Peacock (ed.), *Short Stay Management of Acute Heart Failure*,
Contemporary Cardiology, DOI 10.1007/978-1-61779-627-2_21,
© Springer Science+Business Media, LLC 2012

The annual incidence of sudden cardiac death in the United States is estimated at 0.2% [1]. In patients with inducible dysrhythmias and chronic heart failure due to ischemia (the highest risk subgroup), that incidence climbs to more than 30%. Other high-risk groups include those with a history of cardiac arrest, ventricular tachycardia/ventricular fibrillation (VT/VF) survivors, those with an LV ejection fraction less than 35%, and heart failure patients [2]. In the latter group, SCD comprises about 50% of all deaths [3].

Patients with chronic heart failure who have survived VT/VF, or cardiac arrest, are at high risk for recurrence. Regardless of the degree of underlying structural disease (preserved vs. decreased systolic function) or etiology (ischemic vs. nonischemic cardiomyopathy), an implantable cardioverter-defibrillator (ICD) is recommended when quality of life and prognosis are such that sudden cardiac death prevention is a desirable goal [4]. It should be noted that such secondary prevention is not indicated in all survivors, i.e., patients with poor short- to intermediate-term prognoses will likely not benefit from ICD implantation as death is likely regardless of dysrhythmia protection.

Primary prevention, in contrast, refers to malignant dysrhythmia protection when a sustained VT/VF, or cardiac arrest, has not yet occurred in a patient who is deemed to be at substantial risk. Multiple trials have demonstrated the superiority of ICD over medical therapy for primary prevention of sudden cardiac death in the heart failure population. The Multicenter Automatic Defibrillator Implantation Trial (MADIT I) [5] demonstrated a substantial survival benefit in patients with heart failure (defined as LVEF $\leq$35% and New York Heart Association (NYHA) classes I–III), previous myocardial infarction, and an episode of asymptomatic nonsustained VT that was reproducible during an electrophysiologic study, as compared to nonstandardized medical therapy (hazard ratio (HR) 0.46, 95% confidence interval (CI) 0.26–0.82).

MADIT II continued to focus on ischemic cardiomyopathy (LVEF $\leq$30% and prior myocardial infarction), but removed dysrhythmia as an inclusion criteria [6]. Enrolling 1,232 patients (742 to ICD, 490 to conventional therapy), MADIT II demonstrated a survival benefit in terms of all-cause mortality with the use of primary ICD prophylaxis (HR 0.69, 95% CI 0.51–0.93). Finally, the Sudden Cardiac Death in Heart Failure Trial (SCD-HeFT) compared standard medical therapy plus placebo vs. standard medical therapy plus amiodarone vs. ICD therapy [7]. SCD-HeFT differed from the MADIT trials in allowing nonischemic cardiomyopathy as an inclusion criterion, although substantial systolic dysfunction (LVEF $\leq$35%) and symptomatic heart failure (NYHA II or III) were still required for enrollment. The addition of amiodarone to standard medical therapy did not provide a mortality benefit (HR 1.06 vs. placebo, 97.5% CI 0.86–1.30). Survival was enhanced in the ICD arm (HR 0.77 vs. placebo, 97.5% CI 0.62–0.96), independent of whether cardiomyopathy was ischemic or nonischemic. However, NYHA class at the time of enrollment had an apparent effect on the outcome of each intervention. In those patients with heart failure symptoms on minimal exertion (NYHA III), the use of amiodarone was associated with an increased risk of death (HR 1.44 vs. placebo, 97.5% CI 1.05–1.97), while those with NYHA II continued to show statistical similarity to the placebo group (HR 0.85, 97.5% CI 0.65–1.11). In terms of ICD therapy, the survival benefit was accentuated in the NYHA II group (HR 0.54, 97.5% CI 0.40–0.74), while the survival benefit in NYHA III heart failure patients was not only statistically insignificant, but had changed polarity to the suggestion of harm (HR 1.16 vs. placebo, 97.5% CI 0.84–1.61). These subgroup observations have been viewed as hypothesis generating and not definitive, and the guideline recommendation for primary prevention ICD therapy in heart failure includes NYHA class II and III patients. However, it may be fair to say that patients in the active throes of decompensated heart failure, such as those being managed in the short-stay setting, may not be in optimal condition for immediate device management. After stabilization and treatment, outpatient referral for consideration of prophylactic defibrillator placement would be appropriate.

In addition to delivering shocks to terminate malignant rhythms, implantable cardiac devices may be programmed to manage the beat-to-beat conduction of the failing heart. Prolonged ventricular contraction can exacerbate preexisting cardiomyopathy, resulting in worsening contractile function as well as leading to unfavorable remodeling. The utilization of cardiac resynchronization therapy (CRT) with biventricular pacing is designed to overcome mechanical dyssynchrony by way of controlled synchronous depolarization of both ventricles. This technology has been demonstrated to enhance quality of life, decrease symptoms, and reverse remodeling [8]. The Multicenter InSync Randomized Clinical Evaluation (MIRACLE) trial enrolled 453 subjects with symptomatic heart failure (NYHA III or IV) with ventricular dyssynchrony (QRS ≥130 ms) and impaired systolic function (LVEF ≤35%) [9]. All subjects received an implantable cardiac device with CRT capacity and were randomized to either 6 months of CRT or no pacing. At 6 months, the CRT group had demonstrated significant improvement in NYHA class, 6-minute walk test, and quality of life as measured by the Minnesota Living with Heart Failure Questionnaire. In addition, LVEF improved by a median of 5%, and end diastolic volume decreased in the treatment group. Fewer hospitalizations for heart failure were required in the CRT group as well (83 hospital days vs. 363 hospital days). MIRACLE was not powered for mortality as an endpoint, which was statistically similar between groups at 6 months (HR 0.73 favoring less mortality with CRT, 95% CI 0.34–1.54).

The Comparison of Medical Therapy, Pacing, and Defibrillation in Heart Failure (COMPANION) trial randomized 1,520 patients with NYHA III or IV heart failure, impaired systolic function (LVEF ≤35%), and dysfunctional electrical conduction (QRS ≥120 ms and PR interval ≥150 ms) to CRT with defibrillator (CRT-D), CRT alone, or optimal medical therapy [10]. Although the trial was complicated by a higher than anticipated withdrawal rate from the medical therapy arm, CRT and CRT-D therapies were associated with a substantially decreased rate of the primary endpoint of death or hospitalization (HR 0.8, 95% CI 0.68–0.95). The CRT-D group had a definite reduction in all-cause mortality when compared to the optimal medical therapy group (HR 0.64, 95% CI 0.48–0.86). When Lindenfield et al. performed a focused subgroup analysis examining only those patients with NYHA IV heart failure at the time of enrollment ($n = 217$, or 14% of the COMPANION sample) [11], they found that the risk of the primary endpoint of all-cause death or hospitalization persisted in both CRT and CRT-D groups. This reduction in risk (HR 0.62, 95% CI 0.43–0.90) was driven by a decrease in hospitalization (both all cause and heart failure specific) as all-cause mortality did not show a difference among groups. The importance of this subgroup analysis lies in demonstrating a benefit to the sickest heart failure patients, a population where one could reasonably be concerned that, due to overall decreased life expectancy, device implantation would not produce an appreciable improvement.

The REVERSE, MADIT-CRT, and RAFT trials extended these findings to those patients with heart failure who were only mildly symptomatic. MADIT-CRT demonstrated a 41% decrease in heart failure events in patients with NYHA I or II heart failure who were randomized to cardiac resynchronization with biventricular pacing [12]. Most of the benefit was seen in the subgroup with delayed ventricular depolarization as manifested by a QRS duration ≥150 ms. Although no benefit in mortality was demonstrated (both groups received devices with a defibrillator function), CRT was associated with improved ejection fraction and a decrease in ventricular volumes. RAFT extended these observations in demonstrating a reduction in mortality with CRT in NYHA class II patients [13]. While these mildly symptomatic patients are not those typically seen as requiring management in the short-stay setting, they do eventually progress to more advanced heart failure, have episodes of decompensation, and will increase the need for knowledge of these devices in the ED setting.

To date, CRT has shown little benefit in patients with a narrow QRS complex [14]. It has been suggested that selection of patients with echocardiographic evidence of mechanical dyssynchrony may increase the likelihood that resynchronization therapy will benefit a patient with heart failure and a narrow QRS complex [15]; unfortunately, this contention has not been prospectively borne out [14, 16]. As well, prolonged QRS duration is not a marker for guaranteed improvement, as up to 30% of patients will demonstrate no benefit with CRT [17]. Regardless, multiple clinical trials have consistently demonstrated improvement in quality of life measures as well as survival in patients with severe heart failure, decreased ejection fraction, and electrical evidence of conduction disturbances [9, 10, 12, 18–21]. A large (>1,250 patient) ongoing trial, the EchoCRT study, is evaluating the effects of CRT on outcomes in narrow QRS patients with mechanical dyssynchrony. If positive, we may see many more patients with this implanted cardiac device.

It is not our purpose to suggest that the recognition of implantable device indications and specialist referral for such is the standard of care in the ED or short-stay setting. However, the penetration of these devices in the evidence-based, guideline-recommended population (i.e., those with a class Ia indication) is only about 40–50% [22]. Especially in underserved populations, the medical safety net provided by the ED and the subsequent short-stay setting may represent the best opportunity for appropriate referral for postdischarge device therapies. Even in tertiary centers, standard referral patterns result in missed opportunities to get device-based therapies to at-risk patients [23]; physicians managing heart failure patients in the short-stay setting should be mindful of opportunities and resources that may decrease hospital admission recidivism and improvement in quality of life. As well, we do not mean to imply that if the presence of an indication for device-based therapy exists, then that patient is not appropriate for observation management. Certainly, even if an indication for device therapy exists, a patient who is otherwise appropriate for short-stay management can be referred as an outpatient to the appropriate specialist once the immediate decompensation has been controlled.

Diagnostic Functions

In order for implantable devices to perform the active functions of defibrillation, cardioversion, or pacing, they must record and interpret the patient's intrinsic cardiac rhythm data. Different devices store modestly different parameters, although there are some consistent metrics between devices and manufacturers. In addition to devices that record rate, rhythm, and response data, there are an increasing number of devices that collect advanced telemetry data, including physiological information such as heart rate variability, intrathoracic impedance, and patient activity level. Data from both basic and advanced monitoring parameters may be useful during the initial evaluation of the patient, as well as to the physician caring for the patient in the short-stay unit.

Rhythm Data

Atrial fibrillation is the most common dysrhythmia in patients with chronic heart failure; even patients thought to be maintained in sinus rhythm may experience clinically silent paroxysmal atrial fibrillation episodes [24]. New onset atrial fibrillation may be a worse marker for long-term survival, and many heart failure patients experience worsening symptoms with atrial fibrillation [25]. Conversely, there is evidence that prolonged volume overload can result in atrial tachydysrhythmias, perhaps as a result of electrical instability due to atrial distension [26]. Discovery of atrial fibrillation as a precipitating event could lead to the consideration of several different medical management options that would not have been immediately apparent choices in the absence of such knowledge, such as initiating rate or rhythm controlling pharmacologic agent, starting long-term anticoagulation for stroke prophylaxis, or changing pacemaker programming parameters. In addition to atrial dysrhythmias, VT may also occur without overt clinical symptoms in the setting of chronic heart failure. CRT-based monitoring has shown both malignant ventricular arrhythmias as well as nonsustained VT to be associated with heart failure decompensation, similar to atrial tachydysrhythmias [27–29]. The presence of a high rate of ventricular dysrhythmia in the setting of decompensated heart failure should, of course, prompt optimization of electrolyte abnormalities, as well as consideration for underlying exacerbations of ischemic disease as a potential etiology for the heart failure event. Finally, should the patient have a device not equipped with defibrillation capability, the presence of frequent ventricular tachydysrhythmias should also suggest the need for prompt consultation with the patient's electrophysiologist to consider defibrillator management.

Heart Rate Variability

There is an intrinsic variability in the heart rate of healthy individuals that is a function of compensation for changes in physiologic demand as well as other diurnal patterns. As physiologic stress increases, this variance decreases due to an increase in sympathetic tone and an attenuation of the parasympathetic nervous system [30]. Implantable cardiac devices that monitor atrial depolarization can record atrial rates and calculate the variability in the intrinsic sinoatrial node function. The association between heart rate variability, as monitored by an implantable cardiac device, as a proxy measure for improved heart failure mechanics was established in a secondary analysis of the CRT-based MIRACLE trial [9]. Those patients randomized to active CRT functionality experienced a substantial improvement in heart rate variability, regardless of the use of beta-blocker therapy, that was associated with improvement in multiple echocardiographic indices of cardiac function [31].

Heart rate variability has also been linked as an independent predictor of outcomes, as opposed to a marker of response to therapy, in a prospective observational cohort study of 288 patients receiving a CRT device for NYHA III or IV heart failure coupled with systolic dysfunction (LVEF ≤35%) [32]. In this study, over the course of a year, heart rate variability was significantly lower in patients experiencing hospitalization or death as opposed to those subjects who did not decompensate or had a mild decompensation not requiring hospitalization (74 ± 22 ms vs. 90 ± 22 ms, $p < 0.0001$). The decrease in heart rate variability was notable at a median 16 days prior to hospitalization.

Unfortunately, a decrease in heart rate variability is not specific to acutely decompensated heart failure. Other illnesses and comorbidities that manifest with a ramping up of sympathetic tone also present with a decrease in heart rate variability, such as seen in exacerbation of chronic obstructive pulmonary disease [33] or various infectious states [34]. Examination of all parameters captured by the implantable device will give a fuller understanding of the patient's clinical picture.

Patient Activity

Accelerometers within the implanted device can provide a measurement of hours per day that the patient is moving and presumably physically active, although the actual degree of exertion is not captured with this measurement. As patients become more and more symptomatic with heart failure, exercise intolerance worsens and physical activity decreases [32]. Conversely, a study of patients receiving CRT pacing demonstrated an increase in daily activity levels corresponded to improvements in NYHA class and exercise tolerance (108 ± 81 min/day at baseline vs. 225 ± 140 min/day at 12 weeks, $p < 0.001$) [35]. Patient activity levels have been shown to be less sensitive than decreased heart rate variability in predicting decompensation in the outpatient setting [32], although decreased physical activity levels have been shown to be predictive of subsequent heart failure decompensation within 30 days, when monitored in concert with other implantable device monitoring parameters (HR 5.5, 95% CI 3.4–8.8) [36].

Intrathoracic Impedance

The measurement of intrathoracic impedance utilizes changes in electrical conduction within the cardiopulmonary structures of the chest to gauge fluid overload. As the total amount of tissue fluid increases, resistance (also known as impedance) to conduction of an electrical impulse between a pulse generator and a sensor decreases. Therefore, a low impedance reading is a marker of pulmonic fluid congestion. Intrathoracic impedance determination is made using the pacemaker lead as the pulse generator and the device canister as the receptor. At the time of this writing, the only FDA-approved intrathoracic impedance technology for clinical use is proprietary Medtronic Optivol system, although other investigations are in progress. This system, utilized in conjunction with a CRT or ICD device, provides a fluid index that represents the difference between the daily mean impedance reading and a rolling average of previous daily mean impedance readings. An alarm (currently available only outside of the USA) can notify the patient if the fluid index exceeds a preprogrammed threshold, indicating possible fluid overload.

Intrathoracic impedance has been evaluated as a predictor of heart failure decompensation in the outpatient arena in a number of studies. The proof of concept was established by Yu et al. [37], who demonstrated that impedance dropped an average of 18 days prior to hospitalization for fluid overload and 15 days prior to the onset of worsening symptoms. Impedance values were also inversely correlated with pulmonary capillary wedge pressures obtained upon hospitalization. However, an elevated fluid index was not a perfect predictor of outcomes—a threshold index of 60 ohm days generated a sensitivity for hospitalization of 77% with a false-positive alert rate of 1.5 alerts without subsequent hospitalization per patient-year of observation. Similar performance has been noted in subsequent studies [27, 36, 38, 39].

Of potentially more impact within the acute care setting, Small et al. have demonstrated, in a retrospective analysis of registry data derived from patients with CRT-based intrathoracic impedance monitoring, a low likelihood of hospitalization due to acute heart failure in subjects whose fluid index did not cross the set threshold (0.14 hospitalizations/patient-years vs. 0.76 hospitalizations/patient-years in those patients with multiple threshold crossing events) [40]. It may be that an absence of threshold crossing, or at least a deterioration of the impedance values, may suggest that a dyspneic patient being evaluated in the acute setting has an etiology other than decompensated heart failure for their presenting symptoms.

Pressure Monitoring

Several implantable devices that directly monitor intracardiac pressures are, at the time of this writing, in investigational status. The majority of the current generation of implantable hemodynamic monitors are purely data collection devices, as opposed to acting in combination with a pacemaker or defibrillator, although some have been combined with CRT and/or ICD devices. The HeartPOD system (St. Jude Medical, Minneapolis, MN) utilizes a wired pressure transducer in the left atrium to record cardiac data [41]. The HOMEOSTASIS (Hemodynamically Guided Home Self-Therapy in Severe Heart Failure Patients) trial evaluated the feasibility of providing this data directly to the patient by way of a handheld patient advisory module, which would collect the data from the implant and recommend changes in medication therapy (diuretics or vasodilators) based on algorithms preprogrammed by the physician [42]. The lack of a control group limits the conclusions that can be drawn from this small study ($n=40$); however, given that the programmed algorithms advised medication changes on a frequent basis (53% of days measured), this study provides a strong impetus for moving forward with a controlled trial of patient-facilitated management. That study, the LAPTOP-HF trial, is now ongoing. In addition to the stand-alone HeartPOD system, LAPTOP-HF introduces a combined CRT-ICD-LAP monitoring system into clinical study.

Additional devices under investigation include the CardioMEMS Heart Failure Sensor (CardioMEMS, Atlanta, GA), which uses a pressure transducer implanted in the pulmonary artery with wireless transmission of data to a handheld recorder [43]. In a 550-patient randomized controlled trial, the use of this wireless implantable hemodynamic monitoring system reduced the 6-month rate of heart failure hospitalization by 30% and, over prolonged follow-up averaging 15 months (range 1 day to 30 months), reduced heart failure hospitalizations by 39% [44]. Similarly, the RemonCHF device (Boston Scientific, Natick, MA) measures pulmonary artery pressures by way of a pressure transducer located in the pulmonary artery that provides on-demand interrogation powered by way of ultrasound transmission to and from a handheld unit that can be operated by the patient [45]. These devices are all still in trial stages, but offer exciting potential for patient management.

Finally, the first-generation monitoring system, the Chronicle IHM (Medtronic Inc., Minneapolis, MN), is no longer in active investigation after having been rejected for clinical use by the FDA in 2007. The COMPASS-HF study demonstrated a non-significant reduction in heart failure events (hospitalization or emergency department visits requiring intravenous therapy) in patients receiving device-guided therapy compared to controls [46]. Although the intervention arm experienced fewer events (84 events in 44 patients vs. 113 events in 60 patients in the control arm) over 6 months, this difference was not statistically significant ($p=0.33$).

The Acute Care/Short-Stay Setting

To date, clinical trials of implantable device data have been directed at utilizing these parameters to keep patients from decompensating to the point of requiring emergency department or hospital-based care in the first place. In addition, the interrogation of these devices has generally fallen under the purview of the implanting physician. As a result, there is very little literature available that examines the actual use of device data in the diagnosis and management of decompensated heart failure once the patient has presented to the ED. In terms of preventing ED visits or hospitalization, clinical interventions based on remote monitoring of implantable device data have not yet lived up to expectations, with trials demonstrating neutral results in terms of rates of hospital care [46, 47]. This is frustrating in that it is clearly demonstrable that abnormalities in cardiac parameters are associated with impending heart failure decompensation. Such diverse factors as heart rate variability [32], intrathoracic impedance [37, 38], ambulatory right ventricular pressures [38, 48, 49], and increased atrial tachydysrhythmia burden [26], alone or in various combination [36], are all associated with an increased risk of decompensation, and all can be recorded and transmitted to a clinician remotely.

Once the patient with an implantable cardiac device presents acutely with symptoms such as dyspnea that may be due to heart failure decompensation, several challenges present themselves to the treating physician. First, the doctor must determine if the patient's symptoms are truly due to decompensated heart failure. Given that the patient has severe enough heart failure to warrant placement of an implantable device, one might consider the a priori probability of decompensation to be relatively high. However, the use of implantable device data may either serve as valuable confirmation of the presence of acute heart failure or suggest another pathologic process that is the etiology of the patient's symptoms. However, at this time, no studies have evaluated the diagnostic performance (sensitivity, specificity, positive and negative likelihood ratios) of implantable cardiac device data in differentiating acutely decompensated heart failure from other disease entities that may present in similar fashion.

Once the physician has determined that acute heart failure is present, the next step should be to determine how best to treat the patient. The modalities chosen (diuresis, afterload reduction, inotropic support, and airway intervention) will depend greatly on the perfusion status and the volume status of the patient, as well as the clinical severity of the presentation. Although respiratory compromise and systemic perfusion will be fairly obvious with routine exam, volume status may at times be difficult to discern—especially in the obese. Devices that measure volumetric data, such as intrathoracic impedance or direct atrial pressure monitors, may provide insight into the degree of appropriate diuresis required. This may allow the physician to adequately remove volume while avoiding the complications of overdiuresis and subsequent renal stress.

Finally, in the patient undergoing short-stay management of acute heart failure, it becomes critical to understand why the patient decompensated in the first place. Examination of the longitudinal data contained within the implantable device may provide key insights as to the underlying mechanisms that brought the patient to this state. Rhythm data may indicate increasing frequency of atrial fibrillation, which could require pacemaker reprogramming, pharmacologic management, or even AV nodal ablation to improve hemodynamic function. Rathman et al. have reported the use of device data to uncover monthly cycles of subacute decompensation in a heart failure patient who was running out of medications each month and not resuming them until he had to, due to financial constraints [50]. Given that abnormalities in heart rate variability, patient activity levels, and fluid accumulation precede clinical decompensation by several days [28, 32, 37, 38], going over temporal data with the patient to evaluate medication, diet, and other lifestyle events such as exacerbations of comorbid illnesses may establish a causative link to behaviors or illnesses that led to the acute heart failure syndrome being managed in the short-stay arena.

Unfortunately, these possibilities, although grounded in a solid conceptual framework, have yet to be validated beyond anecdotal experience. As stated previously, the research effort to date has been directed at keeping the patient from requiring acute and short-stay care in the first place. While this is definitely a worthy goal and would benefit the patient, the truth of the matter remains that over one million hospitalizations for heart failure will occur annually [51]. There definitely remains a need for research to establish the additive value of basic and advanced implantable device data for the evaluation and management of the patient with suspected acutely decompensated heart failure. Until such research is established, however, it is certainly reasonable for those of us caring for patients who have this data readily available to evaluate and consider the recorded information in the context of the patient's presentation.

The ability of nonimplanting physicians to view this device data is becoming increasingly available in the ED and short-stay settings. Given the potential for these devices to assist in the acute diagnosis of worsening heart failure and to guide initial therapies, knowledge of the strengths and weaknesses of device-based diagnostics is becoming a must for ED personnel. In the future, it is anticipated that the ED personnel will be among the frontline users of such information.

References

1. Zipes DP, Camm AJ, Borggrefe M, et al. ACC/AHA/ESC 2006 Guidelines for Management of Patients With Ventricular Arrhythmias and the Prevention of Sudden Cardiac Death: a report of the American College of Cardiology/American Heart Association Task Force and the European Society of Cardiology Committee for Practice Guidelines (writing committee to develop Guidelines for Management of Patients With Ventricular Arrhythmias and the Prevention of Sudden Cardiac Death): developed in collaboration with the European Heart Rhythm Association and the Heart Rhythm Society. Circulation. 2006;114:e385–484.
2. Myerburg RJ. Sudden cardiac death: exploring the limits of our knowledge. J Cardiovasc Electrophysiol. 2001;12:369–81.
3. Effect of metoprolol CR/XL in chronic heart failure: Metoprolol CR/XL Randomised Intervention Trial in Congestive Heart Failure (MERIT-HF). Lancet. 1999;353:2001–7.

4. Epstein AE, DiMarco JP, Ellenbogen KA, et al. ACC/AHA/HRS 2008 Guidelines for Device-Based Therapy of Cardiac Rhythm Abnormalities: a report of the American College of Cardiology/American Heart Association Task Force on Practice Guidelines (Writing Committee to Revise the ACC/AHA/NASPE 2002 Guideline Update for Implantation of Cardiac Pacemakers and Antiarrhythmia Devices): developed in collaboration with the American Association for Thoracic Surgery and Society of Thoracic Surgeons. Circulation. 2008; 117:e350–408.

5. Moss AJ, Hall WJ, Cannom DS, et al. Improved survival with an implanted defibrillator in patients with coronary disease at high risk for ventricular arrhythmia. Multicenter Automatic Defibrillator Implantation Trial Investigators. N Engl J Med. 1996;335:1933–40.

6. Moss AJ, Zareba W, Hall WJ, et al. Prophylactic implantation of a defibrillator in patients with myocardial infarction and reduced ejection fraction. N Engl J Med. 2002;346:877–83.

7. Bardy GH, Lee KL, Mark DB, et al. Amiodarone or an implantable cardioverter-defibrillator for congestive heart failure. N Engl J Med. 2005;352:225–37.

8. Solomon SD, Foster E, Bourgoun M, et al. Effect of cardiac resynchronization therapy on reverse remodeling and relation to outcome: multicenter automatic defibrillator implantation trial: cardiac resynchronization therapy. Circulation. 2010;122:985–92.

9. Abraham WT, Fisher WG, Smith AL, et al. Cardiac resynchronization in chronic heart failure. N Engl J Med. 2002;346:1845–53.

10. Bristow MR, Saxon LA, Boehmer J, et al. Cardiac-resynchronization therapy with or without an implantable defibrillator in advanced chronic heart failure. N Engl J Med. 2004;350: 2140–50.

11. Lindenfeld J, Feldman AM, Saxon L, et al. Effects of cardiac resynchronization therapy with or without a defibrillator on survival and hospitalizations in patients with New York Heart Association class IV heart failure. Circulation. 2007;115:204–12.

12. Moss AJ, Hall WJ, Cannom DS, et al. Cardiac-resynchronization therapy for the prevention of heart-failure events. N Engl J Med. 2009;361:1329–38.

13. Tang AS, Wells GA, Talajic M, et al. Cardiac-resynchronization therapy for mild-to-moderate heart failure. N Engl J Med. 2010;363:2385–95.

14. Beshai JF, Grimm RA, Nagueh SF, et al. Cardiac-resynchronization therapy in heart failure with narrow QRS complexes. N Engl J Med. 2007;357:2461–71.

15. van Bommel RJ, Gorcsan III J, Chung ES, et al. Effects of cardiac resynchronisation therapy in patients with heart failure having a narrow QRS Complex enrolled in PROSPECT. Heart. 2010;96:1107–13.

16. Chung ES, Leon AR, Tavazzi L, et al. Results of the Predictors of Response to CRT (PROSPECT) trial. Circulation. 2008;117:2608–16.

17. Bax JJ, Abraham T, Barold SS, et al. Cardiac resynchronization therapy: Part 1–issues before device implantation. J Am Coll Cardiol. 2005;46:2153–67.

18. Young JB, Abraham WT, Smith AL, et al. Combined cardiac resynchronization and implantable cardioversion defibrillation in advanced chronic heart failure: the MIRACLE ICD Trial. JAMA. 2003;289:2685–94.

19. Cleland JG, Daubert JC, Erdmann E, et al. The effect of cardiac resynchronization on morbidity and mortality in heart failure. N Engl J Med. 2005;352:1539–49.

20. Cleland JG, Daubert JC, Erdmann E, et al. Longer-term effects of cardiac resynchronization therapy on mortality in heart failure [the CArdiac REsynchronization-Heart Failure (CARE-HF) trial extension phase]. Eur Heart J. 2006;27:1928–32.

21. Linde C, Abraham WT, Gold MR, et al. Randomized trial of cardiac resynchronization in mildly symptomatic heart failure patients and in asymptomatic patients with left ventricular dysfunction and previous heart failure symptoms. J Am Coll Cardiol. 2008;52:1834–43.

22. Fonarow GC, Yancy CW, Albert NM, et al. Heart failure care in the outpatient cardiology practice setting: findings from IMPROVE HF. Circ Heart Fail. 2008;1:98–106.

23. Bradfield J, Warner A, Bersohn MM. Low referral rate for prophylactic implantation of cardioverter-defibrillators in a tertiary care medical center. Pacing Clin Electrophysiol. 2009;32 Suppl 1:S194–7.

24. Caldwell JC, Contractor H, Petkar S, et al. Atrial fibrillation is under-recognized in chronic heart failure: insights from a heart failure cohort treated with cardiac resynchronization therapy. Europace. 2009;11:1295–300.
25. Wang TJ, Larson MG, Levy D, et al. Temporal relations of atrial fibrillation and congestive heart failure and their joint influence on mortality: the Framingham Heart Study. Circulation. 2003;107:2920–5.
26. Jhanjee R, Templeton GA, Sattiraju S, et al. Relationship of paroxysmal atrial tachyarrhythmias to volume overload: assessment by implanted transpulmonary impedance monitoring. Circ Arrhythm Electrophysiol. 2009;2:488–94.
27. Perego GB, Landolina M, Vergara G, et al. Implantable CRT device diagnostics identify patients with increased risk for heart failure hospitalization. J Interv Card Electrophysiol. 2008;23:235–42.
28. Moore HJ, Peters MN, Franz MR, et al. Intrathoracic impedance preceding ventricular tachyarrhythmia episodes. Pacing Clin Electrophysiol. 2010;33:960–6.
29. Ip JE, Cheung JW, Park D, et al. Temporal associations between thoracic volume overload and malignant ventricular arrhythmias: a study of intrathoracic impedance. J Cardiovasc Electrophysiol. 2010;22(3):293–9.
30. Goldsmith RL, Bigger JT, Bloomfield DM, et al. Long-term carvedilol therapy increases parasympathetic nervous system activity in chronic congestive heart failure. Am J Cardiol. 1997;80:1101–4.
31. Adamson PB, Kleckner KJ, VanHout WL, et al. Cardiac resynchronization therapy improves heart rate variability in patients with symptomatic heart failure. Circulation. 2003;108:266–9.
32. Adamson PB, Smith AL, Abraham WT, et al. Continuous autonomic assessment in patients with symptomatic heart failure: prognostic value of heart rate variability measured by an implanted cardiac resynchronization device. Circulation. 2004;110:2389–94.
33. Camillo CA, Pitta F, Possani HV, et al. Heart rate variability and disease characteristics in patients with COPD. Lung. 2008;186:393–401.
34. Ahmad S, Tejuja A, Newman KD, et al. Clinical review: a review and analysis of heart rate variability and the diagnosis and prognosis of infection. Crit Care. 2009;13:232.
35. Braunschweig F, Mortensen PT, Gras D, et al. Monitoring of physical activity and heart rate variability in patients with chronic heart failure using cardiac resynchronization devices. Am J Cardiol. 2005;95:1104–7.
36. Whellan DJ, Ousdigian KT, Al Khatib SM, et al. Combined heart failure device diagnostics identify patients at higher risk of subsequent heart failure hospitalizations: results from PARTNERS HF (Program to Access and Review Trending Information and Evaluate Correlation to Symptoms in Patients With Heart Failure) study. J Am Coll Cardiol. 2010;55:1803–10.
37. Yu CM, Wang L, Chau E, et al. Intrathoracic impedance monitoring in patients with heart failure: correlation with fluid status and feasibility of early warning preceding hospitalization. Circulation. 2005;112:841–8.
38. Vanderheyden M, Houben R, Verstreken S, et al. Continuous monitoring of intrathoracic impedance and right ventricular pressures in patients with heart failure. Circ Heart Fail. 2010;3:370–7.
39. Catanzariti D, Lunati M, Landolina M, et al. Monitoring intrathoracic impedance with an implantable defibrillator reduces hospitalizations in patients with heart failure. Pacing Clin Electrophysiol. 2009;32:363–70.
40. Small RS, Wickemeyer W, Germany R, et al. Changes in intrathoracic impedance are associated with subsequent risk of hospitalizations for acute decompensated heart failure: clinical utility of implanted device monitoring without a patient alert. J Card Fail. 2009;15:475–81.
41. Ritzema J, Melton IC, Richards AM, et al. Direct left atrial pressure monitoring in ambulatory heart failure patients: initial experience with a new permanent implantable device. Circulation. 2007;116:2952–9.
42. Ritzema J, Troughton R, Melton I, et al. Physician-directed patient self-management of left atrial pressure in advanced chronic heart failure. Circulation. 2010;121:1086–95.

43. Verdejo HE, Castro PF, Concepcion R, et al. Comparison of a radiofrequency-based wireless pressure sensor to swan-ganz catheter and echocardiography for ambulatory assessment of pulmonary artery pressure in heart failure. J Am Coll Cardiol. 2007;50:2375–82.

44. Abraham WT, Adamson PB, Bourge RC, et al. Wireless pulmonary artery haemodynamic monitoring in chronic heart failure: a randomised controlled trial. Lancet. 2011;377:658–66.

45. Hoppe UC, Vanderheyden M, Sievert H, et al. Chronic monitoring of pulmonary artery pressure in patients with severe heart failure: multicentre experience of the monitoring Pulmonary Artery Pressure by Implantable device Responding to Ultrasonic Signal (PAPIRUS) II study. Heart. 2009;95:1091–7.

46. Bourge RC, Abraham WT, Adamson PB, et al. Randomized controlled trial of an implantable continuous hemodynamic monitor in patients with advanced heart failure: the COMPASS-HF study. J Am Coll Cardiol. 2008;51:1073–9.

47. Zile MR, Bourge RC, Bennett TD, et al. Application of implantable hemodynamic monitoring in the management of patients with diastolic heart failure: a subgroup analysis of the COMPASS-HF trial. J Card Fail. 2008;14:816–23.

48. Stevenson LW, Zile M, Bennett TD, et al. Chronic ambulatory intracardiac pressures and future heart failure events. Circ Heart Fail. 2010;3:580–7.

49. Zile MR, Bennett TD, St John SM, et al. Transition from chronic compensated to acute decompensated heart failure: pathophysiological insights obtained from continuous monitoring of intracardiac pressures. Circulation. 2008;118:1433–41.

50. Rathman L. Use of device diagnostics as an educational tool to improve patient adherence. Am J Cardiol. 2007;99:29G–33.

51. Hunt SA, Abraham WT, Chin MH, et al. 2009 focused update incorporated into the ACC/AHA 2005 Guidelines for the Diagnosis and Management of Heart Failure in Adults: a report of the American College of Cardiology Foundation/American Heart Association Task Force on Practice Guidelines: developed in collaboration with the International Society for Heart and Lung Transplantation. Circulation. 2009;119:e391–479.

Chapter 22
Heart Failure and Kidney Disease: Management in the Short-Stay Unit

Shahriar Dadkhah and Korosh Sharain

Background

Heart failure (HF) is one of the fastest growing diagnoses in North America. Approximately 5.8 million Americans have heart failure, and over 600,000 new cases are diagnosed each year [1]. Kidney disease is another rapidly growing diagnosis in North America, with approximately 26 million people in the United States diagnosed with chronic kidney disease (CKD) and 20 million more Americans are at risk for developing CKD [2].

Like heart failure, kidney disease is classified into different stages. Table 22.1 provides the staging classification of kidney function.

Renal function is estimated based on elevated serum creatinine levels or reduced glomerular filtration rate (GFR). The most common calculation is the modification of diet in renal disease (MDRD) formula. Chronic kidney disease is defined as a GFR <60 mL/min/1.73 m^2 and has been associated with increased mortality, adverse cardiovascular events, and hospitalizations [4].

A novel serum marker of GFR, cystatin-C, is beginning to be incorporated into many guidelines. Cystatin-C, which is less influenced by muscle mass than creatinine, has been shown to be superior in estimating GFR and predicting mortality and cardiovascular outcome than serum creatinine [5]. Elevated cystatin-C (>1 mg/L) in persons with GFR >60 mL/min/1.73 m^2 classifies preclinical kidney disease, which signifies an increased risk of cardiovascular disease (CVD) and CKD incidence and death [6]. Since it is a relatively new marker, guidelines and cutoff values have not

S. Dadkhah, MD (✉)
Swedish Covenant Hospital, Chicago, IL, USA
e-mail: dadkhahsc@aol.com

K. Sharain, MA
Stritch School of Medicine, Loyola University Chicago, Chicago, IL, USA

W. Frank Peacock (ed.), *Short Stay Management of Acute Heart Failure*,
Contemporary Cardiology, DOI 10.1007/978-1-61779-627-2_22,
© Springer Science+Business Media, LLC 2012

Table 22.1 Stages of kidney disease

Stage	Description	GFR (mL/min/1.73 m^2)
1	Kidney damage with normal or ↑ GFR	≥90
2	Kidney damage with mild ↓ GFR	60–89
3	Moderate ↓ GFR	30–59
4	Severe ↓ GFR	15–29
5	End-stage renal disease (kidney failure)	<15 or dialysis

National Kidney Foundation [3]
GFR glomerular filtration rate

yet been defined for kidney disease. In one analysis of 3,418 individuals with CKD, serum cystatin-C levels alone estimated GFR as accurately as serum creatinine when adjusted for age, sex, and race [7]. The study concluded that an equation that combines both serum creatinine and cystatin-C for calculating GFR would be the most accurate method for evaluating kidney function.

Interrelationship Between Heart Failure and Kidney Disease

The hemodynamics of the vascular system including blood volume, organ perfusion, and vascular tone depend on the relationship between the heart and the kidneys. These two organ systems are in constant communication through released peptides and other neurohormonal mechanisms. The leading causes of kidney disease are diabetes, hypertension, and CVD; similarly, the leading causes of HF are diabetes, hypertension, coronary artery disease, and kidney disease. The connection between these two pathologies extends beyond risk factors. In fact, kidney disease and heart failure are interrelated such that derangement of one organ consequently promotes derangement of the other. If dysfunction occurs in the intimate relationship between the heart and the kidneys, it is known as the cardiorenal syndrome. Figure 22.1 depicts this relationship.

The overwhelming prevalence of kidney disease in the heart failure population was demonstrated by Smith et al. [8]. In a meta-analysis of 16 studies including 80,098 patients with heart failure, Smith et al. discovered that 63% of the patients with heart failure had concomitant renal impairment (defined as creatinine >1.0 mg/dL, creatinine clearance or estimated GFR <90 mL/min, or cystatin-C >1.03 mg/dL) while 29% had moderate to severe renal impairment (defined as creatinine ≥1.5 mg/dL, creatinine clearance or estimated GFR <53 mL/min, or cystatin-C ≥1.56 mg/dL) [8]. Additionally, Smith et al. demonstrated that mortality increased as renal function decreased [8]. Specifically, there was a 15% increased risk of mortality for every 0.5 mg/dL increase in creatinine and a 7% increased risk of mortality for every 10 mL/min decrease in estimated GFR [8]. With continued advancements in medicine, patients with CVD are surviving longer and thus developing heart failure, similarly, CKD patients are surviving longer, and therefore, it is estimated that patients with combined heart and kidney disease will become even more prevalent.

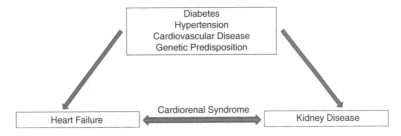

Fig. 22.1 Interrelationship between heart failure and kidney disease

Management of Heart Failure with Concomitant Kidney Disease: Overview

Several studies have demonstrated that renal impairment is strongly associated with outcomes in heart failure patients with systolic and diastolic dysfunction [9]; therefore, it is imperative to treat underlying kidney disease when managing heart failure. In fact, the reversal of renal dysfunction has been shown to improve cardiac function. In a study of 103 hemodialysis patients with heart failure and a left ventricular ejection fraction (LVEF) of ≤40% undergoing renal transplantation had a mean LVEF increase of 20% 1 year post-renal transplantation, increasing from a mean LVEF of 32% to a mean LVEF of 52% [10]. Additionally, 70% of the transplanted patients achieved normalization of cardiac function, defined as an LVEF ≥50% [10]. This data demonstrates that renal insufficiency has a contributory role in heart failure progression. Additionally, a study on 1,906 patients with heart failure concluded that impaired renal function was a better predictor of mortality than either heart failure class or LVEF [11].

It is important to note that the heart is not a victim in this relationship; in fact, the most common cause of mortality in CKD is CVD [12]. Therefore, the treatment of one organ system can dramatically improve the other. Figure 22.2 demonstrates how cardiac dysfunction or renal dysfunction can produce dysfunction in the other organ. Attenuating or even halting the vicious cardiorenal cycle requires therapies that can interrupt the cycle at any point depicted.

Managing heart failure in the emergency department is challenging, but is made even more complex in the setting of kidney disease. It is important to understand the subtle differences when managing this specific patient population compared to heart failure patients alone. The management of cardiorenal syndrome in the emergency department requires individualized therapy. This involves a multifaceted approach in order to optimally manage both the heart failure and the kidney disease. Earlier chapters have indicated the proper management of heart failure in the ED and short-stay unit; therefore, this chapter will focus on the additional therapies recommended for patients with heart failure complicated by underlying kidney disease. Additionally, this chapter will focus on NYHA heart failure classes 1–3 with CKD because NYHA heart failure class 4 and kidney failure patients are considered high risk and are not appropriate for admission to a short-stay observation unit.

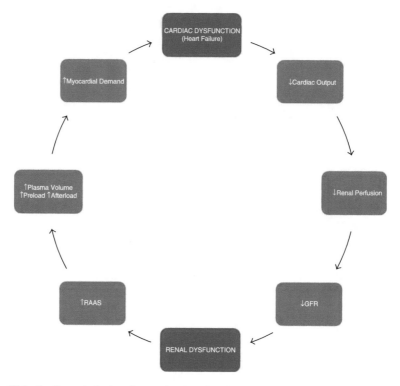

Fig. 22.2 Cardiorenal dysfunction cycle. *RAAS* renin–angiotensin–aldosterone system, *GFR* glomerular filtration rate

It must be noted that although there are well-established guidelines for managing heart failure alone and kidney disease alone, the management of their copresentation in the emergency department remains largely empirical due to the lack of significant randomized clinical trials in this patient population. Thus, most of the following are suggested management options without significant evidence-based guidelines accompanying them.

The management of heart failure in patients with concomitant kidney disease in the short-stay unit requires, first and foremost, the optimal treatment of the acute exacerbation of the heart failure. Therefore, as described in earlier chapters, vasodilators and venodilators must be administered. These drugs reduce systemic vascular resistance and thus reduce the afterload and preload on the heart. Additionally, they decrease the total hydrostatic pressure in the vasculature, thereby reducing pulmonary edema. Diuretics work in a similar fashion, reducing the preload on the heart. Inotropic agents should also be used to improve contractility in order to improve cardiac output.

Biomarkers in Heart Failure with Renal Dysfunction: B-Type Natriuretic Peptide and N-terminal Pro B-type Natriuretic Peptide

The plasma levels of B-type natriuretic peptide (BNP) and N-terminal proBNP (NT-proBNP) are useful markers for the diagnosis and prognosis of heart failure. Since it is the volume overload status on the heart that causes release of these peptides, their levels can be used to aid in diagnosis and prognosis of acute exacerbation of heart failure. Many studies have demonstrated the diagnostic value of BNP and NT-proBNP in heart failure. Unfortunately, the utility of these markers is not as well defined in HF with renal disease. However, BNP and NT-proBNP have been shown to be useful diagnostic and prognostic markers in HF patients with kidney disease, although higher cutoff values are required [13]. Several mechanisms have been proposed for the elevated BNP and NT-proBNP in patients with renal, including reduced renal clearance or increased release by the myocytes possibly due to advanced cardiac damage in renal dysfunction [13]. However, current studies suggest that BNP and NT-proBNP are increased mainly due to cardiac pathology rather than impaired renal clearance [13]. This is supported by another study where NT-proBNP and BNP were significantly higher, while LVEF was lower, in patients with renal dysfunction [14]. Furthermore, this same study demonstrated that BNP and NT-proBNP were independent predictors of 1-year mortality in renal disease patients [14].

Biomarkers in Heart Failure with Renal Dysfunction: Myoglobin, CK-MB, and Troponin

The role of myoglobin in predicting myocardial ischemia is almost nonexistent in renal impairment. Several studies have demonstrated that myoglobin is falsely elevated in renal dysfunction, although CK-MB and troponin are not, due to different clearance mechanisms [15]. This is true for populations in which AMI was ruled in or ruled out [15]. In a study by McCullough et al., myoglobin was falsely elevated 100% of the time in patients with advanced renal function (GFR <47 mL/min) [15]. The recommendation of the use of the multimarker approach still achieves the best negative predictive value [16] for the presence of underlying ACS.

Medical Therapy

In general, medical management of HF with KD requires monitoring of fluid status. This requires physician awareness of the consequences of each drug used on both the HF and the kidney disease. Overly aggressive fluid reduction may damage renal function due to reduced perfusion. Yet increasing plasma volume to improve renal perfusion is detrimental to the heart failure. Therefore, any changes in hemodynamics of this patient population must be closely observed. Fortunately, upon administration in the ED, many of the therapies initiated can be continued and monitored in the short-stay unit.

Diuretics

Diuretics are a mainstay therapy in HF management. Unfortunately, the aggressive use of diuretics can result in worsening renal function via activation of neurohormonal systems. Furosemide is the recommended diuretic due to its proven efficacy. Intravenous administration is most effective due to the reduced bioavailability of oral agents in a hypoperfused edematous small bowel that may be present in heart failure. Diuretic resistance is a common therapeutic roadblock encountered in HF patients with CKD, in which the diuretic response is reduced even with therapeutic doses. Diuretic resistance can be due to reduced renal perfusion, reduced diuretic excretion in the urine, or inadequate dosing [17]. It is suggested that coadministration of loop diuretics along with thiazides can reduce diuretic resistance, but electrolyte levels must be monitored.

Angiotensin Converting Enzyme Inhibitor/Angiotensin Receptor Blocker

The role of angiotensin-converting enzyme inhibitors (ACEI) and angiotensin receptor blockers (ARB) in HF has been well established [18]. Unfortunately, their role in patients with HF and CKD is not well established. This is due to the relatively low number of randomized trials dealing with this patient population and the fear physicians have in exacerbating renal failure and hyperkalemia. Several studies, including that by McAlister et al., demonstrated that patients with renal insufficiency were less likely to receive ACEI, β-blockers, or spironolactone [9]. However, several studies have demonstrated the benefits of ACEI and ARB in this patient population. One analysis of the Minnesota Heart Survey demonstrated a statistically significant reduction in 30-day and 1-year mortality in CHF patients with renal dysfunction not on dialysis who were given ACEI or ARB during their hospital stay [19].

In a review of 12 randomized clinical trials looking at ACEI use in patients with renal insufficiency, the authors demonstrated a 55–75% risk reduction in the progression of renal disease among those on ACEI compared to those not on ACEI [20]. They also concluded that although serum creatinine levels increased by up to 30%, they stabilized within the first 2 months of ACEI administration, and there was long-term preservation of renal function [20]. However, the withdrawal of an ACEI should occur when creatinine rises 30% above baseline or hyperkalemia (>5.6 mmol/L) develops within the first 2 months of ACEI treatment [20]. Another study demonstrated reduced 1-year mortality associated with ACEI and β-blocker use in heart failure patients, even after adjustment for serum creatinine, age, gender, NYHA class, hemoglobin, and other medications [9]. This was true for creatinine clearances <60 mL/min and ≥60 mL/min [9].

Although the use of ACEI and ARBs among patients with renal insufficiency is not established, their role in preserving kidney and heart function has been demonstrated. The use of these medications at low doses along with monitoring of electrolytes in heart failure patients with renal dysfunction should be considered in the short-stay unit and as a discharge medication.

Nesiritide

Nesiritide (synthetic BNP) is an effective vasodilator, diuretic, and RAAS inhibitor, performing these functions without significant reflex tachycardia. Nesiritide's main actions are at the renal level, dilating the afferent arterioles and constricting the efferent arterioles in order to increase intraglomerular pressure and increase GFR [21]. The indirect effects of nesiritide can improve the exacerbation of heart failure as they reduce preload, afterload, and myocardial oxygen consumption through vasodilation and diuresis. Unfortunately, these indirect effects can also lower systemic blood pressure and reduce renal blood flow and GFR [21].

The use of nesiritide for heart failure in renal disease has been constantly debated. Early studies indicated either no difference in kidney function or worsening kidney function with nesiritide use in acute decompensated heart failure versus placebo [22]. A meta-analysis which analyzed heart failure trials using varying doses of nesiritide suggested an increased risk of worsening renal function [23]. The worsening in renal function was linked to nesiritide's hypotensive effects. However, limited control, lack of covariable adjustments, and the fact that some of the reviewed studies used doses of nesiritide higher than those approved for by the FDA [23] question the results of the study.

On the other hand, several studies have demonstrated renal protective effects of nesiritide [24, 25]. Riter et al. demonstrated that low-dose nesiritide in HF and renal dysfunction did not have a significant reduction in systolic blood pressure which was seen with the standard dose [24]. His group showed that nesiritide was actually renal protective in which the low-dose group (2 mcg/kg bolus followed by 0.005 mcg/kg/min and 0.0025 mcg/kg/min without bolus) showed improvement in renal function demonstrated by a decrease in creatinine compared to standard nesiritide doses (2 mcg/kg bolus with an infusion of 0.01 mcg/kg/min). The low-dose group also received less furosemide compared to standard dose nesiritide or no nesiritide group while achieving similar diuresis [24]. Although Riter et al. used a small sample size, the results are promising.

One of the earlier studies to demonstrate the renal protective effects of nesiritide was the NAPA study which evaluated the use of 0.01 mcg/kg of nesiritide without bolus against placebo in postcoronary artery bypass patients [25]. The authors concluded that nesiritide improved renal function postoperatively (measured by a smaller maximal increase in peak creatinine, better preservation of GFR, and greater urine output), reduced hospital length of stay, and decreased mortality at 180 days which they attributed to the improvement of renal function from nesiritide [25]. The VMAC trial demonstrated that compared to placebo, nesiritide resulted in significantly improved hemodynamics in patients with acutely decompensated heart failure [26]. Other results from VMAC included rapid and sustained decreases in cardiac filling pressures and a consistently reduced mean pulmonary capillary wedge pressure with nesiritide use. Nesiritide also significantly reduced patient-reported symptoms and dyspnea at 3 h compared with placebo and the standard of care, nitroglycerin [26].

Most recently, several studies performed by Peacock et al. have demonstrated that the use of nesiritide in the observation unit was safe, reduced hospital admissions, reduced hospital readmission 30 days after discharge, and reduced overall length of stay [27, 28]. Since nesiritide is a synthetic form of the naturally occurring BNP released by the heart, it is self-limiting, and only blood pressure and heart rate need to be monitored [28]. Most recently, the ASCEND-HF trial, which included 7,141 patients, concluded that nesiritide slightly improved shortness of breath, relieved dyspnea, and did not increase the risk of kidney disease compared to placebo in the treatment of heart failure [29].

Anemia Correction

Anemia in CKD has been extensively evaluated. In one study of 5,222 patients with CKD, 48% had anemia, defined as a hemoglobin ≤ 12 g/dL [30], and its prevalence increased from 27% to 76% as GFR decreased from ≥ 60 to <15 mL/min/kg^2 [30]. This is thought to result from a deficiency in erythropoietin due to renal dysfunction. However, the high prevalence of anemia in heart failure patients is a recent finding in cardiology literature. In the OPTIMIZE-HF registry, over half of the 48,612 patients admitted with HF had a hemoglobin <12 g/dL, and 25% had moderate to severe anemia with hemoglobin levels between 5 and 10.7 g/dL [31]. Cardiorenal anemia syndrome is a term used to emphasize the close interaction between these three entities.

Anemia in CHF is associated with increases in mortality, hospitalization, and morbidity rates irrespective of other factors [32]. Additionally, the more severe the anemia in CHF, the more severe the associated mortality, hospitalization, and morbidity [32]. Correction of the anemia with erythropoietin-stimulating agents such as erythropoietin or darbepoetin has been associated with an improvement in renal function, NYHA class, left systolic and diastolic function, quality of life, and reduction in BNP, morbidity, and hospitalization [32]. Yet, anemia is often unrecognized or untreated in CHF. One possible reason is the lack of a universally accepted definition for anemia in the HF population. Additionally, there is uncertainty regarding the most beneficial hemoglobin concentrations that should be achieved with erythropoietin-stimulating-agent treatment for HF. Recent data suggests that the lowest dose of erythropoietic agents that will maintain the hemoglobin level in the 10–12 g/dL range should be used [32].

Patient Education

Approximately one half of heart failure patients are rehospitalized within 6 months due to acute decompensation of their heart failure [33], many of which have underlying renal dysfunction. Patients with heart failure and kidney disease must be educated about how their behaviors and diet influence both their heart and their kidneys. Dietitian counseling and outpatient case manager coordination must be promoted in this patient population. Along with patient education and discharge instructions, institutions are providing patients with a mini booklet similar to the My Medicine List® booklet available through the American Society of Health-System Pharmacists (ASHP). This booklet provides an easy to view and read list of the medications the patient is on, their dosing schedule, what the medication physically looks like, the start date and end date, the reason for the medication (in layman's terms), and the prescribing physician. Patients are instructed to keep this booklet with them as often as possible and bring it with themselves when presenting to the emergency department. Expanding this mini booklet to include additional information such as admission and discharge BNP levels, blood pressure, GFR, creatinine, and ECG can prove to be beneficial for this patient population that has such a high readmission rate. The information on the mini booklet will allow the evaluating emergency physician to compare the current state of the decompensation to previous episodes. This approach can potentially improve door-to-treatment time, reduce length of stay, and improve overall patient care.

References

1. National Chronic Kidney Disease Fact Sheet. http://www.cdc.gov/diabetes/pubs/factsheets/kidney.htm. Accessed 12 Nov 2010.
2. Kidney and urological disease statistics in the United States. http://kidney.niddk.nih.gov/statistics. The National Institute of Diabetes and Digestive and Kidney Diseases (NIDDK). Accessed 12 Nov 2010.
3. Glomerular Filtration Rate. http://www.kidney.org/kidneydisease/ckd/knowGFR.cfm. Accessed 12 Nov 2010.
4. Go AS, Chertow GM, Fan D, et al. Chronic kidney disease and the risks of death, cardiovascular events, and hospitalizations. N Engl J Med. 2004;351:1296–305.
5. Astor BC, Levey AS, Stevens LA, et al. Method of glomerular filtration rate estimation affects prediction of mortality risk. J Am Soc Nephrol. 2009;20:2214–22.
6. Shlipak MG, Katz R, Sarnak MJ, et al. Cystatin C and prognosis for cardiovascular and kidney outcomes in elderly persons without chronic kidney disease. Ann Intern Med. 2006;145:237–46.

7. Stevens LA, Coresh J, Schmid CH, et al. A pooled analysis of 3,418 individuals with CKD. Am J Kidney Dis. 2008;51:395–406.
8. Smith GL, Lichtman JH, Bracken MB, et al. Renal impairment and outcomes in heart failure. J Am Coll Cardiol. 2006;47:1987–96.
9. McAlister FA, Ezekowitz J, Tonelli M, et al. Renal insufficiency and heart failure. Circulation. 2004;109:1004–9.
10. Wali RK, Wang GS, Gottlieb SS, et al. Effect of kidney transplantation on left ventricular systolic function and congestive heart failure in patients with end-stage renal disease. J Am Coll Cardiol. 2005;45:1051–60.
11. Hillege HL, Girbes ARJ, de Kam PJ, et al. Renal function, neurohormonal activation, and survival; in patients with chronic heart failure. Circulation. 2000;102:203–10.
12. The National Kidney Foundation: Kidney Disease Outcomes Quality Initiative. http://www.kidney.org/professionals/kdoqi/guidelines_ckd/p7_risk_g15.htm. Accessed 2 Dec 2010.
13. de Filippi CR, Christenson RH. B-type natriuretic peptide (BNP)/NT-proBNP and renal function: is the controversy over? Clin Chem. 2009;55:1271–3.
14. de Filippi CR, Seliger SL, Maynard S, et al. Impact of renal disease on natriuretic peptide testing for diagnosing decompensated heart failure and predicting mortality. Clin Chem. 2007;53:1511–9.
15. McCullough PA, Nowak RM, Foreback C, et al. Performance of multiple cardiac biomarkers measured in the emergency department in patients with chronic kidney disease and chest pain. Acad Emerg Med. 2002;9:1389–96.
16. Dadkhah S, Sharain K, Sharain R, et al. The value of bedside cardiac multibiomarker assay in rapid and accurate diagnosis of acute coronary syndromes. Crit Pathw Cardiol. 2007;6:76–84.
17. Koniari K, Nikolaou M, Paraskevaidis I, et al. Therapeutic options for the management of the cardiorenal syndrome. Int J Nephrol. 2010;2011:194910.
18. Bonow RO, Bennett S, Casey Jr DE, et al. ACC/AHA clinical performance measures for adults with chronic heart failure: a report of the American college of cardiology/American heart association task force on performance measures (writing committee to develop heart failure clinical performance measures). Circulation. 2005;112:1853–87.
19. Berger AK, Duval S, Manske C, et al. Angiotensin-converting enzyme inhibitors and angiotensin receptor blockers in patients with congestive heart failure and chronic kidney disease. Am Heart J. 2007;153:1064–73.
20. Bakris GL, Weir MR. Angiotensin-converting enzyme inhibitor-associated elevations in serum creatinine. Arch Intern Med. 2000;160:685–93.
21. Witteles RM. Nesiritide, heart failure, and renal dysfunction: irrational exuberance or throwing the baby out with the bathwater. Cardiovasc Drugs Ther. 2009;23:183–6.
22. Wang DJ, Dowling TC, Meadows D, et al. Nesiritide does not improve renal function in patients with chronic heart failure and worsening serum creatinine. Circulation. 2004;110:1620–5.
23. Sackner-Bernstein JD, Skopicki HA, Arronsson KD, et al. Risk of worsening renal function with nesiritide in patients with acutely decompensated heart failure. Circulation. 2005;111:1487–91.
24. Riter HG, Redfield MM, Burnett JC, et al. Nonhypotensive low-dose nesiritide has differential renal effects compared with standard-dose nesiritide in patients with acute decompensated heart failure and renal dysfunction. J Am Coll Cardiol. 2006;47:2334–42.
25. Mentzer RM, Oz MC, Sladen RN, et al. Effects of perioperative nesiritide in patients with left ventricular dysfunction undergoing cardiac surgery. J Am Coll Cardiol. 2007;49:716–26.
26. Publication Committee for the VMAC Investigators. Intravenous nesiritide vs nitroglycerin for treatment of decompensated congestive heart failure. JAMA. 2002;287:1531–40.
27. Peacock WF, Holland R, Gyamarthy R, et al. Observation unit treatment of heart failure with nesiritide: results from the proaction trial. J Emerg Med. 2005;29:243–52.
28. Peacock WF, Emerman CL, Silver MA. Nesiritide added to standard care favorably reduces systolic blood pressure compared with standard care alone in patients with acute decompensated heart failure. Am J Emerg Med. 2005;23:327–31.

29. Hernandez AF. Late-breaking clinical trials presented at the American Heart Association Congress in Chicago 2010: ASCEND-HF. Clin Res Cardiol. 2011;100(1):1–9.
30. McClellan W, Aronoff SL, Bolton WK, et al. The prevalence of anemia in patients with chronic kidney disease. Curr Med Res Opin. 2004;20:1501–10.
31. Young JB, Abraham WT, Albert NM, et al. Relation of low hemoglobin and anemia to morbidity and mortality in patients hospitalized with heart failure (insight from the OPTIMIZE-HF registry). Am J Cardiol. 2008;101:223–30.
32. Silverberg DS, Wexler D, Iaina A, et al. The correction of anemia in patients with the combination of chronic kidney disease and congestive heart failure may prevent progression of both conditions. Clin Exp Nephrol. 2009;13:101–6.
33. American Heart Association. Heart disease and stroke statistics—2005 update. Dallas, TX: American Heart Association; 2005.

Chapter 23
Heart Failure Research in the Emergency Department and Observation Unit

Candace McNaughton, Patricia Fick, and Alan Storrow

Introduction

Acute heart failure syndrome (AHFS) may be defined as *new onset heart failure or a change in chronic heart failure symptoms that requires urgent therapy* [1]. The evaluation and management of emergency department (ED) patients with potential AHFS have remained a significant challenge for decades. Unlike the dramatic advances that have been made in the assessment and treatment of patients with acute coronary syndrome (ACS), the emergency physician's diagnostic, prognostic, and therapeutic tools for heart failure have remained mostly limited. The complexity of the syndrome has led to risk aversion and extremely high admission rates. The need for translating basic science discoveries into clinical research and then into practice changes has never been more compelling. The need for improvement has been highlighted by several recently published guidelines and scientific statements [2–4]. However, it is concerning that these guidelines are not specific to truly acute management, they lack compelling risk stratification tools, and they lack strong evidence for early therapeutics [5].

AHFS is certainly a significant source of morbidity, mortality, and health-care expenditures. In 2006, over one million patients were discharged from the hospital with the primary diagnosis of heart failure after a median length of stay of 4.5 days. These patients bear a 60-day mortality of 10% [6, 7]. Of those patients who present to the ED with acute heart failure, over 80% are admitted [8]. The estimated direct and indirect cost of heart failure in the United States in 2010 was $39.2 billion [9]. Hospitalization accounts for >75% of heart failure care costs, at about $29.6 billion

C. McNaughton, MD (✉) • P. Fick, MD • A. Storrow, MD
Department of Emergency Medicine, Vanderbilt University Medical Center,
Nashville, TN, USA
e-mail: candace.mcnaughton@vanderbilt.edu

W. Frank Peacock (ed.), *Short Stay Management of Acute Heart Failure*,
Contemporary Cardiology, DOI 10.1007/978-1-61779-627-2_23,
© Springer Science+Business Media, LLC 2012

Table 23.1 Similarities and differences between ACS and AHFS resulting in hospitalization in the United States [5]

	ACS	AHFS
Incidence	One million/year	One million/year
Mortality		
Prehospital	High	Unclear
Inhospital	3–4%	3–4%
60–90 days	2%	10%
Targets	Clearly defined (thrombosis)	Unclear
Clinical trial results	Beneficial	Minimal, no benefit, harmful
ACC/AHA guidelines	Level A	Minimal level A/B, mostly C

Reprinted with permission. Circulation 2010;122:1975–1996. ©2010 American Heart Association, Inc. *ACS* acute coronary syndromes, *AHFS* acute heart failure syndromes, *ACC/AHA* american college of cardiology/american heart association

per year or nearly 3% of the total national health-care budget [10, 11]. Compared with ACS, AHFS is generally associated with worse outcomes and much fewer established treatment options (Table 23.1). As the population continues to age and survival from ACSs improves, the prevalence and costs associated with the treatment of AHFS are expected to continue to increase [12].

In its current state, AHFS research is inadequate to meet the needs of patients, providers, and the health-care system. The reasons for this are varied and complex. No cohesive AFHS research agenda exists, patients are typically not recruited while in the ED, and there are no clinical or biochemical agreed-upon therapeutic endpoints to measure success or failure of interventions [13]. For example, while patients with AHFS are often hospitalized due to worsening congestion, many are discharged with persistent signs and symptoms of congestion or high left ventricular filling pressure [14, 15]. Systematic methods for assessing congestion prior to discharge are sorely needed. Additionally, while signs and symptoms of heart failure usually improve during admission, mortality during admission remains high, ranging from 5 to 15% or more [1, 16, 17]. Of those patients who do survive to discharge, a further 10–15% will die within 6–12 weeks and about one-third will be readmitted for multiple reasons, often AHFS [1, 14, 17]. These unacceptable high postdischarge event rates are another important motivator for the interest in ED and observation unit AHFS research. Caregivers and patients need new ways to address these challenges before this enormous resource burden becomes overwhelming.

What Is an Observation Unit?

An observation unit extends care beyond the initial ED visit to determine the need for inpatient admission. Approximately one-third of EDs have an observation unit or are planning one; most are designed to assist in the evaluation of chest pain, asthma, or other well-defined cardiopulmonary conditions. Patients admitted to observation units may lack a definitive diagnosis or may also be in the process of diagnostic evaluation for a specific complaint such as chest pain or abdominal pain [18, 19].

Observation units are tailored to the needs of each hospital and patient population, and therefore, their design and management vary from hospital to hospital. However, the benefits of general observation units are clear: they decrease unnecessary admissions, improve risk management, and improve patient care [20]. In one recent study, the 14-day recidivism for a protocol-driven observation unit designed to treat patients with multiple complaints was 7.9%. Most returns were related to the original chief complaint and took place in the first week following discharge. Painful conditions had the highest recidivism rates [21]. Overall, when treating patients with multiple complaints, observation units result in "lower costs, decreased length of stay, improved use [of] hospital resources, improved patient satisfaction, [and] better diagnostic performance" [21].

Acute Heart Failure Syndromes Research Conducted in the Emergency Department and Observation Units Is Lacking

Even the evaluation of AHFS lacks rigorous data and study. The diagnosis of AHFS is often difficult to make accurately; nearly 20% of AHFS patients are misdiagnosed in the ED [22]. While patients are often admitted for symptoms of congestion, frequently they are discharged without a change in congestion or in weight. "Overall, management of AHFS is challenging given the heterogeneity of the patient population, absence of a universally accepted definition, incomplete understanding of its pathophysiology, and lack of robust evidence-based guidelines" [13]. Clearly, more research is needed to identify patients with AHFS and to measure their clinical improvement [1, 14, 15].

Because ED patients are fundamentally different from patients studied in prior AHFS registries, results drawn from these databases may not be applicable in the ED setting. To date, registry patients have been more likely to be older, female, and have preserved systolic function, and the vast majority of patients were inpatients [23].

Therapy for AHFS has changed little over the past 30 years. New interventions have failed to meet expectations regarding efficacy and safety [24–27]. This is not surprising because, until recently, new therapies have been trialed in subjects enrolled 24–48 h after presentation, long after initial standard therapies were performed and after most patients have experienced significant symptom improvement. Over 70% of patients have already experienced improvement in symptoms from standard therapy within hours of admission, thus studies performed after this initial improvement in symptoms are unlikely to show therapeutic benefit [28].

Much of the standard therapy for AHFS has been used for decades without rigorous study. Indeed, some standard therapies may be harmful. For example, diuretics, which are commonly used to reduce peripheral edema, may be associated with such adverse outcomes such as renal failure and poor perfusion.

In an article discussing the need for more systematic study of AHFS in the ED, the authors note:

> Achievement of symptomatic improvement should not be at the expense of worsened morbidity and mortality. We hypothesize that the "route one travels" to symptomatic improvement is important and may play a role in preserving renal function and hibernating myocardium while avoiding a significant decline in blood pressure. Critical to this hypothesis is an understanding that trial design and timing are as important as the type of intervention…patients should be enrolled when symptoms are maximal, minimizing concomitant therapy, if the effect of a novel agent is to be determined… By discounting initial ED treatment, there is potential for mismatching target enrollment populations with stage-specific symptoms and outcomes [23].

Patients with AHFS spend a significant amount of time in the ED, with an average length of stay of 5 hours. Clearly, these initial hours are of critical importance in the clinical course of AHFS, a time when many of the therapeutic interventions are performed [29]. This should be a focus of research going forward.

In addition to the lack of evidence regarding acute AHFS therapy, risk stratification studies have not defined appropriate discharge criteria for AHFS patients. Without appropriate risk stratification criteria, the vast majority of these patients are admitted to the hospital [30]. "Current therapeutic AHFS guidelines are based on little or no scientific evidence," likely contributing to the 61% 3-month readmission rate reported in one study, for AHFS patients who are discharged from the ED [12].

Mortality, hospital readmission rate, and length of stays are higher for AHFS patients than for ACS patients. Clearly, there is tremendous need for systematic, rigorous AHFS research in the ED. While there are regularly updated guidelines for the care of ACS patients, there is currently limited clinical trial data for usefulness of current AHFS treatment and evaluation strategies in the ED [31].

Benefits of an Observation Unit for Acute Heart Failure Syndromes

The observation unit provides an alternative to inpatient hospitalization for patients with AHFS by allowing for extended diagnostics, risk stratification, therapeutics for acute symptomatology, and protocol-driven disposition decisions (inpatient admission or discharge), all typically within 24 hours. Available data suggests there is no increased risk of death or recidivism, provided appropriate patients are chosen [30]. Particularly for low-to moderate-risk AHFS patients, this strategy has been suggested as safe and cost-effective [30]. The observation unit also allows a more complete acute evaluation and is particularly helpful for those patients whose social situations make it difficult to complete their work-up solely in the ED [32]. Perhaps most importantly, they also provide more time for patient education prior to discharge.

Observation Unit Outcomes

Two preliminary studies have shown no difference in recidivism for AHFS patients admitted to an observation unit when compared with inpatient admission. In one study, the recidivism rate for AHFS evaluated in an observation unit was 19.4%, which was no different from the 30-day readmission rate for the risk-matched inpatient group [21]. A pilot study of AHFS patients assigned to an observation unit rather than inpatient admission found similar rates of recidivism and no deaths. There was a cost saving of $3,600 per patient in the group of AHFS patients admitted to the observation unit [30]. Observation unit admission may be cost-effective for *non-high-risk* AHFS patients [12], and preliminary studies suggest that it may be a safe and efficient alternative to discharge from the ED or inpatient admission.

Emergency Department/Observation Unit Management of Acute Heart Failure Syndromes Can Improve Patient and Physician Satisfaction

In a randomized study comparing patient satisfaction, patients who presented to the ED with low-risk chest pain preferred evaluation in an observation unit over inpatient admission, citing decreased length of stay, increased quality of service, and effective treatment of health problems [33]. Patients evaluated in observation units reported fewer complaints regarding communication, fulfillment of needs, and physical comfort. Physicians and patients alike reported fewer problems with patient communication, total number of problems, physical comfort, patient education, and discharge preparation after admission. These differences were attributed to improved communication, greater physical comfort, and more attention to special needs.

Observation units can provide equivalent, satisfactory care. The authors of this study concluded that "patients who meet study criteria (approximately 17% of the ED chest pain population) [who are] now being referred to inpatient services could be better served by [an] ED-based [observation unit] service" [33].

Emergency Department/Observation Unit Research

As the principle portal for entry for hospitalized patients, the ED or an ED-based observation unit provides the initial point of definitive health-care contact, primary stabilization, and disposition decisions [5]. As key transition points in the continuum of heart failure care, they are ideally suited to address the many current deficiencies in AHFS research. We highlight focused areas in need of future investigation, including diagnostics, risk stratification, and therapy while emphasizing the unique contributions of the ED and observation units.

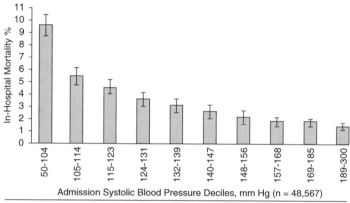

Fig. 23.1 Inhospital mortality rates by admission systolic blood pressure deciles (n=48,567). Reprinted with permission from Gheorghiade et al. [34]. °(2006) American Medical Association. All rights reserved

Initial Evaluation

Many AHFS patients can be categorized phenotypically into hypertensive, normotensive, or hypotensive presentations [31]. Such an approach has been suggested as a start for additional research into optimal treatment strategies [22].

Patients with AHFS who are hypertensive typically experience rapid onset of symptoms, but these symptoms also tend to resolve rapidly with treatment. Often, for these patients, this represents the initial presentation of heart failure. Left ventricular ejection fraction is frequently preserved, and patients present with symptoms of pulmonary vascular congestion without systemic signs of vascular congestion. These patients benefit the most from current acute therapies, and they typically have the lowest mortality of the AHFS presentations.

Patients with AHFS who are normotensive usually develop their symptoms over several days, with progressive worsening of their pulmonary symptoms as well as signs of systemic congestion. These patients are more likely to have depressed left ventricular ejection fraction, and often therapy is less likely to quickly improve symptoms such as dyspnea and lower extremity edema.

Patients with hypotensive AHFS may present in cardiogenic shock, requiring pressors to combat organ hypoperfusion. Although relatively rare (1–8% of heart failure admissions), these patients may require invasive assistive devices to maintain organ perfusion; they also have higher inhospital and postdischarge mortality (Fig. 23.1) [34].

AHFS presentations may be further categorized by comorbidities such as ACS and renal failure as well as by accompanying signs and symptoms such as pulmonary edema (Table 23.2) [5]. Clearly, patients who present with AHFS represent a

Table 23.2 Presenting profiles in emergency department patients with AHFS [5]

Clinical presentation	Incidence[a]	Characteristics	Targets[b] and therapies[c]
Elevated BP (>160 mm Hg)	~25%	Predominantly pulmonary (radiographic/clinical) with or without systemic congestion. Many patients have preserved EF	Target: BP and volume management Therapy: vasodilators (e.g., nitrates[d], nesiritide, nitroprusside) and loop diuretics
Normal or moderately elevated BP	~50%	Develop gradually (days or weeks) and are associated with systemic congestion. Radiographic pulmonary congestion may be minimal in patients with advanced HF	Target: volume management Therapy: loop diuretics ± vasodilators
Low BP (<90 mm Hg)	<8%	Mostly related to low cardiac output and often associated with decreased renal function	Target: cardiac output Therapy: inotropes with vasodilatory properties (e.g., milrinone, dobutamine, levosimendan); consider digoxin (intravenous and/or orally) ± vasopressor medications ± mechanical assist devices (e.g., IABP)
Cardiogenic shock	<1%	Rapid onset. Primarily complicating acute MI, fulminant myocarditis, actue valvular disease	Target: improve cardiac pump function Therapy: inotropes ± vasoactive medications ± mechanical assist devices, corrective surgery
Flash pulmonary edema	3%[c]	Abrupt onset. Often precipitated by severe systemic hypertension. Patients respond readily to vasodilators and diuretics	Target: BP, volume management Therapy: vasodilators, diuretics, invasive or NIV, morphine
ACS and AHFS	~25% of ACS have HF signs/symptoms	Rapid or gradual onset. Many such patients may have signs and symptoms of HF that resolve after resolution of ischemia	Target: coronary thrombosis, plaque stabilization, correction of ischemia Therapy: reperfusion (e.g., PCI, lytics, nitrates, antiplatelet agents)
Isolated right HF from pulmonary HTN or intrinsic RV failure (e.g., infarct) or valvular abnormalities (e.g., tricuspid valve endocarditis)	?	Rapid or gradual onset due to primary or secondary PA hypertension or RV pathology (e.g., RV infarct). Not well characterized with few epidemiological data	Target: PA pressure Therapy: nitrates, epoprostenol, phosphodiesterase inhibitors, endothelin-blocking agents, coronary reperfusion for RV infarcts, valve surgery

(continued)

Table 23.2 (continued)

Clinical presentation	Incidence[a]	Characteristics	Targets[b] and therapies[c]
Postcardiac surgery HF	?	Occurring in patients with or without previous ventricular dysfunction, often related to worsening diastolic function and volume overload immediately after surgery and the subsequent early postoperative interval. Can also be caused by inadequate intraoperative myocardial protection resulting in cardiac injury	Target: volume management, improve cardiac performance (output) Therapy: diuretic or fluid administration (directed by filling pressures and cardiac index), inotropic support, mechanical assistance (IABP, VAD)

Reprinted with permission. Circulation 2010;122:1975–1996. ©2010 American Heart Association, Inc. Original data from Gheorghiade and Pang [13] and Gheorghiade et al [17]

ACS acute coronary syndromes, *AHFS* acute heart failure syndromes, *BP* blood pressure, *EF* ejection fraction, *HF* heart failure, *HTN* hypertension, *IABP* intra-aortic balloon pump, *IACB* intra-aortic balloon counter pulsation, *MI* myocardial infarction, *NIV* non-invasive ventilation, *PA* pulmonary artery, *PCI* percutaneous coronary intervention, *RV* right ventricular, *VAD* ventricular assist device

[a]Of all AHFS admissions

[b]Treating etiology or precipitant is of equal of greater importance (e.g., arrhythmia, ACS, infection)

[c]Represents initial therapies for early management and should be tailored to each patient's unique presentation

[d]Probably preferred in patients with ACS or history of CAD

[e]Its incidence may be related to the definition used (clinical *vs.* radiographic)

heterogeneous population with multiple anatomic and physiologic derangements—it is likely that different patient populations and underlying disease states will respond to with varying degrees of success to different therapeutic interventions.

Diagnostics

Given the complexity of AHFS, it is unsurprising that nearly than 20% of patients with heart failure are misdiagnosed in the ED [22]. The tools currently used to diagnose AHFS are often either unreliable or unacceptably invasive or both. Important clues to the appropriate diagnosis, such as the presence of an S3 heart sound, jugular venous distension, and response to a valsalva maneuver, may be impossible to detect in obese patients or in the loud ED environment [35, 36]. Pulmonary artery catheterization, which can provide objective evidence of acute heart failure, should not be performed in most patients with suspected AHFS because it is invasive, risky, and costly; additionally, recent data suggests it may not be as effective in directing treatment of AHFS as was once thought [37, 38]. Complicating the diagnostic muddle, many of the other readily available diagnostic tests lack sensitivity and specificity or are applied ineffectively. For example, chest X-rays lack congestion in up to 18% of patients with heart failure [39]. The natriuretic peptides B-type natriuretic peptide (BNP) and N-terminal (NT)-proBNP are useful in cases in which there is diagnostic uncertainty after a history, physical exam, and chest X-ray. However, given the potential for variation in clinical history and physical examination combined with the time constraints of the ED, a BNP or NT-proBNP may be sent inappropriately, limiting its usefulness. Additionally, age, sex, renal function, and obesity affect the BNP and NT-proBNP and should be considered in its interpretation [22].

Limited bedside echocardiography performed by emergency medicine physicians is becoming more common, though it has not yet gained widespread acceptance and has yet to be fully studied [22]. Impedance cardiography is another possible diagnostic tool that has yet to be fully evaluated [40]. Clearly, there is dire need for more reliable, sensitive, and specific tests to aid in identifying patients with AHFS; the ED and observation units provide an ideal setting for such research.

Risk Stratification

To date, little prospective research has focused on risk stratification of AHFS patients. In particular, identifying *low-risk* AHFS patients has proven difficult. Most of the available research has focused on high-risk AFHS patients, but those patients who stand to benefit the most from risk stratification may be those low-risk patients who are currently unnecessarily admitted to the hospital. Under the current practice patterns, these unidentified low-risk AHFS patients may undergo unnecessary tests, imaging studies, and procedures; they bear the burden of potentially unwarranted exposure to health-care-acquired infections and medical errors, in addition to higher health-care costs.

A clinical prediction rule was developed in an ED-based study for patients at relatively low risk for short-term complications who were admitted to the hospital for AHFS [34, 41]. However, this rule was designed for benchmarking rather than clinical use, and it is challenging to use at the bedside. Additionally, it has not been tested prospectively or in patients discharged from the ED primarily [42]. This prediction rule serves as a starting point for future risk stratification research.

Therapy

AHFS is a multifaceted disorder, but heterogeneous presentations are often met with homogeneous therapy [5]. Current ED therapy is generally limited to peripheral vasodilators, such as nitroglycerin, angiotensin-converting enzyme (ACE) inhibitors, or angiotensin II receptor blockers, and intravenous diuretics. These therapies are often applied regardless of the underlying cause of the exacerbation. Rarely are comorbid conditions such as ACS, diabetes, and even renal failure taken into account when applying therapeutic interventions. Logically, however, it would seem that patients presenting in heart failure due to low cardiac output would require different therapeutic interventions than patients who present due to diastolic dysfunction or a physiologic imbalanced caused by pneumonia or dietary indiscretion [34, 43].

Even in the case where there is reliable data supporting a therapeutic intervention, the intervention is often not implemented in a systematic manner. Currently available medications known to improve morbidity and mortality from AHFS, such as ACE inhibitors and beta blockers, are often not prescribed to appropriate patients, or patients fail to take prescribed medications. The reasons for these failures are as multifaceted as the causes of AHFS presentations and deserve as much research effort. Future research must focus on safe, effective, and efficient use of existing, proven medications and interventions.

In the same vein, patient education, discharge planning and transition, and medication reconciliation and education should be considered interventions that may have as much, or more, therapeutic benefit as pharmaceuticals. Barriers to self-care that contribute to acute exacerbations of heart failure have not been completely elucidated nor have methods of overcoming these barriers been developed. Potential barriers, including lack of motivation, complex medication regiments, cognitive impairment, low socioeconomic status, low educational level, low health literacy and numeracy levels, and inadequate family and social support, must be rigorously addressed if they are to be effectively overcome.

More than simply providing information, interventions designed to overcome barriers to self-care should improve acquisition of self-management skills or behaviors that are necessary and sufficient to optimize patient outcomes. Research must identify the necessary components to optimize the delivery of care; this will require the involvement of nurses, pharmacists, dieticians, primary care physicians, and case management providers. Interactions between providers should be refined and streamlined. Involvement of family members and caregivers has not yet been studied in great detail but must be explored. Future research should also include targeted transitions from inpatient to outpatient therapies, particularly for those patients who are discharged from the ED [44].

Physicians and practitioners who care for patients with heart failure may have difficulty learning and using the highest quality of care in AHFS management because of the wide range in practice patterns and the lack of supporting evidence. Even when improvements in AHFS management are discovered and generally accepted, the current health-care system requires nearly 20 years to disseminate change [45]. This unnecessary delay can be reduced designing systematic changes that make it easier to incorporate new medical knowledge into daily practice [46]. However, much work in this field remains to be done.

Therapeutic interventions must encompass more than simply adding or changing medications. Future research must include varied combinations of pharmaceutical interventions, old and new, as well as educational, disease-specific, and system-wide changes. Patients, caregivers, and health-care providers need more than new drugs in their arsenal of tools to combat AHFS.

It Is Feasible to Do Research in the Emergency Department and Observation Unit

A clinical network of clinicians and hospitals dedicated to the study of AHFS has been established [23]. This network is made up of expert ED and cardiology physicians who are committed to rigorous research and who have already begun coordinating their research aims. Perceived barriers to AHFS research based in the ED and observation unit, such as a chaotic environment and issues surrounding consent, can be overcome with careful planning and coordination [5]. The infrastructure for continued rigorous research has been laid, but more clinician-scientists are needed to continue and expand the scope of investigation.

Future Directions in the Emergency Department and Observation Units

To date, none of the interventions studied in prospective AHFS clinical trials have been shown to improve inhospital symptoms clinical outcomes when compared with standard care plus placebo. This is likely due to a combination of factors, including the fact that the majority of patients improve even when randomized to standard care plus placebo, clinical outcomes often do not correlate well with targeted hemodynamic changes, the pathophysiological differences between chronic and AHFSs are not well understood, and prior studies have included only drugs initiated hours to days after the initial presentation, thus resulting in "late randomization bias" [17].

The clinical care for patients with AHFS who present to the ED is ripe with opportunities for research and improvement. Which patients with AHFS may be safely discharged? Which patients require observation versus inpatient admission? Risk stratification tools to assist in disposition are clearly needed. For example, a prospective study testing the combination of congestion measurements and their predictive value for rehospitalization could have significant clinical implications [1]. New therapies or innovative use of existing ones should be explored, which will require that the research extend to the most common location for presentation, the ED. This is also an ideal time to evaluate new diagnostics, such as markers of tissue perfusion and ventricular stretch. What are appropriate treatment endpoints for AHFS patients? How can patient education be improved? How can currently accepted treatments be used and implemented more effectively?

Summary

Heart failure is a significant source of morbidity and mortality, and many patients with heart failure symptoms present to the ED for treatment and evaluation. For low-risk patients, initial data suggests that safe and effective evaluation and treatment can be provided in an observation unit. The ED and the observation unit are ideal environments to perform clinical, therapeutic, and epidemiological AHFS research. Future targets for research aims include diagnostics, risk stratification, and therapeutics, including interventions that target the healthcare delivery system as well as pharmaceuticals.

References

1. Gheorghiade M, Follath F, Ponikowski P, et al. Assessing and grading congestion in acute heart failure: a scientific statement from the acute heart failure committee of the heart failure association of the European Society of Cardiology and endorsed by the European Society of Intensive Care Medicine. Eur J Heart Fail. 2010;12:423–33.
2. Hunt SA, Abraham WT, Chin MH, et al. 2009 focused update incorporated into the ACC/AHA 2005 guidelines for the diagnosis and management of heart failure in adults a report of the American College of Cardiology Foundation/American Heart Association Task Force on Practice Guidelines Developed in Collaboration with the International Society for Heart and Lung Transplantation. J Am Coll Cardiol. 2009;53:e1–90.
3. Lindenfeld J, Albert NM, Boehmer JP, et al. HFSA 2010 comprehensive heart failure practice guideline. J Card Fail. 2010;16:e1–194.
4. Peacock WF, Braunwald E, Abraham W, et al. National Heart, Lung, and Blood Institute working group on emergency department management of acute heart failure: research challenges and opportunities. J Am Coll Cardiol. 2010;56:343–51.
5. Weintraub NL, Collins SP, Pang PS, et al. Acute heart failure syndromes: emergency department presentation, treatment, and disposition: current approaches and future aims: a scientific statement from the American Heart Association. Circulation. 2010;122:1975–96.

6. Lloyd-Jones D, Adams RJ, Brown TM, et al. Executive summary: heart disease and stroke statistics–2010 update: a report from the American Heart Association. Circulation. 2010;121: 948–54.
7. Ah A. Heart disease and stroke statistics-2006 update. Dallas, TX: American Heart Association; 2005.
8. Januzzi JL, van Kimmenade R, Lainchbury J, et al. NT-proBNP testing for diagnosis and short-term prognosis in acute destabilized heart failure: an international pooled analysis of 1256 patients: the International Collaborative of NT-proBNP Study. Eur Heart J. 2006;27: 330–7.
9. Lloyd-Jones D, Adams RJ, Brown TM, et al. Heart disease and stroke statistics—2010 update: a report from the American Heart Association. Circulation. 2010;121:e46–215.
10. Hunt SA, Abraham WT, Chin MH, et al. ACC/AHA 2005 guideline update for the diagnosis and management of chronic heart failure in the adult: a report of the American College of Cardiology/American Heart Association Task Force on Practice Guidelines (writing committee to update the 2001 guidelines for the evaluation and management of heart failure): developed in collaboration with the American College of Chest Physicians and the International Society for Heart and Lung Transplantation: endorsed by the Heart Rhythm Society. Circulation. 2005;112:e154–235.
11. Adams Jr KF, Fonarow GC, Emerman CL, et al. Characteristics and outcomes of patients hospitalized for heart failure in the United States: rationale, design, and preliminary observations from the first 100,000 cases in the Acute Decompensated Heart Failure National Registry (ADHERE). Am Heart J. 2005;149:209–16.
12. Collins SP, Schauer DP, Gupta A, Brunner H, Storrow AB, Eckman MH. Cost-effectiveness analysis of ED decision making in patients with non-high-risk heart failure. Am J Emerg Med. 2009;27:293–302.
13. Gheorghiade M, Pang PS. Acute heart failure syndromes. J Am Coll Cardiol. 2009;53: 557–73.
14. O'Connor CM, Stough WG, Gallup DS, Hasselblad V, Gheorghiade M. Demographics, clinical characteristics, and outcomes of patients hospitalized for decompensated heart failure: observations from the IMPACT-HF registry. J Card Fail. 2005;11:200–5.
15. Gheorghiade M, Filippatos G, De Luca L, Burnett J. Congestion in acute heart failure syndromes: an essential target of evaluation and treatment. Am J Med. 2006;119:S3–10.
16. Cleland JG, Swedberg K, Follath F, et al. The EuroHeart Failure Survey programme—a survey on the quality of care among patients with heart failure in Europe. Part 1: patient characteristics and diagnosis. Eur Heart J. 2003;24:442–63.
17. Gheorghiade M, Zannad F, Sopko G, et al. Acute heart failure syndromes: current state and framework for future research. Circulation. 2005;112:3958–68.
18. Mace SE, Graff L, Mikhail M, Ross M. A national survey of observation units in the United States. Am J Emerg Med. 2003;21:529–33.
19. Mace SE, Shah J. Observation medicine in emergency medicine residency programs. Acad Emerg Med. 2002;9:169–71.
20. Leikin JB. The uprooting of observational units from emergency departments: opportunity lost for emergency medicine? Am J Emerg Med. 1988;6:49–51.
21. Ross MA, Hemphill RR, Abramson J, Schwab K, Clark C. The recidivism characteristics of an emergency department observation unit. Ann Emerg Med. 2010;56:34–41.
22. Collins S, Storrow AB, Kirk JD, Pang PS, Diercks DB, Gheorghiade M. Beyond pulmonary edema: diagnostic, risk stratification, and treatment challenges of acute heart failure management in the emergency department. Ann Emerg Med. 2008;51:45–57.
23. Collins SP, Levy PD, Lindsell CJ, et al. The rationale for an acute heart failure syndromes clinical trials network. J Card Fail. 2009;15:467–74.
24. Gheorghiade M, Konstam MA, Burnett Jr JC, et al. Short-term clinical effects of tolvaptan, an oral vasopressin antagonist, in patients hospitalized for heart failure: the EVEREST clinical status trials. JAMA. 2007;297:1332–43.

25. Intravenous nesiritide vs. nitroglycerin for treatment of decompensated congestive heart failure: a randomized controlled trial. JAMA 2002;287:1531–40.
26. Mebazaa A, Nieminen MS, Packer M, et al. Levosimendan vs. dobutamine for patients with acute decompensated heart failure: the SURVIVE randomized trial. JAMA. 2007;297:1883–91.
27. De Luca L, Fonarow GC, Adams Jr KF, et al. Acute heart failure syndromes: clinical scenarios and pathophysiologic targets for therapy. Heart Fail Rev. 2007;12:97–104.
28. Mebazaa A, Pang PS, Tavares M, et al. The impact of early standard therapy on dyspnoea in patients with acute heart failure: the URGENT-dyspnoea study. Eur Heart J. 2010;31:832–41.
29. Han JH, Zhou C, France DJ, et al. The effect of emergency department expansion on emergency department overcrowding. Acad Emerg Med. 2007;14:338–43.
30. Storrow AB, Collins SP, Lyons MS, Wagoner LE, Gibler WB, Lindsell CJ. Emergency department observation of heart failure: preliminary analysis of safety and cost. Congest Heart Fail. 2005;11:68–72.
31. Filippatos G, Zannad F. An introduction to acute heart failure syndromes: definition and classification. Heart Fail Rev. 2007;12:87–90.
32. Peacock WFt, Remer EE, Aponte J, Moffa DA, Emerman CE, Albert NM. Effective observation unit treatment of decompensated heart failure. Congest Heart Fail. 2002;8:68–73.
33. Rydman RJ, Zalenski RJ, Roberts RR, et al. Patient satisfaction with an emergency department chest pain observation unit. Ann Emerg Med. 1997;29:109–15.
34. Gheorghiade M, Abraham WT, Albert NM, et al. Systolic blood pressure at admission, clinical characteristics, and outcomes in patients hospitalized with acute heart failure. JAMA. 2006; 296:2217–26.
35. Stevenson LW, Perloff JK. The limited reliability of physical signs for estimating hemodynamics in chronic heart failure. JAMA. 1989;261:884–8.
36. Marcus GM, Gerber IL, McKeown BH, et al. Association between phonocardiographic third and fourth heart sounds and objective measures of left ventricular function. JAMA. 2005; 293:2238–44.
37. Binanay C, Califf RM, Hasselblad V, et al. Evaluation study of congestive heart failure and pulmonary artery catheterization effectiveness: the ESCAPE trial. JAMA. 2005;294: 1625–33.
38. Shah MR, Hasselblad V, Stevenson LW, et al. Impact of the pulmonary artery catheter in critically ill patients: meta-analysis of randomized clinical trials. JAMA. 2005;294:1664–70.
39. Collins SP, Lindsell CJ, Storrow AB, Abraham WT. Prevalence of negative chest radiography results in the emergency department patient with decompensated heart failure. Ann Emerg Med. 2006;47:13–8.
40. Perego GB, Landolina M, Vergara G, et al. Implantable CRT device diagnostics identify patients with increased risk for heart failure hospitalization. J Interv Card Electrophysiol. 2008;23:235–42.
41. Auble TE, Hsieh M, Gardner W, et al. A prediction rule to identify low-risk patients with heart failure. Acad Emerg Med. 2005;12:514–21.
42. Hsieh M, Auble TE, Yealy DM. Validation of the acute heart failure index. Ann Emerg Med. 2008;51:37–44.
43. Fonarow GC, Abraham WT, Albert NM, et al. Factors identified as precipitating hospital admissions for heart failure and clinical outcomes: findings from OPTIMIZE-HF. Arch Intern Med. 2008;168:847–54.
44. Koelling TM, Johnson ML, Cody RJ, Aaronson KD. Discharge education improves clinical outcomes in patients with chronic heart failure. Circulation. 2005;111:179–85.
45. Balas EA, Boren SA. Managing clinical knowledge for health care improvement. In: Bemmel J, McCray AT, editors. Yearbook of medical informatics 2000: patient-centered systems. Stuttgart: Schattauer Verlagsgsgesellschaft mbH; 2000. p. 65–70.
46. Balas EA, Weingarten S, Garb CT, Blumenthal D, Boren SA, Brown GD. Improving preventive care by prompting physicians. Arch Intern Med. 2000;160:301–8.

Chapter 24
Appendix: Shared Practice Examples

Kay Styer Holmes

The Society of Chest Pain Centers (SCPC) is a nonprofit organization whose mission is to reduce cardiac deaths. SCPC bridges cardiology, emergency medicine, emergency medical services, and other professions focused on the care of the cardiac patient. SCPC promotes a process improvement-based approach, delivered through a heart failure operational model that encompasses the entire facility and is not "brick and mortar."

Heart Failure Accreditation was developed using the principles of improvement science based on research, expert opinion, rational guidelines, and best practice models. The accreditation process helps facilities streamline their processes and improve patient care and financial outcomes.

SCPC's approach to accreditation is radically different from other accreditation organizations that set standards and then measure compliance. SCPC works with facilities to help them improve their processes in a collegial, collaborative, and educational manner. We believe that we best achieve our goal of reducing cardiac deaths by assisting facilities in identifying gaps in their processes and providing resources to improve care.

In this chapter, SCPC provides comprehensive examples from accredited heart failure centers, including EMS protocols, risk stratification tools, flowcharts of processes, treatment protocols, observation services, order sets, and patient education and discharge instructions.

Part I Flowcharts

Figs. 24.1–24.7

K.S. Holmes, RN, BSA, MSA (✉)
Society of Chest Pain Centers, Dublin, OH, USA
e-mail: kholmes@scpcp.org

W. Frank Peacock (ed.), *Short Stay Management of Acute Heart Failure*,
Contemporary Cardiology, DOI 10.1007/978-1-61779-627-2_24,
© Springer Science+Business Media, LLC 2012

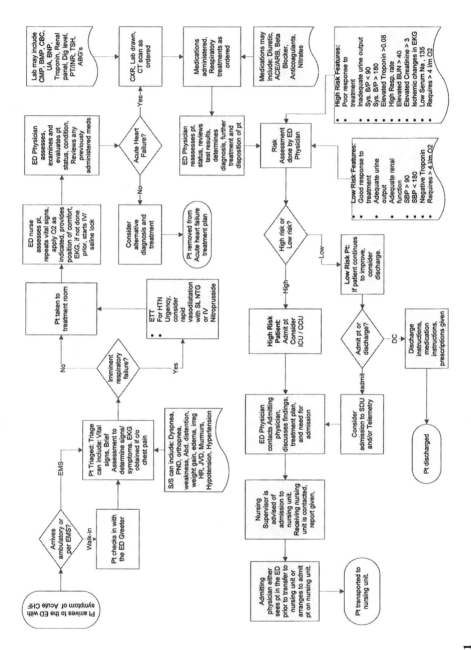

Fig. 24.1

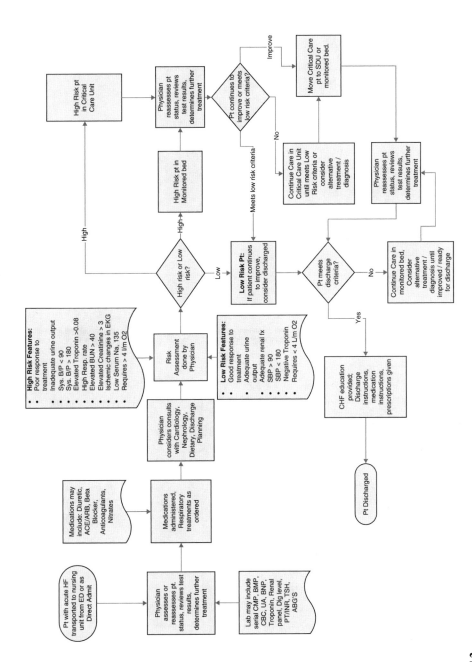

High Risk Features:
- Poor response to treatment
- Inadequate urine output
- Sys. B/P < 90
- Sys. B/P > 180
- Elevated Troponin >0.08
- High Resp. rate
- Elevated BUN > 40
- Elevated Creatinine > 3
- Ischemic changes in EKG
- Low Serum Na. 135
- Requires > 4 l/m O2

Low Risk Features:
- Good response to treatment
- Adequate urine output
- Adequate renal fx
- SBP > 90
- SBP < 180
- Negative Troponin
- Requires < 4 L/m O2

High Risk pt in Critical Care Unit

Physician reassesses pt status, reviews test results, determines further treatment

Pt continues to improve or meets low risk criteria?

Improve — Move Critical Care pt to SDU or monitored bed.

High Risk pt in Monitored bed

No — Continue Care in Critical Care Unit until meets Low Risk criteria or consider alternative treatment / diagnosis

Physician reassesses pt status, reviews test results, determines further treatment

High risk or Low risk?

Meets low risk criteria — **Low Risk Pt:** If patient continues to improve, consider discharged

Low — Pt meets discharge criteria?

No — Continue Care in monitored bed, Consider alternative treatment / diagnosis until improved / ready for discharge

Risk Assessment done by Physician

Physician considers consults with Cardiology, Nephrology, Dietary, Discharge Planning

Yes — CHF education provided; Discharge instructions, medication, instructions, prescriptions given

Pt Discharged

Medications may include: Diuretic, ACE/ARB, Beta Blocker, Anticoagulants, Nitrates

Medications administered, Respiratory treatments as ordered

Pt with acute HF transported to nursing unit from ED or as Direct Admit

Physician assesses or reassesses pt. status, reviews test results, determines further treatment

Lab may include serial CMP, BMP, CBC, UA, BNP, Troponin, Renal panel, Dig level, PT/INR, TSH, ABG'S

Fig. 24.2

**THSW Emergency Department
Heart Failure Protocol (12/5/2009)**

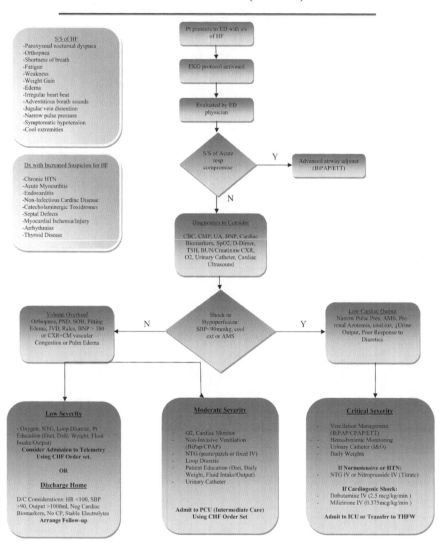

Fig. 24.3

Centinnial Hills Hospital

MEDICAL CENTER

HEART FAILURE PATHWAY DOOR TO DISPOSITION

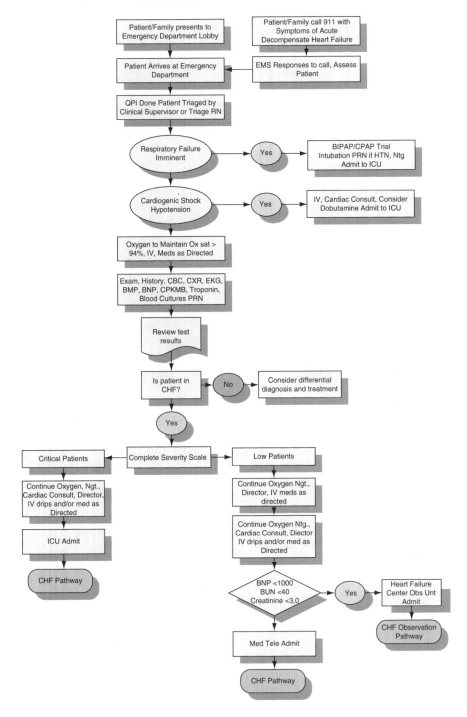

Fig. 24.4

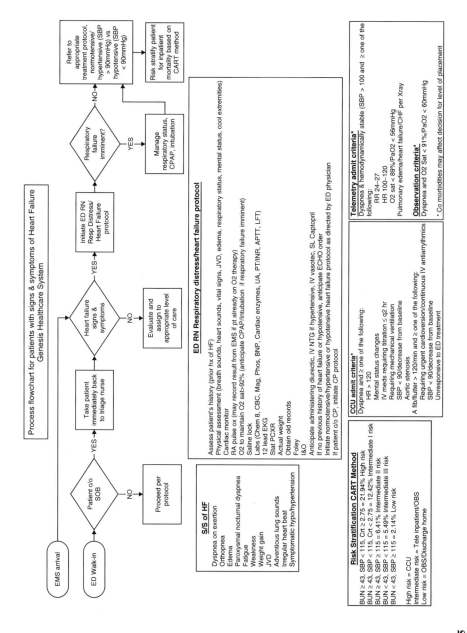

Fig. 24.5

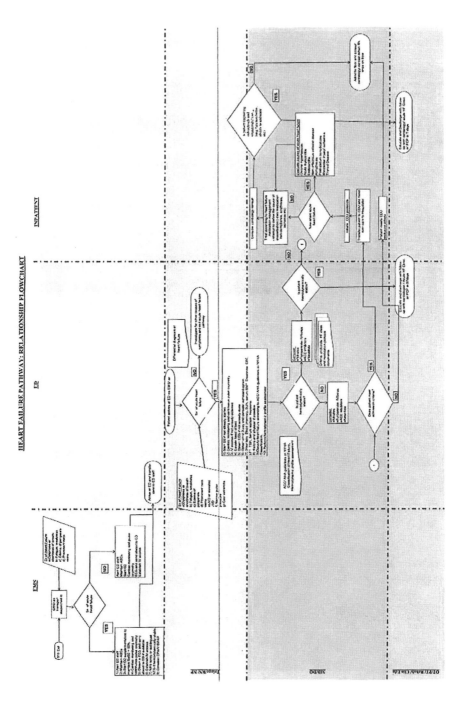

Fig. 24.6

Heart Failure Core Measure Flow

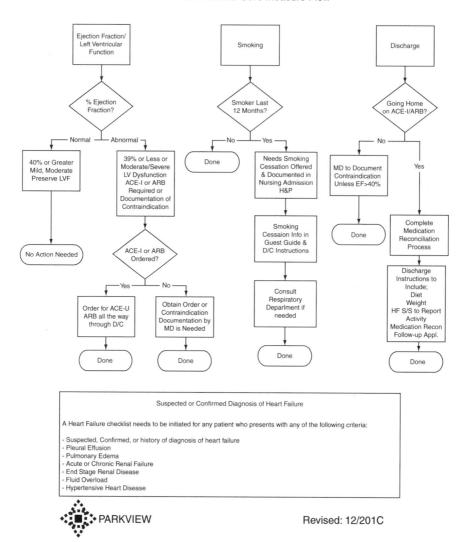

Suspected or Confirmed Diagnosis of Heart Failure

A Heart Failure checklist needs to be initiated for any patient who presents with any of the following criteria:

- Suspected, Confirmed, or history of diagnosis of heart failure
- Pleural Effusion
- Pulmonary Edema
- Acute or Chronic Renal Failure
- End Stage Renal Disease
- Fluid Overload
- Hypertensive Heart Disease

PARKVIEW   Revised: 12/201C

Fig. 24.7

Part II Order Sets and Treatment Protocols

Figs. 24.8–24.16

<table>
<tr><td colspan="2" rowspan="2"></td><td style="text-align:center">Stormont-Vail
Health*Care*</td><td></td></tr>
<tr><td style="text-align:center">Draft 5/7/10</td><td></td></tr>
</table>

In accordance with Medical Staff formulary policy, authorization is given for dispensing medications by generic name unless "No Sub" is written next to each product desired by brand name only.

Date Ordered	Time	Medication or Order	R,	Noted Initials
		HEART FAILURE STANDARD ORDERS		
		Allergies:		
		Reason for Admission (Check all that apply) ( ) New HF ( ) Noncompliance, meds ( ) Noncompliance, diet ( ) Volume overloaded ( ) Arrhythmias ( ) Exacerbation of HF ( ) Refractory HF ( ) Over-diuresis ( ) Other _____		
		1. Diagnosis: Heart Failure		
		2. Status: ( ) Inpatient ( ) Observation Telemetry Orders: ( ) Yes ( ) No		
		3. Vital signs every 4 hours _____		
		4. Weight upon admission and daily: _____		
		5. Record all Intake and Output		
		6. Activity level: ( ) Bed rest ( ) Bathroom w/assistance ( ) Chair ( ) Up ad lib		
		7. Diet ( ) 2000 mg Na with 2000ml fluid restriction ( ) Additional restrictions: _____		
		8. Echocardiogram if not done in previous 6 months ( ) Yes ( ) No If done in previous 6 months, obtain OLD REPORT. CHF History: LV ejection fractions <40%: ( ) Yes ( ) No ( ) Unknown		
		9. Admission EKG, Fasting Lipid Profile, Comprehensive Metabolic Panel (COMP) ( ) Chest x-ray ( ) TSH w/reflex to FT4 ( ) PT/INR ( ) CPK/MB and Troponin I ( ) Digoxin level ( ) APTT ( ) Mg ( ) CBC w/diff ( ) BNP		
		10. Daily Basic Profile x 3 days		
		11. IV Vasodilating Agents ( ) Nesiritide 2 mcg/kg. Bolus over 1 minute, with 0.01 mcg/kg/minute gtt in dedicated line. (Only if SBP ≥90 mmHg.) Do not use with any other vasodilating IV agents. ( ) Nitroglycerin – start at 3 mcg/minute to 5 mcg/minute and titrate to maintain SBP ≥90 mmHg.		

Physician's signature must accompany each entry, including standing orders: Date and hour for instituting and discontinuing order must be recorded.

PHYSICIAN'S ORDERS

Fig. 24.8

Stormont-Vail
Health *Care*

Draft 5/7/10

In accordance with Medical Staff formulary policy, authorization is given for dispensing medications by generic name unless "No Sub" is written next to each product desired by brand name only.

Date Ordered	Time	Medication or Order	Rx	Noted Initials
		HEART FAILURE STANDARD ORDERS		
		12. IV Inotropes (if clinical signs and symptoms of low cardiac output):		
		13. Diuretics (example: Furosemide, Torsemide, Metolazone, HCTZ)		
		14. Potassium Replacement (KCL or KCL elixir) K+ Level _____		
		MANDATORY MEDICATION – GIVE UNLESS CONTRAINDICATED		
		15. **ACE Inhibitors** (example: Enalapril, Lisinopril, Captopril, or Ramapril) Patient has contraindication to ACE Inhibitor of: - BP _____ - Allergy _____ - Electrolyte Abnormality _____ - Other _____ Drug: _____ Dose: _____ Route: _____ Frequency: _____		
		16. **Angiotension Receptor Blockers (ARB)** (example: Olmesartan (Benicar) or Losartan (Cozaar) Patient has contraindication to ARB of: - BP _____ - Allergy _____ - Electrolyte Abnormality _____ - Other _____ Drug: _____ Dose: _____ Route: _____ Frequency: _____		

Physician's signature must accompany each entry, including standing orders: Date and hour for instituting and discontinuing order must be recorded.

ZZ-117   Rev.:   Page 2 of 3

PHYSICIAN'S ORDERS

Fig. 24.8 (continued)

Stormont-Vail HealthCare

Draft 5/7/10

In accordance with Medical Staff formulary policy, authorization is given for dispensing medications by generic name unless "No Sub" is written next to each product desired by brand name only.

Date Ordered	Time	Medication or Order	R.	Noted Initials
		HEART FAILURE STANDARD ORDERS		
		17. **Beta Blockers** (Bisoprolol, Carvedilol, or Metroprolol Extended Release – example: Toprol XL) Patient has contraindication to Beta Blocker of: - BP _____ - Allergy _____ - High Degree AV Block _____ - Severe Asthma _____ - Other _____ Drug: _____ Dose: _____ Route: _____ Frequency: _____		
		18. Additional Therapies (example: Digoxin, ECASA, or Spironolactone (Aldactone)		
		19. Lovenox 40 mg subcutaneous daily		
		20. Notify Heart Failure Nurse at 354-6237		
		21. Initiate Dietary Education Consult		
		22. Patient Education Provide patient with: • Smoking cessation information, as appropriate • Heart Failure Information		
		23. Follow-up appointment for ≤ 7 days post-discharge with: ( ) Cardiologist **OR** ( ) Primary Care Physician **OR** ( ) Cotton-O'Neil Heart Improvement Center (HIC) at 270-4243		
		24. Update pneumococal and seasonal influenza vaccinations regardless of age.		

Physician's signature must accompany each entry, including standing orders: Date and hour for instituting and discontinuing order must be recorded.

ZZ-117   Rev.:   Page 3 of 3

PHYSICIAN'S ORDERS

Fig. 24.8 (continued)

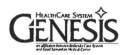

Normotensive/Hypertensive (SBP > 90) Heart Failure ED Treatment Protocol

OXYGEN THERAPY
- O2 to maintain O2 sat > 92%

IV
- Saline lock

XRAY
- STAT PCXR

EKG
- EKG now.

LABS
- Chem 8, CBC, Mag, Phos, BNP, Cardiac enzymes, UA, PT/INR, APTT, LFT

NITRATES
- Anticipate Nitroglycerin 50mg/250 ml D5W IV @ _____ mcg/min

DIURETICS
- Anticipate Furosemide IV 2 x daily PO dose or 40mg if furosemide naive

ACE INHIBITORS
- Anticipate Vasotec 1.25mg IV or Captopril 25mg sublingual

NURSING INTERVENTIONS
- Actual weight
- Foley
- I&O

ECHO
- If new onset, anticipate Echo order
- Obtain most recent echo results and place results on chart
- Anticipate new Echo if most recent one > 6 months ago or recent event
- Echo staff on call after 5pm and on weekends for emergencies.

PLAN OF CARE
- If prompt diuresis and patient stable and feeling much improved, consider discharge from ED with follow-up with PCP within 3 days and provide heart failure discharge instructions.
- If prompt diuresis, but patient not much improved, consider admit to OBS/tele based on clinical presentation and CART risk score
- If inadequate diuresis, give additional diuretic, consider admit to tele/CCU based on clinical presentation and CART risk score.

CONSULTS
- Cardiology consult if new onset

Fig. 24.9

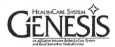

Hypotensive (SBP < 90) Heart Failure ED Treatment Protocol

OXYGEN THERAPY
- O2 to maintain O2 sat > 92%

IV
- Saline lock or IVF if intravascular depleted

XRAY
- STAT PCXR

EKG
- EKG now.

LABS
- Chem 8, CBC, Mag, Phos, BNP, Cardiac enzymes, UA, PT/INR, APTT, LFT

DIURETICS
- Anticipate Furosemide IV (gentle diuresis)

NURSING INTERVENTIONS
- Actual weight
- Foley
- I&O

ECHO
- If new onset, anticipate Echo order
- Obtain most recent echo results and place results on chart
- Anticipater new Echo if most recent one > 6 months ago or recent event
- Echo staff on call after 5pm and on weekends for emergencies

PLAN OF CARE
- Identify and treat cause for hypotension, i.e. MI, cardiogenic shock, GI bleed. Stat Echo may be indicated.

CONSULTS
- Appropriate consult to treat cause of hypotension, if identified
- Cardiology consult if new onset

Fig. 24.10

Date Time	Noted By	Yes Initiate Order	**59309 ED HEART FAILURE ORDERS**	Order Completed
℞ Quality/Core Measure		☒	⬅⋯ **NOTE: ONLY ORDERS MARKED WITH "X" WILL BE INITIATED**	
			DIAGNOSIS: Acute Decompensated Heart Failure	
			NURSING:	
		☒	1. Weigh patient (in ED if possible).	
		☒	2. Record all intake and output.	
		☒	3. Establish Saline lock.	
		☒	4. Urinary catheter to gravity.	
		☒	5. Assess response to diuretic in 2 hours. If urine output is less than 1000 ml with normal renal function or less than 800 with renal insufficiency, consider Natrecor (nesiritide) therapy.	
			CARDIOPULMONARY:	
		☒	6. Check oxygen saturation.	
		☐	7. BiPAP/CPAP Settings: _____	
		☒	8. Initiate nasal oxygen at 2 liters/min to keep saturation greater than 92%.	
		☒	9. Continuous cardiac monitoring.	
			LABS: If not already done.	
		☐	10. ☐Cardiac Profile ☐Glucose ☐Chem 6 ☐Magnesium ☐Phosphorus ☐ABG ☐PT/INR ☐PTT ☐D-Dimer ☐CPK ☐BNP-if not on nesiritide ☐Dig level-if on Digoxin	
			SPECIAL TESTS:	
		☒	11. 12 Lead EKG	
		☐	12. Chest X-ray ☐PA & LAT ☐Portable	
		☒	13. Echocardiogram with ejection fraction if not done in last 6 months.	
			ALLERGIES:	
		☒	14. Complete and send "Patient Allergies" form to Pharmacy on admission.	
			IV:	
		☐	15. IV _____ at _____ ml/hr. ☐Bolus: _____	
			MEDICATIONS:	
		☐	16. Enteric Coated Aspirin 325 mg by mouth once STAT.	
		☐	17. Enteric Coated Aspirin 81 mg by mouth once STAT.	

Clinician Signature: _____   Time: _____

☐TO ☐WO _____   ☐R/V Date: _____

Time: _____   Place Patient ID Label Here

Physician Signature: _____   Date: _____

*Unless identified as an exception, any order for a drug identified by its proprietary name MAY be filled with its formulary identical.   Filed By: (Pharmacy)

Parkview Hospital
2200 Randallia Drive
Fort Wayne, IN 46805   ORD-59309 (3/16/2010) Page 1 of 2   MDORDER

Fig. 24.11

+   +

Date Time	Noted By	Yes Initiate Order	59309 ED HEART FAILURE ORDERS	Order Completed
Quality/Core Measure		☒	← ⋯ NOTE: ONLY ORDERS MARKED WITH "X" WILL BE INITIATED	
			Diuretic:	
		❑	18. Lasix (furosemide) 40 mg IV push over 2 minutes times 1 dose.	
		❑	19. Lasix (furosemide) 80 mg IV push over 2 minutes times 1 dose.	
		❑	20. Other: _____	
			Chest Pain:	
		❑	21. Nitroglycerin 0.4 mg sublingual for anginal chest pain. May repeat every 5 minutes times 2. *Do not use if SBP is less than or equal to 90.*	
		❑	22. Morphine _____ mg IV every _____ hours prn pain. (Normal dose 2 mg every 4 hours)	
			Vasodilators:	
		❑	23. Natrecor (nesiritide) 2 mcg/kg IV bolus over 1 minute once then 0.01 mcg/kg/min continuous infusion. Prime IV tubing with 25 ml of infusion prior to giving bolus or starting infusion. *Do not use if SBP is less than or equal to 90.*	
		❑	24. Nitroglycerin IV infusion at _____ mcg/min (5-50 mcg/min). *Hold if SBP is less than ____*	
			Nitrates:	
		❑	25. Nitroglycerin 2% ointment _____ inches topically once. Remove in 12 hours. *Hold if SBP is less than ____*	
			Inotropes: Hold if systolic blood pressure is less than _____	
		❑	26. Primacor (milrinone) 50 mcg/kg IV bolus.	
		❑	27. Primacor (milrinone) IV at _____ mcg/min (Normal range 0.375-0.75 mcg/kg/min).	
		❑	28. Dobutrex (dobutamine) IV at _____ mcg/min (Normal range 2-10 mcg/kg/min).	
		❑	29. Dopamine (dopamine hydrochloride) IV at _____ mcg/kg/min (Normal range 5-20 mcg/kg/min).	
		❑	30. Lanoxin (digoxin) _____ mg once. ❑ by mouth ❑ IV	
			Electrolyte Replacement:	
		❑	31. Potassium Chloride _____ meq IVPB once. Maximum rate of infusion 10 mEq/hr for unmonitored patients or 20 mEq/hr for monitored patients.	
		❑	32. Potassium Chloride _____ mEq (tabs) by mouth once.	
		❑	33. Potassium Chloride _____ mEq (elixir) by mouth once.	
		❑	34. Magnesium Sulfate _____ gm IVPB over _____ hours once.	
			ADDITIONAL ORDERS:	

Clinician Signature:	Time: _____	
❑TO ❑WO _____	❑R/V Date: _____	Place Patient ID Label Here
	Time: _____	
Physician Signature: _____	Date: _____	

*Unless identified as an exception, any order for a drug identified by its proprietary name MAY be filled with its formulary identical.   Filled By: (Pharmacy)

Parkview Hospital
2200 Randallia Drive
Fort Wayne, IN 46805   ORD-59309 (3/16/2010) Page2 of 2   MDORDER

Fig. 24.12

MAURY REGIONAL
MEDICAL CENTER   CONGESTIVE HEART FAILURE PATIENT LANGUAGE MAP

Patient Label

Each person is unique and this plan may vary to best suit your individual needs

	Day 1	Day 2	Day 3
GOALS AND OUTCOMES	Breathe easier	Breathe easier while out of bed Understand diet	Breathe easier with activity Know all your discharge instructions
NURSING CARE AND TREATMENTS	Vital signs at least every 4 hours Lung sounds every shift Weigh on admission Heart monitor If needed: Oxygen Measure Oxygen level Blood work Chest X-Ray (CXR) Echocardiogram (Ultrasound of heart) Track what you are eating and drinking	Vital signs every 4 hours Lung sounds every shift Weigh in AM Heart monitor If needed: Oxygen Measure Oxygen level Blood work CXR Echocardiogram if not done already Help the nurse track what you are eating and drinking	Vital signs every 4 hours Lung sounds every shift Weigh in AM and track Heart monitor If needed: Stop Oxygen Measure Oxygen level Blood work CXR Echocardiogram if not done already Help the nurse track what you are eating and drinking
DIET	Low salt diet Fluids restricted as ordered Dietitian to visit	Dietitian to visit if not already done yesterday	Any questions? Ask your nurse Review discharge instructions
ACTIVITY	Walk to bathroom with assistance	Sit up in chair for 30 minutes 3 times per day Ambulate in room	------>Ambulate in hall with increased independence
MEDICATIONS	IV medications	IV/oral medications	Oral medications If you have any questions about your medications, ask your Nurse
DISCHARGE PLANNING AND TEACHING	The nurse will ask questions about your home situation to see if you qualify for help at home. Begin CHF teaching booklet, view CHF education channel	A Care manager will visit you to see if you need equipment or more help at home Continued CHF teaching/view CHF educational channel	If you have concerns about going home, tell your nurse and your care manager ------>

Fig. 24.13

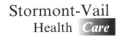

Stormont-Vail
Health *Care*

2 minute hemodynamic profile assessment

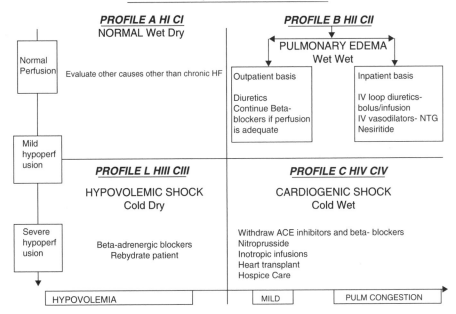

PROFILE A HI CI
NORMAL Wet Dry

Normal Perfusion

Evaluate other causes other than chronic HF

PROFILE B HII CII
PULMONARY EDEMA
Wet Wet

Outpatient basis

Diuretics
Continue Beta-blockers if perfusion is adequate

Inpatient basis

IV loop diuretics-bolus/infusion
IV vasodilators- NTG
Nesiritide

Mild hypoperfusion

PROFILE L HIII CIII
HYPOVOLEMIC SHOCK
Cold Dry

PROFILE C HIV CIV
CARDIOGENIC SHOCK
Cold Wet

Severe hypoperfusion

Beta-adrenergic blockers
Rebydrate patient

Withdraw ACE inhibitors and beta- blockers
Nitroprusside
Inotropic infusions
Heart transplant
Hospice Care

HYPOVOLEMIA   MILD   PULM CONGESTION

Fig. 24.14

Stormont-Vail
Health *Care*

USE OF BIOCHEMICAL MARKERS IN THE INITIAL EVALUATION OF HEART FAILURE

Recommendations for use biochemical markers for diagnosis of Heart Failure

Class I
1. BNP or NT-proBNP testing can be used in the acute setting to rule out or to confirm the diagnosis of heart failure among patients presenting with ambiguous signs and symptoms. (Level of Evidence: A)

Class IIa
1. BNP and NT-proBNP testing can be helpful to exclude the diagnosis of heart failure among patients with signs and symptoms suspicious of heart failure in the non-acute setting. (Level of Evidence: C)

Class III
1. In diagnosing patients with heart failure, routine blood BNP or NT-proBNP testing for patients with an obvious clinical diagnosis of heart failure is not recommended. (Level of Evidence: C)
2. In diagnosing patients with heart failure, blood BNP or NT-proBNP testing should not be used to replace conventional clinical evaluation or assessment of the degree of left ventricular structural or functional abnormalities (e.g., echocardiography, invasive hemodynamic assessment). (Level of Evidence: C)

USE OF BIOCHEMICAL MARKERS IN RISK STRATIFICATION OF HEART FAILURE
Recommendations for use of biochemical markers for risk stratification of Heart Failure

Class IIa
1. Blood BNP or NT-proBNP testing can provide a useful addition to clinical assessment in selected situations when additional risk stratification is required. (Level of Evidence: A)
2. Serial blood BNP or NT-proBNP concentrations may be used to track changes in risk profile and clinical status among patients with heart failure in selected situations where additional risk stratification is required. (Level of Evidence: B)

Class IIb
1.Cardiac troponin testing can identify patients with heart failure at increased risk beyond the setting of acute coronary syndromes. (Level of Evidence: B)

Class III
1. Routine blood biomarker testing for the *sole* purpose of risk stratification in patients with heart failure is not warranted (Level of Evidence: B)

USE OF BIOCHEMICAL MARKERS IN SCREENING SOR CARDIAC DYSFUNCTION
Recommendations for use of BNP and NT-proBNP in screening of Heart Failure

Class IIb
1. Blood BNP or NT-proBNP testing can be helpful to identify selected patients with left ventricular systolic dysfunction in the post-infarction setting or to identify patients at high risk of developing heart failure (e.g., history of myocardial infarction, diabetes mellitus). However, the diagnostic ranges and cost-effectiveness in different populations remain controversial. (Level of Evidence: B)

Class III

Fig. 24.15

CHF OBSERVATION PATHWAY PHYSICIANS ORDER SET

PROMOTE PATIENT SAFETYI

1) Indicate <u>REASONS FOR USE</u> for all PRN medication orders   2) Do <u>NOT</u> use these dangerous abbreviations:

AMISSION STATUS OF PATIENT:		HEIGHT:	WEIGHT:
ALLERGIES: 1.	2.	3.	☐ None
DIAGNOSIS:			

Date	Time	
		Place pt. in: OBSERVATION TELEMETRY

Admitting physician Name: _____ Admit Time _____

Cardiologist: _____

1. Transfer to Heart Failure Center (HFC)
2. Risk Stratification: ☐ Low Risk   ☐ High Risk
3. Diet: ☐ NPO for testing p Midnight   ☐ 2gm Na, Low Cholesterol   ☐ Cardiac Prudent
   ☐ Fluid Restriction   ☐ 1½ liters/24 hours   ☐ 2 liters/24 hours
4. Strict Intake and Output
5. Weight patient upon arrival to HFC: _____   ☐ lbs   ☐ kgs
6. Activity as tolerated
7. Bathroom privileges
8. Saline lock with NS flushes every 8 hours and as needed
9. VS every 1 hr X 1, then every 4 hrs. Notify MD of chest pain, shortness of breath, nausea or vomiting, diaphoresis.
10. Titrate oxygen to keep SaO2 greater than 93%
11. Continuous Pulse Ox Monitoring
12. Telemetry Continuous Cardiac Monitoring. Notify physician of any ST sigment changes
13. Tests: a) ABG on Room Air on admit and 20 hours after admit or prior to discharge.
   b) EKG PRN for chest pain
   c) If NOT done in the ED: ☐ DO ALL OF THE FOLLOWING LABS
      ☐ CXR PA And LAT (if patient unable to tolerate, do portable CXR)
      ☐ CBC   ☐ Troponin   ☐ BNP   ☐ Magnesium
      ☐ Digoxin Level (if patient previously on Digoxin)   ☐ Serum pregnancy if appropriate
      ☐ Basic Metabolic Panel   ☐ PT/INR   ☐ EKG   ☐ TSH
      ☐ CPK-MB   ☐ Lipids Panel   ☐ Liver Panel   ☐ Free T3 & T4
   d) CPK-MB in 2 hours and 6 hours from the first draw
   e) Troponin in 2 hours and 6 hours from the first draw
   f) 2D Echocardiogram with Doppler (if not performed in the fast 6 months)
      Interpreting Cardiologist: _____
      (If EF less than or equal to 40%, call Primary MD regarding ACE or if unable to tolerate:
      ARB medication order)
      Obtain and place previous Echo on Chart
14. Medications: _____
   ☐ Asprin 325 mg by mouth every day
   ☐ Nitroglycerin paste_____inch to Anterior Chest Wall every 6 hours (Discontinue 2 hours prior to stress test)
   ☐ Albuterol 2.5 mg SVN every 6 hours PRN for wheezing
   ☐ Tylenol 650mg by mouth every 4 hours PRN for headache
   ☐ Zofran 4mg IV every 6 hours PRN for Nausea
   ☐ Magnesium Oxide 400mg by mouth Daily PRN for Magnesium less than 1.8; times 1 dose
   ☐ K-Dur 40mEg by mouth Daily PRN for Potassium less than 3.6; times 1 dose
   ☐ STAT EKG with Chest Pain
   ☐ Nitroglycerin 0.4mg sublingual every 5min if patient develops chest pain, give until chest pain relieved. (Max dose of 3 tabs)   Hold if Systolic BP < 110
   ☐ Betablocker: _____
   ☐ Ace: _____

MSO₄ → MSO_4

MgSO₄ → $MgSO_4$

LEADING DECIMAL

TRAILING ZEROS

ORDERS: AUTHORIZATION IS GIVEN TO DISPENSE A THERAPUETIC EQUIVALENT UNLESS NOTED. NON.FORMULARY DRUGS MAY REQUIRE 48 HOURS TO OBTAIN.

BAR CODE		PATIENT IDENTIFICATION
P00010-Physician Orders	**CHF OBSERVATION PATHWAY PHYSICIAN ORDER SET** Page 1 of 3 (PMM#DRAFT) (R 12/09) (IKON COPY CENTER)	

Fig. 24.16

CHF OBSERVATION PATHWAY PHYSICIANS ORDER SET

PROMOTE PATIENT SAFETYI

1) Indicale REASONS FOR USE for all PRN medication orders   2) DO NOT use these dangerous abbreviations:

AMISSION STATUS OF PATIENT:		HEIGHT:	WEIGHT:	U
ALLERGIES: 1.	2.	3.	☐ None	
DIAGNOSIS:				

Date	Time		
		15. Stress Test (if Cardiac exzymos are within normal limits) ☐ Exercise Treadmill Stress Test with Nuclear Imaging ☐ Exercise Treadmill Stress Test without Nuclear Imaging ☐ Dobutamine Stress Test (if patient has asthma or COPD) ☐ Persantine Stress Test ☐ Lexiscan Stress Test Intrepreting Cardiologist:_____ call results of stress test to Attending Physician. 16. Referrals: ☐ Dietary Consult for Cardiac Diet education or per physician order ☐ Social Services Consult for discharge needs ☐ Prior to discharge, notify Primary Care Physician and obtain follow-up appointment 17. Heart Failure Educational Information to be given to the patient upon arrival to the Heart Failure Center 18. Smoking Cessation Screening and Counseling to be done by Primary RN or designee.	IU QD QOD MS MSO_4 $MgSO_4$ LEADING DECIMAL TRAILING ZEROS	

_____   _____   _____
Physician Signature   Print Name or License #   Date / Time

ORDERS: AUTHORIZATION IS GIVEN TO DISPENSE A THERAPUETIC EQUIVALENT UNLESS NOTED. NON-FORMULARY DRUGS MAY REQUIRE 48 HOURS TO OBTAIN.

BAR CODE		PATIENT IDENTIFICATION
* PO0010* PO0010 - Physician Orders	CHF OBSERVATION PATHWAY PHYSICIAN ORDER SET Page 2 of 2 (PMMM# DRAFT) (R 12/09) (IKON COPY CENTER)	

Fig. 24.16 (continued)

Part III Policy, Clinical and Operational examples

Figs. 24.17–24.20

Department:		Version: 1	Page 1 of 2
PATIENT CARE SERVICES		Original Date:	
Category:		Last Review/Revised Date: 01/07/2010	
		Approved By: PCS DIRECTORS	
Title: Heart Failure Policy			

Printed copies are for reference only. Please refer to the electronic copy for the latest version.

POLICY:
The following policy is implemented on patients who present with signs and symptoms suggestive of new acute heart failure or exacerbation of chronic heart failure.

ASSESSMENT:
1. Vital signs upon admission then per floor protocol or physician order.
2. Observe the patient every 12 hours or more frequently if indicated for the following:
   a. Dyspnea
   b. Activity intolerance
   c. Orthopnea or difficulty sleeping
   d. Edema
   e. Fatigue
   f. Tachycardia and/or presence of a 3rd heart sound (S_3)
   g. Jugular venous distention
   h. Lung sounds
   i. Abdominal distention/bloating, nausea, abdominal pain, and/or poor appetite.
3. Weight patient daily.
4. Identify oxygen needs.
5. Monitor intake and output.
6. Presence of pacemaker and/or ICD.

PATIENT CARE MANAGEMENT:
1. Monitor vital signs and SaO_2 and provide oxygen if needed.
2. Elevate the HOB for patient comfort.
3. Anticipate potential need for additional respiratory needs (i.e. BIPAP) and/or transfer to ICU or telemetry.
4. Assess need for telemetry monitoring and intermittent needle.
5. Refer to NYHA and ACC/AHA Class Heart Failure Guide in Clinicomp Reference Library.
6. Dietary consult.
7. Consider PT/OT consult.
8. Consult Cardiac Rehab Phase I.
9. Ensure patient has follow up appointment within one week of discharge with licensed practitioner or physician.
10. Monitor lab values as ordered:
    a. CBC, UA, electrolytes including Ca^{2+}, and Mg^{2+}, BUN, creatinine, BNP, lipid panel, LFT's, thyroid
    b. Daily Basic Panel X3 days.
11. Review diagnostic studies as ordered:
    a. CXR
    b. Echcardiogram including left ventricular assessment
    c. Cardiac catheterization report or stress test
    d. EKG.
12. Review medication regimen as ordered. Administer and monitor the patient's response to:
    a. Diuretic
    b. ACE inhibitors

Fig. 24.17

  c. ARB's
  d. Beta blockers
  e. Nitrates
  f. Aspirin??

PATIENT /SO EDUCATION:
1. Medications
2. Diet and fluid intake (<2 liters/day unless otherwise specified by the physician)
3. Activity
4. Weight monitoring (daily weights)
5. Alcohol use
6. Smoking cessation
7. When to call the physician
8. Managing Heart Failure Booklet and review with patient/SO
9. Symptom monitoring
10. Avoid temperature extremes
11. Follow up appointment with a licensed practitioner or physician on a regular basics.

REPORTABLE CONDITIONS:
1. Weight gain of >1 kg/day or >2-3 kg/week
2. Occurrence of chest pain
3. Urinary output <30 ml/hr
4. Increased oxygen demands or increased shortness of breath and/or activity intolerance
5. Adventitious lung sounds (i.e. crackles, wheezing)
6. Tachycardia and/or presence of S_3 and/or abnormal vital signs
7. Abnormal labs
8. Abnormal diagnostic studies
9. Onset of JVD, increased abdominal distention, pain, bloating, or nausea.

REFERENCES:
American Heart Association of Heart Failure Nurses
http://www.AAHFN.org/assets/Comprehensive Assessment and Symptoms of HF-CASH.pdf

U.S. Department of Health and Human Services
http://www.hospitalcompare.hhs.gov/Hospital/Static/About-
HospQuality.asp?dest=NAV%7CHome%7CAbout%7CQualityMeasures

Fig. 24.17 (continued)

Centennial Hills Hospital

███████ ⁀ₘ MEDICAL CENTER

Cardiac Observation Unit (COU)
Operational Guidelines

Patient Admission Process:

- Upon patient arrival: Introduce yourself, orient the patient and family to their room, secure belongings, and explain the admission process.
- Verify that telemetry monitoring is in place. If not, apply monitoring and verify rhythm with telemetry technician.
- Provide the patient with the appropriate education packet (Heart Failure or Chest Pain) and discuss their plan of care.
- Discuss dietary restrictions. Patients may be NPO, on a fluid restriction, on a low-fat or low-sodium diet. It is important that patients and family members understand these restrictions.
- Most patients will have a stress test ordered. If so, Check for timing of NPO and caffeine restrictions and explain restrictions to patients and family members, This is a good time to discuss what is expected before, during, and after a stress test (if ordered).
- Obtain a full set of vital signs. Perform patient assessment.
- Smoking cessation information and counseling should be given to all patients as well as any dietary and nutrition information. These topics will be rienforced prior to discharge.
- Assess for and initiate referrals to address nutrition and/or social service needs.

Upon Admission Completion and During Stay:

- Monitor timed blood draws. Verify that all tests are accurately ordered. In verifying stress test orders, make sure the appropriate type of stress test has been entered. Review test results upon completion and place in patient chart. Notify physician as appropriate to update on test results.

Fig. 24.18

- Please make sure there is a cardiologist assigned to read your patient's EKG and/or stress test.
- The Primary Nurse should follow up on patient's stress test results. Results are usually available 1-2 hours after test completion. Please call Radiology for results if you have not received them within this time.
- If a stress test is positive, the physician should be called for notification and an upgrade order.
- Complete all required documentation
  - ○ Kardex
  - ○ Medication Administration Record (MAR)
  - ○ Observation Documentation Form
  - ○ Medication Reconciliation Form
- Verify that all orders have been scanned to pharmacy.
- Remember that all COU patients are 23-hour observation patients. It is the Primary Nurse's responsibility to monitor the length of stay and communicate it in communication hand-offs. Test results should be monitored and results communicated to the patient's physician efficiently so disposition decisions can be made in a timely manner. If the patient is nearing the 23-hour mark and a disposition decision has not been reached, the physician needs to be contacted to inquire about disposition or an upgrade order.

- If a patient is upgraded to a full admission, the House Supervisor must be notified. Admitting staff must be notified as well and a copy of the upgrade order faxed to admitting.

Discharge Process

- Physicians should be notified if patient's meet established discharge criteria (refer to discharge criteria).
- Upon discharge, the appropriate education information and discharge instructions should be provided and reviewed with the patient and their family (if indicated). A reconciled medication list should be provided.
- Follow-up appointments should be discussed and arranged for patients. Arrangements to fax pertinent records (EKG, echo, stress test, labs) to the patient's PMD should be made.
- Please make sure you fill out the COU log completely.

Fig. 24.18 (continued)

CONTINUOUS POSITIVE AIRWAY PRESSURE
(CPAP) GUIDE.

Continuous positive Airway Pressure has been shown to rapidly improve vital signs, gas exchange, reduce the work of breathing, decrease the sense of dyspnea, and decrease the need for endotracheal intubation in patients who suffer from shortness of breath, from asthma, COPD, pulmaonary edema, CHF. CPAP improves hemodynamics by reducing left ventricular preload and afterload.

I. INDICATIONS

    A. Any patient who is in respiratory distress with signs and symptoms consistent with asthma, COPD, pulmonary edema, CHF, or pneumonia and who is

        1) Awake and able to follow commands
        2) Is over 12 yrs old and is able to fit the CPAP mask
        3) Has the ability to maintain an open airway
        4) And exhibits two or more of the following:
        1. a respiratory rate greater than 25 breaths per minute
        2. SPO2 of less than 94% at any time.
        3. use of accessory muscles during respirations.

II. Contraindications

    A. Patient is in respiratory arrest/apneic
    B. Patient is suspected of having a pneumothorax or has suffered trauma to the chest
    C. Patient has a tracheostomy.
    D. Patient is actively vomiting or has upper GI bleeding

III. Procedure

    A. Explain the procedure to the patient.
    B. Ensure adequate oxygen supply to ventilation device.
    C. Place the patient on continuous pulse oximetry.
    D. Place the patient on cardiac monitor and record rhythm strips with vital signs.
    E. Place the delivery device over the mouth and nose.
    F. Secure the mask with provided straps or other provided devices.
    G. Use up to 10cm H20 of peep valve.
    H. Check for air leaks.
    I. Monitor and document the patient's respiratory response to treatment.
    J. Check and document the patient's respiratory response to treatment.
    K. Administer appropriate medication as certified (nebulized Albuterol f or COPD/Asthms)
    L. Continue to coach patient to keep the mask in place and readjust as needed.
    M. If respiratory status deteriorates, remove device and consider intermittent positive ventilation via BVM and/or placement of non-visualized airway or endotracheal intubation.

IV. REMOVAL PROCEDURE.

Fig. 24.19

A. CPAP therapy needs to be continuous and should not be removed unless the patient can not tolerate the mask or experiences respiratory arrest or begins to vomit.

B. Intermittent positive pressure ventilation with a Bag- valve -mask, placement of a non-visualized airway and/or endotracheal intubation should be considered if the patient is removed from CPAP therapy.

V. Special Notes,

A. Do not remove CPAP until hospital therapy is ready to be placed on patient.

B. Watch patient for gast ric distention, which can result in vomiting.

C. Procedure may be performed on patient with Do Not Resuscitate Order.

D. Due to changes in preload and afterload of the heart during CPAP therapy, a complete set of vital signs must be obtained every 5 minutes.

Fig. 24.19 (continued)

Parkview Hospital	CARDIOPULMONARY SERVICES
Policy & Procedure Title: BI-LEVEL POSITIVE AIRWAY PRESSURE (BIPAP)	
CATEGORY: CLINICAL - CRITICAL CARE	

I.   **POLICY STATEMENT:** Noninvasive delivery of gas at a positive inspiratory and/or expiratory pressure per face mask, nasal mask or nasal pillows for the purpose of augmenting ventilation in the spontaneous breathing patient.

II. **QUALIFICATIONS:** When ordered by a physician, BiPAP may be initiated by any RCP oriented to the procedure.

III. **INDICATIONS:**
   1. Acute obstructive sleep apnea.
   2. Neuromuscular diseases with impending acute ventilatory failure (pH<7.35,PaC02>50).
   3. Chronic obstructive pulmonary diseases with impending acute ventilatory failure.
   4. Hypoxemia refractory to increasing Fi02.
   5. Impending ventilatory failure.
      NOTE: BIPAP will rarely, if ever, be successful with patients who are less than fully cooperative.

IV. **CONTRAINDICATIONS:**
   1. Preexisting pneumothorax or pneumomediastinum.
   1. Hypotension due to or associated with intravascular volume depletion.
   2. Pre-existing bullous lung disease may represent a contraindication.
   3. Pneumocephalus has been reported in patients with elevated ICP.
   4. Facial/skull fractures, as well as patients with elevated ICP
   5. Post operative patients who have recently under gone abdominal surgery may not be appropriate candidates for BIPAP or nasal CPAP.

V.   **PREPARATION:**   Gather the following equipment:
   1. Nasal mask, full face mask or nasal pillows.
   2. Head gear.
   3. BiPAP ventilatory support system.
   4. Smooth bore inner diameter corrugated tubing.
   5. Bacteria filter.
   6. Flowmeter
   7. O2 analyzer (preferably analog/non-digital).
   8. O2 supply tubing.
   9. Continuous oximeter, if not already ordered. (Not required if BIPAP is for comfort measures only and alarms are a nuisance.)
   10. Ventilator flowsheet.

Origination Date: August, 1994	Original Source: Technical Specialist
Revision Date: October 2010	Source of Revision: Clinical Supervisor
	Authorized by: CRAIG TRAXLER

Fig. 24.20

Parkview Hospital	CARDIOPULMONARY SERVICES
Policy & Procedure Title: BI-LEVEL POSITIVE AIRWAY PRESSURE (BIPAP) CATEGORY: CLINICAL - CRITICAL CARE	

VI.   **PROCEDURE:**
1.   Place BiPAP at patient's bedside.
2.   Explain device, and reassure patient as necessary.
3.   Attach bacterial filter to patient gas outlet of BiPAP machine.
4.   Connect bleed-in adapter(s) to filter.
5.   Connect O2 supply tubing to O2 flowmeter.
6.   Connect corrugated tubing to bleed- in adapter.
7.   Attach mask and head gear to corrugated tubing.
8.   Verify patient exhalation port.
9.   Set mode on machine panel.
10.   Set IPAP (Inspiratory Positive Airway Pressure) and EPAP (Expiratory Positive Airway Pressure).
      Note: Manufacturer's recommendation is that IPAP be set at least 4 cwp above EPAP.
11.   Adjust oxygen "bleed-in" gas flow to ordered flowrate.
12.   Place mask and head gear on patient. Do not obstruct exhalaton port.
13.   Turn on machine.
14.   Adjust head gear fit to maintain ordered settings on manometer, being careful not to over tighten the mask.
15.   Initiate ventilator flow sheet and document in Carecast. (In Critical Care units, document in Chart +.)

VII.   **RT TO MANAGE/RESCUE PROTOCOL:**

In the event of a physician order for BIPAP without specific settings or an order for R.T. to manage, the following is to be initiated.

A.   Indications for protocol may include:
1.   PH < 7.35 with a $PaCO_2$ > 45 mm Hg
2.   RR > 24
3. PaO_2/FiO_2 < 200
4.   Hypoxemia refractory to increasing FiO_2
5.   Respiratory distress
6.   Abdominal paradox
7.   Use of accessory muscles, abnormal for patient.

Origination Date: August, 1994	Original Source: Technical Specialist
Revision Date: October 2010	Source of Revision: Clinical Supervisor
	Authorized by: CRAIG TRAXLER

Page 2 of 5

Fig. 24.20   (continued)

Parkview Hospital	CARDIOPULMONARY SERVICES
Policy & Procedure Title: BI-LEVEL POSITIVE AIRWAY PRESSURE (BIPAP) CATEGORY: CLINICAL - CRITICAL CARE	

B. Settings:
  A. Mode- Spontaneous/Timed
  B. Initial IPAP 10 cm H_2O – titrate to achieve an average exhaled tidal volume of 6 x patient's ideal body wt. in kg (not to exceed 16 cm H_2O unless Resource Person is notified.)
      (See Predicted Body Weight Calculations Chart.)
  C. Initial EPAP of 4 cm H_2O
  D. Rate - Set at a minimum of 8 BPM, may titrate up to 2-5 less than patient's spontaneous rate.
  E. Initial FiO_2 – set to approximate amount required prior to initiating BIPAP and titrate to maintain SpO_2 of 89% to 94%.

C. ABG Results:
    ABG's may be drawn prn.
  1. If ABG is improved, continue with same settings and monitor the patient.
  2. No improvement of pH and/or $PaCO_2$ – Increase IPAP in increments of 2-3 cmH_2O.
  3. No improvement of PaO_2 - increase FiO_2 by 10% or 2-3 liter increments until improvement is noted. Patient may require more than one oxygen bleed in. At that point increase the EPAP 1-2 cmH_2O (remember to increase the IPAP also to maintain same level of PS). Note: Quantum: Maximum FiO_2 is approximately 0.65 . Vision: Maximum FiO_2 is 1.00.
  4. If pH or PaO_2 are found to be significantly worsening, or vital signs or general patient status are continuing to deteriorate, the physician shall be notified for further guidance and/or orders.

VIII. DOCUMENTATION: The following parameters must be documented:
  1. Time
  2. Mode
  3. IPAP reading
  4. EPAP reading
  5. Mandatory rate (if ordered)
  6. Total rate
  7. FiO_2

Origination Date: August, 1994	Original Source: Technical Specialist
Revision Date: October 2010	Source of Revision: Clinical Supervisor
	Authorized by: CRAIG TRAXLER

Page 3 of 5

Fig. 24.20 (continued)

Parkview Hospital	CARDIOPULMONARY SERVICES
Policy & Procedure Title: BI-LEVEL POSITIVE AIRWAY PRESSURE (BIPAP) CATEGORY: CLINICAL - CRITICAL CARE	

       8.   Gas flow bleed in
       9.   Vital signs (HR, B/P, if monitored)
     10. SpO_2

IX.   SPECIAL CONSIDERATIONS:

1. Precise control of FiO_2 is difficult to achieve with many models of BIPAP/CPAP machine.
2. When analyzing, the FiO_2 reading will fluctuate significantly with the patient's VE and breathing pattern. (It is much easier to determine a "ballpark" FiO_2 using an analog analyzer, due to its slower response time.)
3. If delivering a high FiO_2 (>60%) or the patient desaturates when the mask is removed, aerosolized medication should be given "in line". Otherwise, turn machine off, and give treatments utilizing routine procedures.
4. Experience has shown that the best results occur when trial periods of 30 minutes or longer, are attempted on two or three occasions prior to their first overnight trial. Patients who are gradually acclimated to this device in the above mentioned fashion do-considerably better than those who's initial exposure/trial is initiated at bedtime.
5. Patients should refrain from eating 1-2 hours prior to the application of the BIPAP system.
6. Heat moisture exchangers (HME) should not be used with the BIPAP system. Testing has shown that the HME may interfere with the ability of the BIPAP system to maintain the prescribed pressures.
7. Supplemental humidification, if necessary, can be provided by a passover humidifier for 2-3 days. Often the patient's mucociliary blanket appears to adapt to the new conditions. Pediatric patients usually will required humidification.
8. Oximetry should be performed prior to the initiation of this therapy as well as when the BIPAP system is in place. The oximeter will not only aid in the titration of the oxygen but will serve as tool to monitor the effectiveness of this therapy.
9. Although no reports of gastric distension or aspiration have been reported, the most common complication has been abrasion of the

Origination Date: August, 1994	Original Source: Technical Specialist
Revision Date: October 2010	Source of Revision: Clinical Supervisor
	Authorized by: CRAIG TRAXLER

Fig. 24.20 (continued)

Parkview Hospital	CARDIOPULMONARY SERVICES
Policy & Procedure Title: BI-LEVEL POSITIVE AIRWAY PRESSURE (BIPAP) CATEGORY: CLINICAL - CRITICAL CARE	

bridge of the nose. Application of wound-care dressing appears to eliminate this problem.

X.   AUTOMATIC DISCONTINUATION:

If the patient has refused to wear BIPAP for 24 hours, the unit will be discontinued and removed from the patient's room. A notation will be made by the RCP in the Progress Notes of the patient's chart.
An order for "BIPAP prn " does not require that the machine be in the patient's room.

XI.   INFECTION CONTROL:

1.   After therapy is discontinued, dispose of all "single patient use" items. Clean BIPAP machine with a surface disinfectant (i.e. TOR or Cavicide).

2.   Corrugated tubing, mask, and head gear are all nondisposable. Wash these items with detergent (i.e.: Manu-Klenz). Submerge in Cidex for appropriate length of time, rinse thoroughly with water, and dry in "clean" drier.

3.   Air intake filters should be cleaned after each patient or every 7 days.

Origination Date: August, 1994	Original Source: Technical Specialist
Revision Date: October 2010	Source of Revision: Clinical Supervisor
	Authorized by: CRAIG TRAXLER

Page 5 of 5

Fig. 24.20 (continued)

Part IV Patient Discharge Instructions

Figs. 24.21–24.23

STOP

HEART FAILURE

DISCHARGE TIMEOUT

All heart failure patients or any patients with heart failure on the admission orders, heart failure mentioned in the progress notes or receiving treatment for heart failure (IV lasix, etc) must meet the following Core Measures prior to discharge.

Has your patient received the following?:

HF-1. Discharge instructions that include instructions on:

	Yes	No
Activity	☐ Yes	☐ No
Diet (low sodium)	☐ Yes	☐ No
Follow up appt scheduled (within 7 days)	☐ Yes	☐ No
Medication list	☐ Yes	☐ No
Symptom guide (what to do if symptoms return)	☐ Yes	☐ No
Weight monitoring	☐ Yes	☐ No

* If any No, please explain why: _____

HF-2. Evaluation of LVS (left ventricular systolic) function   ☐ Yes   ☐ No
(Look at H&P, progress notes, consults, echo report for EF%)

* If No, is patient scheduled for one as an outpatient? _____

HF-3. ACEI or ARB for LVSD (left ventricular systolic dysfunction, EF < 40%) prescribed at discharge or reason not ordered is documented by Dr. ☐ Yes   ☐ No
(Look at H&P, progress notes, consults) **Patient's EF%** _____

* If No, you must contact the discharging Dr for med order or reason why not ordered and write as an order.

HF-4. Adult Smoking cessation advice/counseling provided   ☐ Yes ☐ No ☐ NA

Please complete prior to discharge and place in Heart Failure Folder at nurses station.

Fig. 24.21

CHF PATHWAY INITIAL QUESTIONS
YES - NO QUESTIONS
1. Do you have a bathroom scales?
2. Have you been weighed in the past week?
3. Do you weigh yourself the same time each day?
4. Are you following a low salt diet?
5. Do you have all of your medications at home?
6. Are you taking the medications as written on the discharge instruction sheet?
7. Do you have a home health nurse?
8. Did you find the CHF teaching that you received in the hospital beneficial?

DATE DESCRIPTIONS
1. Date of follow-up with primary care physician.
2. Date of follow-up with specialist.

MULTIPLE CHOICE
1. How often do you weigh yourself?
   - Daily
   - Weekly
   - 2 times per week
   - 3 times per week
   - Monthly
   - Never
2. Describe your weight the last three times you were weighed.
   - Remains the same
   - Increasing with each weight
   - Decreasing with each weight
   - Fluctuates within 2 pounds of each weight
   - Fluctuates greater than 2 pounds of each weight
3. Name two symptoms of when you should call your doctor between scheduled visits.
   - Upper abdominal pain
   - Bloated feeling
   - Breathing difficulties
   - Dry cough
   - Swelling or edema
   - Increased fatigue
   - Increased urination at night
   - Increased weakness

FREE FORM DESCRIPTIONS

1. If your weight increased over two pounds in one day or five pounds in a week what would you do?
2. Patient comments.
3. Nurse comments.

Fig. 24.22

HEART FAILURE DISCHARGE CHECK LIST

Date of Arrival: _____   Time of Arrival: _____   Admitting MD: _____

Key for Using Checklist:	√ = complete, indicator met X = complete, indicator not me *= Indicates Core Measures Requirement	Date Completed	Documentation: Location / Comments	Initials
☐	*Smoking cessation counseling (for cigarettes only) This applies to any patient who has smoked a cigarette within the past year. In case of conflicting documentation, assume patient is a smoker.			
☐	*Assessment and documentation of LVSF (left ventricular systolic function) is in medical record. If LVSF assessment completed previously, place in medical record. If physician has reason for not performing or plans to do as an outpatient document in medical record.			
☐ OR AND	*ACEI or ARB prescribed for LVSD (EF less than 40% or documentation of Moderate to Severe Systolic Dysfunction) prior to discharge. →Document Contraindication to ACEI in medical record →Document Contraindication to ARB in medical record.			
☐	*Discharge Instructions have been taught to the patient or caregiver and evidence of the teaching Documented in the Medical Record includes:			
	☐ *Diet Check if Ordered: ☐ 2 Gram Sodium ☐ Fluid restriction if indicated			
	☐ *Activity			
	☐ *Follow-up information with physician			
	☐ *What to do if symptoms worsen or do not improve (include specific signs and symptoms of heart failure)			
	☐ *Daily weight monitoring			
	☐ *Heart Failure specific education			
	☐ *Medications: A complete list of medications, including PRN's, over the counter and herbals must be listed on Discharge Instruction Form given to the patient or caregiver. Inappropriate and unacceptable documentation includes: medications as at home, resume meds as before, continue same meds,etc. and must be clarified with the physician.			
	Check only if Ordered – AHA / ACC Recommendations			
☐	Beta blocker (if LVSD or symptomatic exacerbation of heart failure during chronic maintenance treatment).			
☐	Aldosterone antagonist (if LVSD and moderate-severe HF symptoms)			

ACE-Inhibitor				Angiotensin II Receptor Blockers / Antagonists			
Formulary		Non-Formulary		Formulary		Non-Formulary	
Benazepril	Lotensin®	Moexipril	Univasc®	Losartan	Cozaar®	Irbesartan	Avapro®
Captopril	Capoten®	Perindopril	Aceon®	Valsartan	Diovan®	Irbesartan /	Avalide®
Enalapril	Vasotec®	Trandolapril	Mavik®	Candesartan	Atacand®	HCTZ	
Fosinopril	Monopril®			Olmesartan	Benicar®		
Lisinopril	Prinivil®			Telmisartan	Micardis®		
Quinapril	Accupril®						
Ramipril	Altace®						

Initials Legend:

Initials	Name	Initials	Name

Discharge Nurse: _____   Nurse Manager / Designee: _____

THIS FORM IS NOT PART OF THE OFFICIAL MEDICAL RECORD. RETURN COMPLETED FORM TO NURSE MANAGER

Apply Patient Label Here
Revised 3/2010

Fig. 24.23

Part V Patient Education

Figs. 24.24–24.28

CONGESTIVE HEART FAILURE DISCHARGE TEACHING INSTRUCTIONS

Topic	Instructions
CHF	• The heart pumps oxygen and nutrients to the body. • Congestive Heart Failure (CHF) is a weakening of the heart muscle and the heart is not working as efficiently. • This causes back up of blood in the chambers of the heart that are weakened, and the veins that return blood to the heart from the rest of the body. • The pooling of blood leads to congestion of surrounding tissue and organs and the development of symptoms such as leg edema or swelling, nausea or bloating (bowel edema), shortness of breath due to lung edema.
Weight Monitoring	• Weight yourself each day at the same time with the same amount of clothing on. • Notify your doctor if there is a 3 pound increase in one day, or a 5 pound increase in one week.
Smoking Cessation	• **Do not smoke or use other tobacco products.** Tobacco is probably the single most dangerous thing you can do to your health. Nicotine robs the heart of oxygen and constricts blood vessels, which raises heart rate and blood pressure. If you smoke or use tobacco products, discuss alternatives with your doctor. The most important thing is that you continue to try to quit until you are successfull • **Nevada Tobacco Users Helpline**- (702) 877-0684 Toll Free 1-888-866-6642
Diet/Nutrition	• Limit your salt inlake. Too much salt will cause swelling and could make it harder for you to breathe. Use salt substitutes **only** in your doctor approves. • Follow any diet instructions given to you by your doctor or the dietitian including how much salt you are allowed each day. • If you are overweight, talk to your doctor about a weight reduction plan. • You may need to limit the amount of fluids you drink. *Remember*: Things that melt (ice cream, Jell-O, Ice) still count as fluids.
Activity	• Remain physically active following your doctor's instructions about exercise and activity • Rest often. Any time you become even a little tired or short of breath, SIT DOWN and rest. • Plan your activities to include rest periods. • Keep your feel and legs elevated while sitting. Do not dangle them. • Take note of your breathing pattern and how well you tolerate activity.

Call your doctor if:	• **Return to this facility immediately or contact your doctor if you begin to have any of the following:**
	  ⇨ Trouble breathing, especially at rest or when lying flat in bed.
	  ⇨ Waking up out of breath at night.
	  ⇨ Frequent dry, hacking cough, especially when lying down.
	  ⇨ Feeling tired, weak, faint, or dizzy.
	  ⇨ Swollen feet, ankles, or legs.
	  ⇨ Nausea, with stomach swelling, pain and tenderness.

Medications	• Your doctor may prescribe one or a combination of medications for you. • You MUST take medicine every day to treat congestive heart failure. Be sure to take medicines, **exactly as your doctor tells you: no more, no less.** • Skipping doses or not refilling a prescription could cause serious problems. Do not stop taking your medicine without talking to your doctor first. • Medicines sometime cause side effects like causing you to cough or the bathroom more often. If you have side effects or questions or believe the medicine is not helping you, **Call your doctor.**
Follow-up	• Be sure and schedule a follow-up appointment with your primary care doctor or any specialists as instructed.
Additional Instructions	• Avoid People with colds or the flu. • Keep all appointments • Work with your doctor. To get the most benefit from your healthcare, you need to take an active role. • Visit your doctor regularly, take notes and ask questions.

By signing, I acknowledge that I have reviewed the above information with my nurse.

_____   _____
Patient Signature   Date

BAR CODE		PATIENT IDENTIFICATION
‖‖‖‖‖‖‖‖‖‖‖‖‖‖‖‖‖‖‖ DC0010 - Discharge Instructions	**Centennial Hills Hospital** ◼◼◼◼**MEDICAL CENTER** **CONGESTIVE HEART FAILURE** **DISCHARGE TEACHING INSTRUCTIONS** (PMM# 78584653) (R 1/08) (IKON COPY CENTER) ORIGINAL - MEDICAL RECORDS CANARY - PATIENT	

Fig. 24.24

GENESIS HEALTHCARE SYSTEM
CONGESTIVE HEART FAILURE
PATIENT EDUCATION ON HOSPITAL STAY

3 DAY TIMEFRAME	DAY 1	DAY 2	DAY 3
Activity	Bedrest May use bedside commode	Up as needed	Up as needed
Treatment Diagnosis	Chest X-Ray Oxygen Heart monitor Lab work Weight Measure intake/output of fluids	Echocardiogram, if needed Oxygen, if needed Measure intake/output of fluids Weight	Chest X-Ray, if needed Oxygen, if needed Measure intake/output of fluids If you do not have scales at home, notify nursing staff
Nutrition	Low Salt Diet	Low Salt Diet	Low Salt Diet
Medication	IV medications	IV medications	Medication by mouth
Education	Congestive Heart Failure education package received.	Ask nursing staff if questions regarding education packet.	

Fig. 24.25

bolsford
general
hospital

YOUR GUIDE TO
THE NEW FOOD LABEL

The new food label will carry an up-to-date, easier-to-use nutrition information guide, to be required on almost all packaged foods (compared to about 60 percent of products until now). The guide will serve as a key to help in planning a healthy diet.

Serving sizes are now more consistent across product lines, stated in both household and metric measures, and reflect the amounts people actually eat.

The list of nutrients covers those most important to the health of today's consumers, most of whom need to worry about getting to much of certain items (fat, for example), rather than too few vitamins or minerals, as in the past.

The label will now tell the number of calories per gram of fat, carbohydrates, and protein.

Nutrition Facts

Serving Size ½ cup (114g)
Servings Per Container: 4

Amount Per Serving

Calories 90	Calories From Fat 30

	% Daily Value*
Total Fat 3g	5%
Saturated Fat 0g	0%
Cholesterol 0mg	0%
Sodium 300mg	13%
Total Carbohydrate 13g	4%
Dietary Fiber 3g	12%
Sugars 3g	
Protein 3g	

Vitamin A	80%	•	Vitamin C	2%
Calcium	4%	•	Iron	4%

• Precent Daily Values are based on a 2,000 calorie diet. Your daily values may be higher or lower depending on your calorie needs:

		Calories	2,000	2,500
Total Fat	Less than		65g	80g
Sat Fat	Less than		20g	25g
Cholesterol	Less than		300mg	300mg
Sodium	Less than		2,400mg	2,400mg
Total Carbohydrate			300g	375g
Fiber			25g	30g

Calories per gram:
Fat 9   •   Carbohydrates 4   •   Protein 4

New title signals that the label contains the newly required information.

Calories from fat are now shown on the label to help consumers meet dierary guidelines that recommend people get no more than 30 percent of their calories from fat.

% Daily Value shows how a food fits into the overall daily diet.

Daily Values are also something new, Some are maximums, as with fat (65 grams or less); others are minimums, as with carbohydrates (300 grams or more). The daily value on the label are based on a daily diet of 2,000 and 2,500 calories. Individuals should adjust the values to fit their own calorie intake.

Fig. 24.26

GENERAL GUIDELINES TO LABEL READING

1. Legal Definitions for the following terms:

Sodium Free – less than 5 mg per standard serving, can't contain any sodium chloride
(also known as table salt)
Very Low Sodium – 35mg or less sodium per standard serving
Low Sodium – 140 mg or less per standard serving
Reduced Sodium – At least 25% less sodium than in regular food
Light in Sodium – 50% less sodium per standard serving than in regular food
Unsalted or No Salt Added – No salt added in the processing, STILL has sodium
AND it may contain a substantial amount
Lightly Salted – 50% less added sodium than is normally added. This product
Will state NOT a low sodium food if that criteria is not met.

2. Nutrition Label

This will state the sodium content of foods, in milligrams (mg) per serving

3. Suggestions To Reading The Food Label

1. Look at the number of servings in the given package
   (i.e. – If you were reading the back of a soup can, it would state how many servings
   are in that can under the heading "serving")
2. Now you want to determine how much of that product you will eat
3. You then want to look at how much sodium is in EACH serving
4. REMEMBER that the label ONLY records the amount PER SERVING.
5. If you are going to consume the entire package and there are three servings, you will
   need to multiply the milligrams of sodium stated times three
   (i.e.- If the label states there is 100mg of sodium in one serving, and there are three
   servings in the box, and you wish to eat the entire box, you will want to take 100mg
   and multiply this times 3. This will let you know that there is 300mg of sodium in the
   box)

4. To Choose Appropriate Foods, You Will Want To Look For Foods That Contain 200mg Sodium or Less Per Serving

If you are consciously reading labels aim for no more than 700mg of sodium per
meal

Fig. 24.26 (continued)

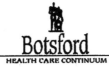

Botsford
HEALTH CARE CONTINUUM

COMMON QUESTIONS ASKED ABOUT THE
2 GRAM SODIUM DIET

1. WHAT IS SODIUM?
    This is an essential mineral to the body. It helps the body regulate fluid balance.

2. WHY IS IT IMPORTANT THAT I REDUCE MY SODIUM INTAKE?
    Under certain conditions, such as heart disease, high blood pressure, and renal disease, the intake of excess sodium can cause the body to retain too much fluid. Every time you eat extra sodium, water is drawn out of the body's tissues to dilute it, causing more fluid buildup. In summary, living with these conditions is MUCH easier when you follow these sodium guidelines.

3. WHAT HAPPENS WHEN THERE IS FLUID BUILDUP IN MY BODY?
    This means you experience more swelling (edema), and an increase in shortness of breath. And with more fluid, it is more difficult for the body to absorb your medications, so therefore your medicine becomes less effective.

4. WHERE IS SODIUM FOUND?
    Sodium is found naturally in every food we eat. However, most of the sodium in our diet is added, usually as table salt. It is also found in many baking ingredients and medications. This information will provide you with guidelines to reducing your overall sodium intake.

Fig. 24.27

WHAT ARE THE BASIC GUIDELINES FOR THIS DIET?

1. **DO NOT** USE TABLE SALT!
   Table salt is 40% sodium. JUST ONE TEASPOON contains 2300mg (2.3 grams) of sodium. This is more than the sodium level prescribed by your physician.

2. **DO NOT** ADD SALT IN COOKING! *(THIS CAN BE ELIMINATED FROM ANY RECIPE EXCEPT ONE CONTAINING YEAST)*

3. **DO** READ FOOD LABELS TO MONITOR YOUR SODIUM INTAKE.

4. **LIMIT** THE USE OF COMMERCIALLY PREPARED CONDIMENTS OR SALAD DRESSINGS, UNLESS THE PRODUCT STATES "NO SALT ADDED.
   (or 1 serving contains less than 200 mg)

5. **DO** PURCHASE A LOW SODIUM COOKBOOK TO PROVIDE GUIDELINES TO COOKING MEALS LOW SODIUM AND PALATABLE

6. **DO** MAKE USE OF HERBS AND SPICES INSTEAD OF SALT

7. **DO** FOLLOW THE "DINING OUT" GUIDELINES INCLUDED IN THIS BOOKLET.

8. **DO** KEEP THIS BOOK NEAR YOUR KITCHEN AS A GUIDE AND A REMINDER!

9. **WEIGH YOURSELF OFTEN, AS SUGGESTED BY YOUR DOCTOR TO MONITOR FOR EXCESS FLUID GAINS!!**

10. **CALL YOU DIETITIAN SHOULD _ANY_ QUESTIONS ARISE REGARDING YOUR DIET AS PRESCRIBED. A DIETITIAN CAN BE REACHED BY CALLING 248-471-8221.**

Fig. 24.27 (continued)

SODIUM CONTENT IN COMMON FOODS

***FOODS WITH O-200 MG SODIUM PER SERVING *ARE ACCEPTABLE* ***FOODS WITH MORE THAN 200 MG PER SERVING *ARE NOT ACCEPTABLE*

SEASONINGS   **SODIUM CONTENT**
1 TSP GARLIC POWDER   (1 MG SODIUM)
1 TBSP HORSERADISH, PREPARED   (165 MG SODIUM)
1 TSP GARLIC SALT   (2050 MG SODIUM)
1 TSP SALT   (2132 MG SODIUM)

CONDIMENTS
1 TSP MUSTARD   (65 MG SODIUM)
1 TBSP LOW SODIUM KETCHUP   (90 MG SODIUM)
1 TSP BARBECUE SAUCE   (127 MG SODIUM)
1 TBSP. KETCHUP   (178 MG SODIUM)
1 TBSP LITE SOY SAUCE   (600 MG SODIUM)
1 TBSP REGULAR SOY SAOUCE   (1029 MG SODIUM)

CHEESE
1 OUNCE CREAM CHEESE   (85 MG SODIUM)
1 OUNCE BRICK CHEESE   (159 MG SODIUM)
1 OUNCE MUENSTER CHEESE   (178 MG SODIUM)
1 CUP RICOTTA CHEESE   (208 MG SODIUM)
1 OUNCE BLUE CHEESE   (394 MG SODIUM)
1 OUNCE ROQUEFORT CHEESE   (512 MG SODIUM)
1 CUP COTTAGE CHEESE   (918 MG SODIUM)

BEVERAGES
REGULAR SODA   (10 MG SODIUM)
DIET SODA   (30 MG SODIUM)
MILK, 8 OUNCES   (120 MG SODIUM)
COCOA MIX   (201 MG SODIUM)
BUTTERMILK   (257 MG SODIUM)

MEATS
FISH, BAKED, 3 OUNCES   (54 MG SODIUM)
BEEF, 3 OUNCES   (55 MG SODIUM)
EGGS   (63 MG SODIUM)
CHICKEN, ½ BREAST   (69 MG SODIUM)
SHRIMP, 3 OUNCES, RAW   (126 MG SODIUM)
FRIED FISH, 3 OUNCES   (238 MG SODIUM)
CORNED BEEF, 3 OUNCES   (972 MG SODIUM)

Fig. 24.27 (continued)

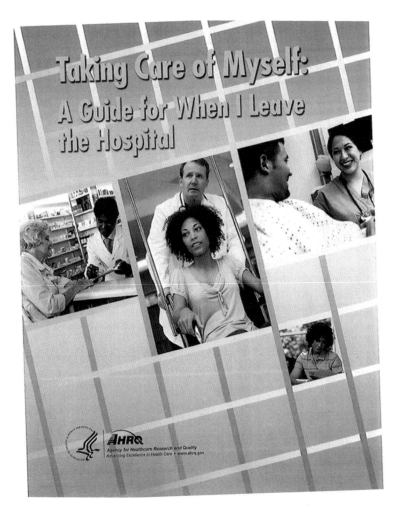

Fig. 24.28

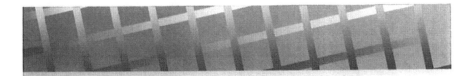

To use this guide you should:

- Talk with the hospital staff about each of the items that are listed in the guide.

- Take the completed guide home with you. It will help you to take care of yourself when you go home.

- Share the guide with your family members and others who want to help you. The guide will help them know how to help take care of you.

- Bring the guide to all of your doctor appointments so the doctor knows what you have been doing to care for yourself since you left the hospital.

This guide is adapted from *Project Re-Engineered Discharge (RED)*, which was funded by AHRQ and conducted by Brian Jack, M.D., and colleagues at Boston University Medical Center. Additional tools for implementing Project RED are currently being developed.

Fig. 24.28 (continued)

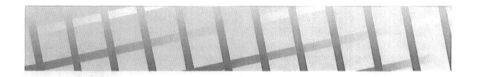

Taking Care of Myself:
A Guide for When I Leave the Hospital

When you leave the hospital, there are a lot of things you need to do to take care of yourself. You need to see your doctor, take your medicines, exercise, eat healthy foods, and know whom to call with questions or problems. This guide helps you keep track of all the things you need to do.

My name: _____

When I'm leaving the hospital _____

If I have questions or problems, I should call:

_____

Phone number: _____

If I have a serious health problem, I should call:

_____

Phone number: _____

Bring this plan to all your medical appointments.

1

Fig. 24.28 (continued)